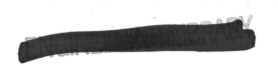

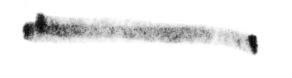

Handbook of
Injury and
Violence Prevention

Handbook of
Injury and
Violence Prevention

Edited by

Lynda S. Doll
Sandra E. Bonzo
David A. Sleet

and

James A. Mercy

Elizabeth N. Haas

Managing Editor

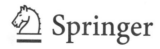 Springer

Lynda S. Doll, Sandra E. Bonzo, James A. Mercy,
and David A. Sleet
Centers for Disease Control and Prevention
National Center for Injury Prevention and Control
Atlanta, GA 30341
USA

Library of Congress Control Number: 2005934788

ISBN-10: 0-387-25924-4   e-ISBN-10: 0-387-29457-0
ISBN-13: 978-0387-25924-6   e-ISBN-13: 978-0387-29457-5

Printed on acid-free paper.

The information provided in this book does not necessarily represent the official views or policies of
the U.S. Department of Health and Human Services (HHS) and the Centers for Disease Control and
Prevention (CDC). The inclusion of individuals, programs, or organizations in this book do not constitute endorsement by the federal government, HHS, or CDC.

9 8 7 6 5 4 3 2

springer.com

Foreword

We live in challenging times and our attention becomes focused on the public health threats that lead daily news reports. Yet, there is one health threat that the public has accepted as *fait accompli*—injuries. Injuries kill more Americans in their first three decades of life than any other cause of death. In fact, injuries—both unintentional and those caused by acts of violence—are among the top 10 killers for Americans of all ages. However, injuries do not have to be an accepted risk of living. Lives can be saved and disabilities prevented. That is why I am pleased to present the *Handbook of Injury and Violence Prevention*. This comprehensive manual details injury and violence interventions that have proven to work effectively with vulnerable populations across all stages of life. It will benefit practitioners who manage, implement, or evaluate injury or violence prevention programs; policymakers who influence injury or violence prevention through legislation and other policies; university faculty who teach course work in injury and violence prevention; and graduate students preparing to work in or with injury or violence prevention programs.

Much effort has gone into making this manual a useful reference tool. In addition to providing information on a wide range of health threats and prevention strategies, the manual summarizes trends, controversies, future research, and training issues for injury and violence prevention. The appendices also contain a wealth of valuable resources.

The *Handbook of Injury and Violence Prevention* is a "must read" for all who strive to make our world safer and healthier.

Julie Louise Gerberding, MD, MPH Director,
Centers for Disease Control and Prevention
Atlanta, Georgia

Acknowledgments

We thank the many authors who contributed to this book for sharing their research and expertise in injury and violence prevention and control to make this handbook possible. They are among a small but growing number of researchers and practitioners devoted to uncovering "what works" in injury and violence prevention. Their commitment, enthusiasm, and persistence in documenting the impact of their own work and the work of others will surely benefit the growing support for injury prevention as an integral part of public health.

Lynda Doll expresses her gratitude to the CDC Injury Center for providing time and resources in preparing this book and, in particular, her coeditors, Sandra Bonzo, James Mercy, and David Sleet, who have worked diligently to bring together what we hope is a useful resource for our colleagues in injury and violence research and practice. To Elizabeth Haas, our managing editor, whose commitment, careful attention to editorial detail, and management of the many logistics associated with manuscript development and review were absolutely essential to the success of this project. To her colleagues, Sue Binder and Ileana Arias, who provided excellent counsel throughout this project. To her family, Ted and Jennifer Doll and Abigail Devine, who have been so wonderfully supportive and patient throughout her career and to her granddaughters, Ansley and Halle, for whose future we write this book.

Sandra Bonzo acknowledges all of the past, current, and future inspirational and passionate researchers and practitioners in the field of injury prevention and control. Change can not occur without you. To the National Center for Injury Prevention and Control's Office of Communication Resources staff, thank you for all we accomplished together. My utmost gratitude to my parents and family for their unwavering support and encouragement to make a difference.

James Mercy acknowledges the growing numbers of violence prevention researchers and practitioners across the world and the staff in the Division of Violence Prevention at CDC for their contributions to both the theory and evidence that underlie the information provided in this handbook. And also to his wife, family, and many colleagues at CDC and elsewhere for their support and encouragement in highlighting violence as a public health problem and efforts to document the impact of violence prevention on individuals, families, and society.

David Sleet acknowledges the scientific staff in the Division of Unintentional Injury Prevention at CDC, its director Dr. Christine Branche, and others in the injury research and practice community for contributing the evidence base for interventions included in this handbook. To colleagues in the social and behavioral sciences who have helped us shape new approaches to interventions for injury control. To H.H. Leonards and Ted and Hannah Spero at the Mansion on 0 Street for providing "Simple Things" and a tranquil environment for writing and editing. And to his late parents, Marshall and Anna Mae Sleet, and to his vibrant wife, Louise Gobron, who gave up her weekends to allow us to work on this book.

Finally, we thank Bill Tucker, Executive Editor, and Louise Farkas, Senior Production Editor, and the entire editorial staff at Springer who encouraged us to write this book and helped bring it to completion. This book might never have been published without their support and guidance.

Lynda S. Doll
Sandra E. Bonzo
James A. Mercy
David A. Sleet
April, 2006

Contributors

Joseph L. Annest, PhD, Director, Office of Statistics and Programming, CDC National Center for Injury Prevention and Control, Atlanta, GA 30341, lannest@cdc.gov

Ileana Arias, PhD, Director, CDC National Center for Injury Prevention and Control, Atlanta, GA 30341, iarias@cdc.gov

Charlene K. Baker, PhD, Health Scientist, CDC National Center for Injury Prevention and Control, Atlanta, GA 30341, cbaker@cdc.gov

Michael F. Ballesteros, PhD, Epidemiologist, CDC National Center for Injury Prevention and Control, Atlanta, GA 30341, mballesteros@cdc.gov

Erin L. Bauer, Fellow/Dept. Criminology and Criminal Justice, University of Maryland, College Park, MD 21104, ebauer@crim.umd.edu

Elizabeth E. Bennett, MPH, CHES, Patient/Family Communications and Education Manager, Children's Hospital and Medical Center, Seattle, WA 98145, Elizabeth.bennett@seattlechildrens.org

Lawrence R. Berger, MD, MPH, Academic Director, Indian Health Service Injury Prevention Program, Albuquerque, NM 87106, bergerlaw@msn.com

Sandra E. Bonzo, MLIS, Deputy Director, Office of Communication Resources, CDC National Center for Injury Prevention and Control, Atlanta, GA 30341, sbonzo@cdc.gov

Christine M. Branche, PhD, Director, Division of Unintentional Injury Prevention, CDC National Center for Injury Prevention and Control, Atlanta, GA 30341, cbranche@cdc.gov

Kimberley E. Brice, BSBA, Statistical Programming Assistant, CDC National Center for Injury Prevention and Control, Atlanta, GA 30341, kbrice@cdc.gov

Alison M. Brodie, Project Manager, Queensland University of Technology, Kelvin Grove, QLD 4059 Australia, a.brodie@qut.edu.au

Christy L. Cechman, DC, Contract Research Librarian, CDC National Center for Injury Prevention and Control, Atlanta, GA 30341, ccechman@cdc.gov

Phaedra S. Corso, PhD, Health Economist, CDC National Center for Injury Prevention and Control, Atlanta, GA 30341, pcorso@cdc.gov

Andrew L. Dannenberg, MD, MPH, Association Director for Science, Division of Emergency and Environmental Health Science, CDC National Center for Environmental Health, Atlanta, GA 30341, adannenberg7@cdc.gov

Deborah A. Daro, PhD, Research Fellow, Associate Professor, University of Chicago, Chicago, IL 60637, ddaro@uchicago.edu

Ann M. Dellinger, PhD, Team Leader, Motor Vehicle Injury Prevention Team, CDC National Center for Injury Prevention and Control, Atlanta, GA 30341, adellinger@cdc.gov

Lynda S. Doll, PhD, Associate Director for Science, CDC National Center for Injury Prevention and Control, Atlanta, GA 30341, ldoll1@cdc.gov

Rob J. Donovan, PhD, Professor-Centre for Behavioral Research in Cancer Control, Curtin University, Perth, Western Australia, rdonovan@cc.curtin.edu.au

Randy W. Elder, PhD, Senior Service Fellow, CDC National Center for Injury Prevention and Control, Atlanta, GA 30341, relder1@cdc.gov

Mark J. Francas, MA, National Director of TNS Social Research, Shenton Park WA Australia, mark.francas@tns-global.com

Kimberley E. Freire, MPH, Doctoral Candidate-Health Behavior and Health Education, University of North Carolina, Chapel Hill, NC 27599, freire@email.unc.edu

Howard Frumpkin, MD, DrPH, Director, CDC National Center for Environmental Health and Agency for Toxic Substances & Disease Registries, CDC, Atlanta, GA 30341 Hfrumpkin@cdc.gov

Andrea C. Gielen, ScD, ScM, Director, Center for Injury Research and Policy, Johns Hopkins University, Bloomberg School of Public Health, Baltimore, MD 21205, agielen@jhsph.edu

Julie Gilchrist, MD, Medical Epidemiologist, Home and Recreation Team, CDC National Center for Injury Prevention and Control, Atlanta, GA 30341, jgilchrist@cdc.gov

Denise C. Gottfredson, PhD, Professor of Criminology and Criminal Justice, University of Maryland, College Park, MD 21104, dgottfredson@crim.umd.edu

David C. Grossman, PhD, MPH, Medical Director, Preventive Care, Director, Group Health Cooperative, Seattle, WA 98101, navajo@u.washington.edu

Robin H. Gurwitch, PhD, Associate Professor, Department of Pediatrics, University of Oklahoma Health Sciences Center, Oklahoma City, OK 73117, robin-gurwitch@ouhsc.edu

Nadine Henley, PhD, Professor of Social Marketing, Edith Cowan University, Joondalup Western Australia 6027, n.henley@ecu.edu.au

Ralph W. Hingson, PhD, IPA and Director for Research, National Institute on Alcohol and Alcoholism, National Institutes of Health, Bethesda, MD 20892, rhingson@mail.nih.gov

Arthur L. Kellerman, MD, MPH, Department of Emergency Medicine, Emory University Atlanta, GA 30322, akell01@emory.edu

Richard W. Klomp, CDC National Center for Injury Prevention and Control, Atlanta, GA 30341, rklomp@cdc.gov

Kerry L. Knox, PhD, Assistant Professor, University of Rochester School of Medicine, Rochester, NY14624, Kerry_Knox@URMC.Rochester.edu

Matthew W. Kreuter, PhD, MPH, Associate Professor and Director, Saint Louis University, St. Louis, MO 63104, kreuter@slu.edu

Mark S. Lachs, MD, MPH, Professor of Medicine, Co-Chief of the Division of Geriatrics and Gerontology, Cornell University, New York, NY 10021, mslachs@med.cornell.edu

Karin A. Mack, PhD, Behavioral Scientist-Unintentional Injury, CDC National Center for Injury Prevention and Control, Atlanta, GA 30341, kmack@cdc.gov

Sue Mallonee, RN, MPH, Director of Science, Oklahoma State Department of Health, Oklahoma City, OK 73117, SueM@Health.State.ok.us

Stephen W. Marshall, PhD, Assistant Professor, Department of Epidemiology, University of North Carolina, Chapel Hill, NC 27599, Smarshall@unc.edu

Karen P. McCurdy, PhD, Assistant Professor, Human Development & Family Studies, University of Rhode Island, Kingston, RI 02881, kmccurdy@uri.edu

James A. Mercy, PhD, Associate Director of Science, Division of Violence Prevention, CDC National Center for Injury Prevention and Control, Atlanta, GA 30341, jmercy@cdc.gov

Steven E. Mock, PhD, Project Director, Lighthouse International, New York, NY 10022, smock@lighthouse.org

Katrin U. Mueller-Johnson, PhD, Department of Human Development, Cornell University, Ithaca, NY 14853, kum2@cornell.edu

Lydia N. O'Donnell, EdD, Senior Scientist, Education Development Center, Inc., Newton, MA 02458, lo'donnell@edc.org

Brian F. Oldenburg, PhD, Professor and Regional Director, Queensland University of Technology/Asia Pacific Academic Consortium for Public Health, Kelvin Grove QLD 4059 Australia, b.oldenburg@qut.edu.au

Sharyn E. Parks, MPH, Epidemiologist, East Pittsburgh, PA 15112, sep19@pitt.edu

Corinne L. Peek-Asa, PhD, Professor, College of Public Health-University of Iowa, Director, Iowa Injury Prevention Research Center, Iowa City, IA 52242, Corinne-peek-asa@uiowa.edu

Betty J. Pfefferbaum, MD, JD, Paul and Ruth Jonas Chair, Department of Psychiatry and Behavioral Science, University of Oklahoma Health Sciences Center; Director, Terrorism and Disaster Branch-National Center for Child Traumatic Stress, Oklahoma City, OK 73190, betty-pfefferbaum@ouhsc.edu

Rose L. Pfefferbaum, PhD, MPH, Director, Terrorism and Disaster Preparedness, Phoenix College, Phoenix, AZ 85013, rose.pfefferbaum@pcmail.maricopa.edu

Karl A. Pillemer, PhD, Professor, Department of Human Development, Cornell University, Ithaca, NY 14853, kap6@cornell.edu

Ronald J. Prinz, PhD, Carolina Distinguished Professor, Psychology Department, University of South Carolina, Columbia, SC 29208, prinz@sc.edu

Linda Quan, MD, Director, Emergency Services, Children's Hospital and Medical Center-University of Washington, Seattle, WA 98105, lquan@u.washington.edu

Dori B. Reissman, MD, MPH, CDR, U.S. Public Health Service/Senior Advisor for Emergency Preparedness and Mental Health, CDC National Center for Injury Prevention and Control, Atlanta, GA 30341, dreissman@cdc.gov

Caryll F. Rinehart, Senior Program Analyst, CDC National Center for Injury Prevention and Control, Atlanta, GA 30341, crinehart@cdc.gov

Frederick P. Rivara, MD, MPH, Professor of Pediatrics, University of Washingon, Seattle, WA 98104, fpr@u.washington.edu

Laurence Z. Rubenstein, MD, Director, Geriatric Center, Veterans Affairs Medical Center-UCLA School of Medicine, Sepulveda, CA 91343, laurence.rubenstein@med.va.gov

Carol W. Runyan, PhD, MPH, Director, UNC Injury Prevention Research Center, Professor of Health Behavior and Health Education, Chapel Hill, NC 27599, carol_runyan@unc.edu

Gitanjali Saluja, PhD, Research Fellow, Division of Epidemiology, National Institute for Child Health and Human Development, Bethesda, MD 20892, salujag@mail.nih.gov

Richard W. Sattin, MD, FACP, Associate Director for Science, Division of Injury Response, CDC National Center for Injury Prevention and Control, Atlanta, GA 30341, rsattin@cdc.gov

Janet S. Saul, PhD, Team Leader, Research Synthesis and Application Team, CDC National Center for Injury Prevention and Control, Atlanta, GA 30341, jsaul@cdc.gov

Paul A. Schewe, PhD, University of Illinois at Chicago, Chicago, IL 60607, schewepa@uic.edu

Vicky Scott, Senior Advisor on Falls Prevention, Ministry of Health Services, Victoria British Columbia, Canada, vicky.scott@gems1.gov.bc.ca

Ruth A. Shults, PhD, MPH, Senior Epidemiologist, Division of Unintentional Injury, CDC National Center for Injury Prevention and Control, Atlanta, GA 30341, rshults@cdc.gov

David A. Sleet, PhD, Associate Director for Science, Division of Unintentional Injury Prevention, CDC National Center for Injury Prevention and Control, Atlanta, GA 30341, dsleet@cdc.gov

Ellen D. Sogolow, PhD, Team Leader, Home and Recreation Team, CDC National Center for Injury Prevention and Control, Atlanta, GA 30341, esogolow@cdc.gov

Lorann Stallones, PhD, MPH, Professor and Director, Colorado Injury Control Research Center, University of Colorado, Fort Collins, CO 80523, lorann@colostate.edu

Catherine E. Staunton, MD, King County Department of Public Health, Seattle, WA 98102, jaicat@earthlink.net

Malinda Steenkamp, M.Phil, Associate Service Fellow, Etiology and Surveillance Branch, CDC National Center for Injury Prevention and Control, Atlanta, GA 30341, msteenkamp@cdc.gov

Judy A. Stevens, PhD, Senior Epidemiologist, Division of Unintentional Injury, CDC National Center for Injury Prevention and Control, Atlanta, GA 30341, jstevens@cdc.gov

J. Jill Suitor, PhD, Sociology Professor, Purdue University, West Lafayette, IN 47907, jsuitor@purdue.edu

Monica H. Swahn, PhD, Epidemiologist, Division of Violence Prevention, CDC National Center for Injury Prevention and Control, Atlanta, GA 30341, mswahn@cdc.gov

Sallie R. Thoreson, MS, Injury Epidemiologist, Colorado Department of Public Health and Environment, Grand Junction, CO 81501, sallie.thoreson@state.co.us

Lynne J. Warda, MD, FRCPC, Medical Director, IMPACT-The Injury Prevention Centre of Children's Hospital, Winnipeg, Manitoba, Canada, lwarda@mts.net

Daniel J. Whitaker, PhD, Team Leader, Development and Efficacy Research Team, CDC National Center for Injury Prevention and Control, Atlanta, GA 30341, dwhitaker@cdc.gov

Renee F. Wilson-Simmons, DrPH, Senior Scientist, Education Development Center, Inc., Ocean, NJ 07712, rwilson@edc.org

Contents

PART IV: INTERVENTIONS IN THE FIELD

PART V: DISSEMINATION AND ADOPTION OF EFFECTIVE INTERVENTIONS AND POLICIES

APPENDICES

Part **I**

Introduction

Chapter 1

The Epidemiology and Costs of Unintentional and Violent Injuries

Richard W. Sattin and Phaedra S. Corso

1.1. INTRODUCTION

Injuries are the number one killer of children and young adults in the United States (Centers for Disease Control and Prevention [CDC], 2005). More than 28 million injuries serious enough to require emergency medical care occur annually (CDC, 2005). The lives of millions of others have been dramatically affected by injuries to themselves or someone they love. Injury leads to pathological conditions and impaired physiological functioning that can affect any part, organ, or system of an individual and can have both short-term and long-term effects (Sattin, 1992). Due to the potential extensive nature of injuries, outcomes depend on a broad continuum of multidisciplinary care.

Injury has been described, until recently, as the "neglected disease" because it occurs in such great numbers but has been tacitly accepted as a normal occurrence of living in a modern society (Committee on Trauma, and Committee on Shock, Division of Medical Sciences, National Academy of Sciences/National Research Council [Committee on Trauma], 1966). However, the 1985 report *Injury in America* noted that a public health approach similar to that used for other diseases could lead to significant reduction in injuries (Committee on Trauma Research, Commission on Life Sciences, National Research Council and the Institute of Medicine [Committee on Trauma Research], 1985).

Injuries can be viewed as a problem in medical ecology—that is, as a relationship between a person (the host), an agent, and the environment (Haddon, 1970; Haddon & Baker, 1981; Sattin, 1992). The underlying agent of injury is not a microbe or carcinogen but energy, most often in the form of mechanical force (Haddon, 1970). The dose of energy received; the dose's distribution, duration, and rapidity; and the individual's response to the transfer of the energy can determine if a physical injury occurs or is prevented (Committee on Trauma Research, 1985). For example, a large mechanical energy load quickly transmitted to a hip during a fall involving an older person may lead to a fracture. If that same energy load could be dissipated through use of energy-absorbing flooring or mats or through hip pads or other new technologies, the fracture that occurred during the fall could have been prevented. Likewise, exercises leading to strengthening of the lower extremities or to improving gait and balance among older persons could lead to preventing the fall itself (AGS Panel on Falls Prevention [AGS], 2001) or to improving reflexes that would lead to dissipating the energy or changing the location of that energy to a more forgiving body area.

The basic injury paradigm of host, agent, and environment mentioned above needs to include energy tranference by perpetrators, the threat of energy transference by potential perpetrators of violence, and the effect of the social as well as physical environment. Victims of violence can experience physical injury; adverse mental health consequences such as depression, anxiety, and low self-esteem; and harmful physical health consequences such as suicide attempts, cardiovascular disease, and substance abuse (National Center for Injury Prevention and Control [NCIPC], 2002). Any of these consequences can lead to hospitalization, disability, or death. Programs and policies that provide counseling for batterers, improve parenting skills, or prevent dating violence, intervene with perpetrators and potential perpetrators before the violence occurs or recurs can prevent energy or threat of energy transference. In some social contexts, intimate partner violence, sexual violence, and child maltreatment are considered normative behavior (NCIPC, 2002). To design effective interventions, researchers must first identify the particular social norms and beliefs that support these types of violence and then find ways to alter or replace them with ones that prevent violence. Even when such violent behaviors are not considered "acceptable," cultural attitudes and beliefs may exacerbate these problems by blaming victims or by supporting attitudes and behaviors that create social atmospheres conducive to, or tolerant of, such violence (NCIPC, 2002).

The classification of injury poses a number of epidemiological issues. One can classify injuries by the actual nature of the injury (e.g., fracture of the hip, traumatic brain injury, splenic rupture), by the mechanism of the injury (e.g., fall, motor vehicle, poisoning), and by the intent (e.g., unintentional, intentional, undetermined). If one classifies by the nature of the injury, then one needs to decide to analyze by the number of injuries or the number of injurious episodes or both, and the choice of the denominator is critical. The mechanism and intent of the injury is useful in quantifying the problem of falls, motor-vehicle crashes, suicide, domestic violence, and so forth in the community, and that information can be used to implement effective intervention strategies. However, sometimes a fall, motor-vehicle incident, or suicide attempt, occurs that does not lead to physical injury. These incidents are important, though, because opportunities for preventing future injuries may be lost. For example, a person involved in an alcohol-related motor-vehicle crash who is brought to an emergency department but who has sustained no physical injury might benefit from counseling on alcohol use before being discharged from the emergency department (Hungerford & Pollock, 2002). Finally, definitions of some mechanisms of injury can vary significantly. For example, most definitions of a fall are clinically or research oriented, are subjective, and are likely to miss a substantial number of falls (Sattin, 1992). Even though the number of falls can be ascertained from medical records and by using the *International Classification of*

Diseases's external causes of injuries (E-codes), falls have been shown to be significantly underreported using such data sources (Fife, 1987).

Despite these issues, injury epidemiology has shown significant progress over the last several decades and has led to a better understanding of mechanisms, behavior, and prevention strategies. Motor vehicle safety has improved through the development and use of safety equipment, the enactment and enforcement of traffic safety laws, and the changes in driver behavior (CDC, 1999). Although the design of safety equipment in motor vehicles was based primarily on biomechanical data, epidemiological analysis of crash data was critical in defining the problems, determining high-risk populations, and identifying solutions to improve safety behavior. The benefits of using bicycle helmets to prevent death and disability among youth was demonstrated through epidemiological analysis (Thompson, Rivara, & Thompson, 1989). The idea that violence is a public health issue is now largely accepted based on epidemiological analyses begun in the 1980s (Mercy & O'Carroll, 1988). As the field of injury continues to grow; and as new events unfold, new aspects of injury present challenges that can be addressed through epidemiological analyses. For example, the events of September 11, 2001, showed that the care of the acutely injured during a terrorist event is a critical role for public health and that better, compatible data systems are needed to evaluate and improve the effectiveness of trauma care (CDC, 2002a, 2002b; NCIPC, 2005).

1.2.   METHODS

In this chapter, we report the incidence and costs of injuries stratified by age group, sex, mechanism (e.g., falls, motor vehicle), and intent (e.g., intentional or unintentional). Throughout, we include unique injury episodes occurring in 2000 (the most current year for which data are available), meaning that if someone suffered multiple injuries (e.g., a hip fracture and a wrist fracture) in one event (e.g., a fall), the episode would be counted only once. For readability, we use the terms *persons injured* and *number of injuries* synonymously to refer to injury episodes.

Given space limitations, we have chosen not to include, beyond basic mechanisms, the epidemiology of specific injury problems, such as drowning, fires, motor vehicles, sports injuries, falls, child maltreatment, youth violence, intimate partner violence, elder abuse, suicide, sexual violence, and firearms. We do provide references to these topics for the interested reader (Table 1.1).

The incidence and cost estimates presented in this chapter are divided into two mutually exclusive categories that reflect the highest level of treatment for an injury, as a proxy for severity: (1) injury resulting in death, including deaths occurring within and outside a health care setting, and (2) nonfatal injuries, including injuries resulting in hospitalization with survival to discharge and injuries requiring medical attention without hospitalization (e.g., injuries requiring an emergency department visit, an office visit, or a hospital outpatient visit). Injuries that were not severe enough to result in medical attention are not included in our calculations. We sum the incidence and costs of fatal and nonfatal injuries to quantify total lifetime medical costs.

Incidence data used to develop these estimates were taken from a variety of sources. Fatal injury counts were taken from the 2000 National Vital Statistics System (NVSS) data. We used the 2000 Healthcare Cost and Utilization Project— Nationwide Inpatient Sample (HCUP-NIS) to estimate the incidence of nonfatal

Table 1.1. References to Detailed Epidemiologic Descriptions of Specific Injury Problems

Specific Injury Problems	Reference(s)
Drowning	Quan, L., & Cummings, P. (2003). Characteristics of drowning by different age groups. *Injury Prevention, 9* (2), 163–168.
	Centers for Disease Control and Prevention. (2004). Nonfatal and fatal drownings in recreational water settings—United States, 2001–2002. *Morbidity and Mortality Weekly Report, 53,* 447–452.
Falls	Tideiksaar, R. (2002). *Falls in Older People: Prevention & Management.* Baltimore, Health Professionals Press.
	Rubenstein, L. Z., & Josephson, K. R. (2002). The epidemiology of falls and syncope. *Clinics in Geriatric Medicine, 18* (2), 141–158.
Fires	Warda, L., Tenenbein, M., & Moffatt, M. E. K. (1999). House fire injury prevention update. Part 1. A review of risk factors for fatal and non-fatal house fire injury. *Injury Prevention, 5,* 145–150.
Motor vehicles	National Highway Traffic Safety Administration. (2005). *Traffic safety facts 2003: A compilation of motor vehicle crash data from the Fatality Analysis Reporting System and the General Estimates System.* (Report No. DOT HS 809-775). Washington, DC: U.S. Department of Transportation.
Sports injuries	Caine, D. J., & Maffulli, N. (Eds.). (2005). *Epidemiology of pediatric sports injuries: Vol. 48. Individual sports.* Farmington, CT: S. Karger.
	Maffulli, N., & Caine, D. J. (Eds.). (2005). *Epidemiology of pediatric sports injuries: vol. 49. Team sports.* Farmington, CT: S. Karger.
Interpersonal violence, sexual violence	Tjaden, P., & Thoennes, N. (2000). *Extent, nature, and consequences of intimate partner violence: Findings from the National Violence against Women Survey* (NCJ 181867). Washington, DC: U.S. Department of Justice, Office of Justice Programs, National Institute of Justice.
	Paulozzi, L. J., Saltzman, L. E., Thompson, M. P., Holmgreen, P. (2001). Surveillance for homicide among intimate partners—United States, 1981–1998. (2001).*MMWR Surveillance Summaries, 50,* (no. SS-3), 1–15.
Youth violence	*Youth Violence: A Report of the Surgeon General. Surgeon General's Office, Public Health Service.* (2001). Retrieved July 5, 2005, from www.hhs. gov/surgeongeneral/library/youthviolence.
Suicide	Goldsmith, S. K., Pellmar, T. C., Kleinman, A. M., & Bunney, W. E. (Eds.). Committee on Pathophysiology & Prevention of Adolescent & Adult Suicide, Board on Neuroscience and Behavioral Health (2002). *Reducing suicide: A national imperative.* Washington, DC: National Academy of Sciences.
Child maltreatment	Department of Health and Human Services, Administration on Children, Youth, and Families (2005). *Child maltreatment 2003.* Washington DC: U.S. Government Printing Office. Retrieved April 5, 2005, from www.acf.hhs.gov/programs/cb/publications/cm03.pdf.

injuries resulting in hospitalization. We estimated the incidence of nonfatal, non-admitted medically treated injuries using the 1999 Medical Expenditure Panel Survey (MEPS), the 2001 National Electronic Injury Surveillance System—All Injury Program (NEISS-AIP), the 1999 and 2000 National Hospital and Ambulatory Medical Care Survey (NHAMCS), and the 1999 and 2000 National Ambulatory Medical Care Survey (NAMCS).

Incidence of injury episodes and corresponding rates apply to the civilian, noninstitutionalized U.S. population ($n = 276,410,000$). *Incidence,* as defined in this analysis, addresses injury resulting in the use of medical care as the primary outcome only and does not necessarily reflect the many other adverse sequelae and other long-term health consequences that can and do result from physical injury to society, families, and communities. For example, incidence data that are missing include use of mental-health services that were not identified as injury related but were needed due to the psychological trauma of injury. Based on a survey of mental health providers, Cohen and Miller (1998) estimated that 3.4 million physical and sexual assaults resulted in mental health treatment, often without treatment in other medical settings. These treatment episodes are unlikely to be coded as injury related. Likewise, injuries resulting in the use of nontraditional health care services (e.g., chiropractors, acupuncturists, and alternative medicine providers) are not included in this analysis.

We computed unit costs for injuries by the same strata identified for incidence, separately for fatal and nonfatal injuries. Costs, presented in 2000 U.S. dollars, include all those direct medical expenditures required in the use of health care services and losses in productivity. Medical expenditures include costs associated with inpatient admissions, emergency department (ED) care, outpatient services, rehabilitation costs, transport, coroner/medical examiner, long-term care for permanent disability, and nursing home costs. Productivity losses include short- and long-term losses in wages and household productivity. All future costs were converted to present value using a 3% discount rate.

Productivity losses were also estimated separately for fatal and nonfatal injuries using the same strata identified earlier. For someone of a given sex and age who sustained a fatal injury, we summed the product of the sex-specific probability of surviving to each subsequent year of age and sex-specific expected earnings for someone in that age bracket (using 10-year age brackets) (Haddix, Teutsch, & Corso, 2003). Earnings at future ages, including salary and the value of fringe benefits, were adjusted upward to account for a historical 1% productivity growth rate (Haddix et al., 2003) and then discounted to present value using the 3% discount rate. Parallel calculations valued lost household work, again using unit costs by age group and sex.

For nonfatal injuries, productivity loss equals the sum of the value of wage and household work lost due to short-term disability in the acute recovery phase and, for the subset of injuries that cause lasting impairments that restrict work choices or preclude return to work, the value of wage and household work lost due to permanent or long-term disability. A more complete description of the data and methods used to calculate these estimates will be available soon (Finkelstein, Corso, & Miller, 2006).

We also provide incidence of injury death by race, ethnicity, and sex for injuries overall and by intent for the year 2000, based on a different data source than the stratifications described above—that is, from the Web-Based Injury Statistics Query and Reporting System (WISQARS) (CDC, 2005). Cost-of-injury estimates for race or ethnicity were not calculated for this chapter because of limited information.

1.3. RESULTS

1.3.1. Total Injury Incidence and Cost

In 2000, injuries in the United States resulted in approximately 149,000 fatalities and nearly 50 million nonfatal injuries (Table 1.2). Of the nonfatal injuries, 1.9 million resulted in hospitalization, and 48.1 million resulted in nonhospitalized treatment episodes. This sums to a total of 50.1 million injury episodes in 2000, or

Table 1.2. The Incidence, Rate (per 100,000), and Total Lifetime Costs for Injuries by Age and Sex, 2000

	Incidence						Costs (in Millions)		
	Fatal	Rate*	Nonfatal	Rate*	Total	Rate*	Medical Costs	Productivity Losses	Total
Total	149,075	54	49,978,023	18,081	50,127,098	18,135	$80,248	$326,042	$406,289
0–4	3,532	18	3,423,039	17,385	3,426,571	17,403	3,729	12,264	15,992
5–14	3,741	9	7,942,051	19,239	7,945,792	19,249	8,170	26,400	34,569
15–24	23,698	63	8,794,716	23,540	8,818,414	23,604	12,895	66,940	79,835
25–44	48,487	59	15,504,520	18,759	15,553,007	18,818	22,704	141,188	163,892
45–64	31,935	53	8,782,618	14,696	8,814,553	14,750	14,278	66,311	80,589
65–74	10,595	60	2,368,679	13,428	2,379,274	13,488	5,865	7,541	13,406
75+	27,087	179	3,162,399	20,888	3,189,486	21,067	12,608	5,399	18,007
Male	103,900	77	26,461,330	19,659	26,565,230	19,736	$44,445	$238,688	$283,133
0–4	2,059	20	2,076,975	20,224	2,079,034	20,244	2,438	8,733	11,170
5–14	2,397	11	4,539,032	21,676	4,541,429	21,688	4,973	18,810	23,783
15–24	18,609	98	5,110,966	26,928	5,129,575	27,026	8,346	52,930	61,276
25–44	37,126	92	8,516,730	21,123	8,553,856	21,215	14,033	107,019	121,052
45–64	23,313	81	4,185,422	14,477	4,208,735	14,558	7,999	45,612	53,611
65–74	6,916	87	1,048,797	13,129	1,055,713	13,215	2,704	3,873	6,578
75+	13,480	228	983,409	16,599	996,889	16,827	3,952	1,712	5,663
Female	45,175	32	23,516,693	16,584	23,561,868	16,616	$35,803	$87,353	$123,156
0–4	1,473	16	1,346,065	14,295	1,347,538	14,311	1,291	3,531	4,822
5–14	1,344	7	3,403,019	16,731	3,404,363	16,737	3,197	7,589	10,786
15–24	5,089	28	3,683,750	20,031	3,688,839	20,059	4,549	14,010	18,559
25–44	11,361	27	6,987,790	16,508	6,999,151	16,535	8,671	34,169	42,840
45–64	8,622	28	4,597,196	14,902	4,605,818	14,930	6,279	20,699	26,978
65–74	3,679	38	1,319,882	13,673	1,323,561	13,711	3,160	3,668	6,828
75+	13,607	148	2,178,990	23,636	2,192,597	23,783	8,656	3,687	12,343

*Rate per 100,000 people.

18 injuries requiring medical attention per every 100 civilian, noninstitutionalized U.S. residents. Injuries that occurred in 2000 will cost the U.S. health care system $80.2 billion in medical care costs, with an additional cost of $326 billion in productivity losses.

1.3.2.   Overall Age and Sex Patterns

The overall number of injuries among males (26.6 million) was only slightly higher than that among females (23.6 million) (Table 1.2). Taking into account population size, the overall rate of injuries for males was 19,736 per 100,000 people and that for females was 16,616 per 100,000 people. Of the total injuries in 2000, almost one third (15.6 million) occurred among 25- to 44-year-olds, but this age group also represents approximately one third of the U.S. population. In comparison, 15- to 24-year-olds represent only 14% of the U.S. population but accounted for 18% of injuries. Thus those aged 15–24 years, with 8.8 million injuries, had the highest *rate* of injuries, 23,604 per 100,000 persons; the second-highest rate, 21,067 per 100,000 people, occurred among those aged 75 years or older; and the third-highest rate, 19,249 per 100,000 people, occurred among those aged 5–14 years. These high injury rates across different age groups reveal that, unlike chronic conditions (e.g., heart disease, diabetes, and osteoarthritis), which disproportionately affect the elderly, injuries affect both the young and the old alike. Thus it is possible that the economic burden of injuries is much larger than that for many chronic conditions because injuries are more likely to affect people during their peak earning years.

The highest rate of injury fatalities, 179 per 100,000, occurred among people aged 75 years and older (Table 1.2), and was nearly three times greater than the next highest rate, 63 per 100,000, which occurred among those aged 15–24 years. Males in every age group were more likely to sustain a fatal injury than females. The overall rate of injury fatalities among males (77 per 100,000) was more than double that among females (32 per 100,000). Injuries among males accounted for $44.4 billion, or approximately 55% of all medical costs for injuries; injuries among females accounted for $35.8 billion, or approximately 45% of all medical costs for injuries (Table 1.2). This cost distribution is similar to the incidence distribution. When productivity losses are included in lifetime costs, males had more than a twofold increased cost overall than females, $283 billion vs. $123 billion. From ages 0 through 64 years, males had between a twofold and threefold greater lifetime cost than females of similar ages. For ages 65 years and older, females had higher lifetime costs of injury than males. This is due, in part, to the higher rate of nonfatal injuries in females aged 75 years and older (23,636 per 100,000) compared to males of the same age (16,599 per 100,000). Those aged 25–44 years accounted for $22.7 billion, or nearly 30% of injury-attributable medical costs. This age group also represents 30% of the U.S. population and accounted for 30% of all injuries. In contrast, those aged greater than 75 years (representing 5% of the population) accounted for only 6% of all injuries, yet they represent 16% (or $12.6 billion) of the medical costs for injuries. This likely reflects the frail nature of elderly persons and their inability to recover as quickly from an injury compared to their younger counterparts. About 79% of injury-attributable medical costs among people aged 75 years or older resulted from fatal (3%) and hospitalized injuries (76%) (results not shown). In contrast, only 15% of the medical costs for injuries among people aged 5–14 years resulted from fatal (<1%) and hospitalized injuries (14.6%).

Conversely, the percentage of medical costs attributable to nonhospitalized injuries decreased as age increased.

1.3.3.   Race and Ethnicity Patterns

For males, African Americans had the highest age-adjusted rate of injury fatality, 107.4 per 100,000 people, followed by American Indian/Alaska Native (AI/AN), 100.55 per 100,000, by Whites, 75.5 per 100,000 and by Asian/Pacific Islanders, 36.8 per 100,000 (data not shown). Non-Hispanic males had a higher age-adjusted rate of injury fatality, 53.3 per 100,000, than Hispanic males, 44.4 per 100,000. Males had consistently higher fatality rates than females regardless of race or ethnicity: 3.5 times higher in African Americans, 2.6 times higher in Whites, 2.4 times higher in AI/AN, 2.0 times higher in Asian/Pacific Islanders, and 3.2 times higher in Hispanics. AI/AN males had the highest age-adjusted rate of unintentional injury fatality, 71.0 per 100,000, followed by African Americans, 58.3 per 100,000, by Whites, 49.2 per 100,000, and by Asian/Pacific Islanders, 23.2 per 100,000. Hispanic males had a lower age-adjusted rate of unintentional injury fatality than non-Hispanic males, 44.6 per 100,000 vs. 49.6 per 100,000. African American males had nearly twice the rate of violence-related fatalities than AI/AN and White males, 46.0 per 100,000 vs. 27.0 per 100,000 and 24.4 per 100,000, respectively, and more than three times the fatality rate than Asian/Pacific Islanders, 13.0 per 100,000 people. Hispanic males had a slightly lower rate of death from violence, 13.5 per 100,000, than non-Hispanic males, 16.7 per 100,000.

1.3.4.   Injury Mechanisms

The two leading mechanisms of fatal injuries were motor vehicles and firearms, accounting for 43,802 and 28,722 deaths (16 and 10 per 100,000 people), respectively (Table 1.3). These two mechanisms were responsible for nearly half (49%) of all injury fatalities. In contrast, falls caused both the highest incidence (11.6 million or 23%) and rate (4,180 per 100,000) of nonfatal injuries. Being struck by or against an object (10.7 million) and motor vehicles (5 million) were the next most likely mechanisms for nonfatal injury. Treatment for falls ($26.9 billion) and motor vehicle incidents ($14 billion) represented roughly half of injury-attributable medical costs. Yet, these two mechanisms represented only one third of injury incidence. Thus falls and motor-vehicle incidents represent a disproportionate fraction of medical costs, reflecting the severity of resultant injuries (i.e., injuries caused by these mechanisms are more likely to result in a fatality or hospitalization). In contrast, struck by/against injuries, which accounted for 21% of all injuries in 2000, represented only 14% of medical costs for injuries.

Injuries categorized as "other" resulted from varied mechanisms. For fatal injuries, these mechanisms, representing 20% of fatal injuries, primarily included inhalation/suffocation (8% of all deaths) and unspecified (7% of all deaths) (results not shown). Of the 16.5 million nonfatal other injuries, overexertion accounted for nearly 5.2 million (32%), other specified accounted for 4.3 million (26%), and bites/stings accounted for 3.3 million (20%). Of the other nonfatal injuries resulting in hospitalization (representing 16% of all hospitalized injuries), the mechanisms were largely related to other specified or unspecified mechanisms (50%), overexertion (14%), and other transport (13%).

Table 1.3. Total Lifetime Costs for Injuries, by Mechanism, 2000

| | Incidence | | | | | | Costs (in Millions) | | |
	Fatal	Rate*	Nonfatal	Rate*	Total	Rate*	Medical Costs	Productivity Losses	Total
Total	149,075	54	49,978,023	18,081	50,127,098	18,135	$80,248	$326,042	$406,289
Motor vehicle/other road user	43,802	16	4,966,637	1,797	5,010,439	1,813	14,026	75,130	89,156
Falls	14,052	5	11,552,690	4,180	11,566,742	4,185	26,892	54,028	80,920
Struck by/against	1,301	0	10,672,879	3,861	10,674,180	3,862	11,028	37,104	48,132
Cut/pierce	2,293	1	4,121,792	1,491	4,124,085	1,492	3,662	12,664	16,326
Fire/burn	3,922	1	770,454	279	774,376	280	1,345	6,202	7,546
Poisoning	20,261	7	1,247,204	451	1,267,465	459	2,236	23,707	25,944
Drowning/submersion	4,168	2	5,915	2	10,083	4	95	5,215	5,310
Firearm/gunshot	28,722	10	102,291	37	131,013	47	1,225	35,226	36,451
Other	30,554	11	16,538,162	5,983	16,568,716	5,994	19,738	76,767	96,505
Male	103,900	77	26,461,332	19,659	26,565,232	19,736	44,445	238,688	283,133
Motor vehicle/other road user	29,686	22	2,521,644	1,873	2,551,330	1,895	8,713	55,214	63,927
Falls	7,647	6	5,194,029	3,859	5,201,676	3,865	11,778	31,824	43,602
Struck by/against	1,109	1	6,659,192	4,947	6,660,301	4,948	7,493	29,123	36,617
Cut/pierce	1,678	1	2,600,406	1,932	2,602,084	1,933	2,442	9,775	12,217
Fire/burn	2,333	2	369,655	275	371,988	276	764	4,078	4,842
Poisoning	13,721	10	575,179	427	588,900	438	1,063	18,319	19,382
Drowning/submersion	3,198	2	3,818	3	7,016	5	61	4,389	4,450
Firearm/gunshot	24,638	18	92,391	69	117,029	87	1,081	31,809	32,890
Other	19,890	15	8,445,018	6,274	8,464,908	6,289	11,050	54,157	65,207
Female	45,175	32	23,516,693	16,584	23,561,868	16,616	35,803	87,353	123,156
Motor vehicle/other road user	14,166	10	2,444,939	1,724	2,459,105	1,734	5,313	19,916	25,229
Falls	6,405	5	6,358,661	4,484	6,365,066	4,489	15,114	22,204	37,318
Struck by/against	192	0	4,013,688	2,831	4,013,880	2,831	3,535	7,981	11,516
Cut/pierce	615	0	1,521,386	1,073	1,522,001	1,073	1,221	2,889	4,109
Fire/burn	1,589	1	400,800	283	402,389	284	581	2,124	2,704
Poisoning	6,540	5	672,025	474	678,565	479	1,173	5,388	6,562
Drowning/submersion	970	1	2,097	1	3,067	2	34	825	859
Firearm/gunshot	4,084	3	9,900	7	13,984	10	144	3,417	3,561
Other	10,664	8	8,093,143	5,707	8,103,807	5,715	8,688	22,610	31,298

*Rate per 100,000 people.

Males had a higher incidence and rate of fatal injuries than females, regardless of mechanism (Table 1.3). This difference was particularly pronounced for motor-vehicle-related and firearm-related fatal injuries. The rate of fatal motor-vehicle-related injuries among males (22 per 100,000 people) was more than double that among females (10 per 100,000); the rate of fatal firearm injuries among males (18 per 100,000) was six times that among females (3 per 100,000).

Males had a higher incidence and rate of nonfatal injuries than females from all mechanisms except falls, fires/burns, and poisoning (Table 1.3). Of all fall-related nonfatal injuries, 55% occurred among females, at a rate of 4,484 per 100,000 females. This rate was 16% higher than the rate of nonfatal fall injuries among males (3,859 per 100,000 males). The rate of nonfatal fires/burns was 3% higher for females compared to males, and the rate of nonfatal poisoning was 11% higher. The largest difference in overall incidence of injuries between males and females by mechanism was for firearm-related injuries, with males suffering 90% of these injuries. The rate of firearm injuries among males, 87 per 100,000 people, was almost nine times more than that for females, 10 per 100,000. With the exception of falls (44%) and poisonings (48%), males accounted for more than half of the medical costs associated with each injury mechanism. The medical costs associated with struck by/against and cut/pierce injuries among males were double those for females; the medical costs associated with firearm injuries among males were more than seven times those for females. These cost disparities, however, were largely driven by a higher incidence of these injuries among males.

1.3.5. Injury-Related Hospitalizations

As a percentage of all injuries, fatal injuries accounted for 0.3% of the total, hospitalized or ED-treated injuries accounted for 59%, and injuries seen in an outpatient setting or during a doctor's visit accounted for the remaining incidences (Table 1.4). Medical costs were greatest for hospitalized ($33.7 billion) and for ED-treated ($31.8 billion) injuries. However, when productivity losses were added to direct medical costs, fatal injuries accounted for the greatest costs ($143 billion), followed by ED-treated injuries ($99 billion). Females accounted for 968,000 (52%) of hospitalizations, but males had higher incidence counts and rates of hospitalization for all mechanisms other than falls and poisonings (data not shown). The rate of fall-related hospitalized injuries among females (386 per 100,000) was 69% higher than that among males (228 per 100,000), and that of poisonings (91 per 100,000) was 36% higher than that among males (67 per 100,000). Males had higher hospitalized injury rates than females for motor vehicles (125 per 100,000 vs. 76 per 100,000), for struck by/against (50 per 100,000 vs. 13 per 100,000), for cut/pierce (37 per 100,000 vs. 15 per 100,000), for fire/burn (11 per 100,000 vs. 7 per 100,000), for drowning/submersion (2 per 100,000 vs. 1 per 100,000), and for firearm/gunshot (20 per 100,000 vs. 2 per 100,000). For females, both the highest number (408,000, or 42%) and the highest rate of injury hospitalizations occurred among those aged 75 years and older. In fact, the rate of injury hospitalizations (4.4 per 100 people) among older females was nearly four times greater than that among any other age group. For males, although the highest number of injury hospitalizations (272,000, or 30%) occurred among those 25–44 years old, the highest *rate* of injury hospitalizations (2.5 per 100 people) occurred among those aged 75 years or older.

Table 1.4. The Incidence, Rate (per 100,000), and Total Lifetime Costs of Injuries by Treatment Location, 2000

	Incidence						Costs (in Millions)		
	Fatal	Rate*	Nonfatal	Rate*	Total	Rate*	Medical Costs	Productivity Losses	Total
	149,075	54	49,978,023	18,081	50,127,098	18,135	$80,248	$326,041	$406,289
Fatal	149,075	54	—	—	149,129	54	1,113	142,041	143,154
Hospital	—	—	1,869,857	676	1,869,857	676	33,737	58,716	92,453
Emergency department treated	—	—	27,928,975	10,104	27,928,975	10,104	31,804	67,288	99,092
Outpatient	—	—	590,554	214	590,554	214	526	1,553	2,079
Medical dotor visit	—	—	19,588,637	7,087	19,588,637	7,087	13,068	56,443	69,511

*Rate per 100,000 people.

For hospitalized injuries, males accounted for a greater percentage of attributable medical costs than did females for all age groups younger than 65 years (data not shown). Comparing the distribution of injury-attributable medical costs with that of injury incidence, except for males aged 0–4 and 5–14 years, males accounted for a greater percentage of medical costs than similarly aged females for hospitalized injuries than they accounted for the incidence of hospitalized injuries. In particular, males aged 15–24, 25–44, and 45–64 years accounted for 74%, 71%, and 62% of medical costs for hospitalized injuries, but only 65%, 63%, and 54% of hospitalized injuries. This may indicate that hospitalized injuries among males in these age groups are, on average, more severe or more difficult to treat than injuries among same-age females. For nonhospitalized injuries, the medical cost distribution between males and females in all age groups is nearly identical to the corresponding incidence distribution.

The rate of fall-related hospitalized injuries (309 per 100,000 people) was more than three times greater than any other specified mechanism category, followed by motor vehicles (100 per 100,000) and poisonings (79 per 100,000) (data not shown). In contrast to all nonfatal injuries for which people aged 15–24 years had the highest rate, people aged 75 years or older had the highest rate of hospitalized injuries (3,663 per 100,000 people), more than three times that of any other age group (data not shown). People aged 75 years and older accounted for nearly 555,000 injury hospitalizations, or 30% of the total injury hospitalizations. The increased rate of serious injuries (i.e., fatal and hospitalized injuries) among older persons compared to other age groups may be due in part to underlying co-morbid conditions, poorer gait and balance, and loss of elasticity of tissues and organs.

1.3.6. Intentionality

According to the data sources used to develop these estimates, nearly two thirds of all injury fatalities were reported as unintentional, resulting in more than $74 billion in medical costs alone (Table 1.5). Of fatalities owing to intentional causes, 64% were suicides (29,416) and 36% were homicides (16,830). Whereas less than 1% of unintentional injuries were fatal, 9% of self-inflicted injuries were fatal. Males accounted for 80% of self-inflicted injury fatalities, 65% of unintentional injury fatalities, 77% of assault fatalities, and 97% of military/legal fatalities (results not shown). For nonfatal injuries, 95% (or 47.4 million) were due to unintended mechanisms. The rate of unintentional nonfatal injuries for males, 18,635 per 100,000 persons, was 18% greater than that for females, at 15,722 per 100,000 people (results not shown). The rate of assault-related nonfatal injuries among males, 885 per 100,000, was 26% higher than the rate among females, at 703 per 100,000. Females, on the other hand, accounted for 59% of self-inflicted nonfatal injuries, at a rate of 122 per 100,000, which was 36% greater than that for males, at 90 per 100,000.

1.4. CONCLUSION

Injuries represent a substantial burden to society. As we have shown in this chapter, the burden can be considered in several ways: by incidence, defined as total or fatal versus nonfatal; by incidence rates; or by total costs, defined by medical costs

Table 1.5. The Incidence, Rate (per 100,000), and Total Lifetime Costs of Injuries by Intent, 2000

	Incidence						Costs (in Millions)		
	Fatal	Rate*	Nonfatal	Rate*	Total	Rate*	Medical Costs	Productivity Losses	Total
Total	149,075	54	49,978,023	18,081	50,127,098	18,135	$80,248	$326,040	$406,289
Unintentional	98,622	36	47,375,945	17,140	47,474,567	17,175	74,145	255,159	329,304
Self-inflicted	29,416	11	294,636	107	324,052	117	1,364	31,994	33,358
Assault	16,830	6	2,187,268	791	2,204,098	797	4,277	32,826	37,103
Legal/military	377	0	61,899	22	62,276	23	110	743	853
Undetermined	3,830	1	58,278	21	62,108	22	351	5,319	5,670

*Rate per 100,000 people.

and losses in productivity. How one defines *burden* determines which stratification of injury is most burdensome. For example, Table 1.6 shows that motor vehicles, falls, and struck by/against, consistently rank as the top three mechanisms for causing the highest burden, with some variation in how burden is defined. Motor vehicles led to the highest fatality burden among all age and sex groups except for those aged 75 years or more, for which falls was the highest. However, for nonfatal injuries, falls and struck by/against injuries had the highest burden for most age and sex groups. Motor vehicles led to the highest total cost overall, but variations in costs by mechanism and by type of costs existed among different population groups.

Table 1.6. Mechanism* Resulting in Highest Injury Burden by Age and Sex, 2000

	Incidence			Costs (In Millions)		
	Fatal	Nonfatal	Total	Medical	Productivity†	Total
ALL	MV 43,802	Falls 11,552,690	Falls 11,566,742	Falls $26,892	MV $75,130	MV $89,156
0–4	MV 835	Falls 1,312,815	Falls 1,312,865	Falls $1,610	Falls $3,754	Falls $5,364
5–14	MV 1,821	Struck By/Against‡ 2,675,579	Struck By/Against 2,675,620	Struck By/Against $2,401	Falls $7,921	Falls $10,261
15–24	MV 10,534	Struck By/Against 2,644,560	Struck By/Against 2,644,709	MV $3,587	MV $22,875	MV $26,462
25–44	MV 14,053	Struck By/Against 2,932,759	Struck By/Against 2,933,206	MV $5,039	MV $32,627	MV $37,666
45–64	MV 9,001	Falls 2,037,076	Falls 2,039,087	Falls $4,466	Falls $14,021	Falls $18,487
65–74	MV 3,069	Falls 806,803	Falls 808,504	Falls $3,259	Falls $3,095	Falls $6,354
75+	Falls 8,695	Falls 1,785,175	Falls 1,793,870	Falls $9,611	Falls $3,246	Falls $12,857
Males	MV 29,686	Falls 5,194,029	Falls 5,201,676	Falls $11,778	MV $55,214	MV $63,927
0–4	MV 463	Falls 758,672	Falls 758,705	Falls $1,100	Falls $2,611	Falls $3,711
5–14	MV 1,065	Struck By/Against 1,915,521	Struck By/Against 1,915,551	Struck By/Against $1,805	Struck By/Against $6,110	Struck By/Against $7,915
15–24	MV 7,474	Struck By/Against 1,670,280	Struck By/Against 1,670,414	MV $2,284	MV $17,187	MV $19,471
25–44	MV 10,246	Struck By/Against 1,760,230	Struck By/Against 1,760,629	MV $3,192	MV $24,483	MV $27,675
45–64	MV 6,149	Struck By/Against 800,933	Struck By/Against 801,316	Falls $2,177	MV $8,473	MV $10,035
65–74	MV 1,824	Falls 313,270	Falls 314,288	Falls $1,201	Falls $1,270	Falls $2,471

Table 1.6. *Continued*

	Incidence			Costs (In Millions)		
	Fatal MV	Nonfatal Falls	Total Falls	Medical Falls	Productivity† MV	Total MV
75+	Falls 3,781	Falls 489,793	Falls 493,574	Falls $2,648	Falls $817	Falls $3,465
Females	MV 14,116	Falls 6,358,661	Falls 6,365,066	Falls $15,114	Falls $22,204	Falls $37,318
0–4	MV 372	Falls 554,143	Falls 554,160	Falls $510	Falls $1,143	Falls $1,653
5–14	MV 756	Falls 927,694	Falls 927,704	Falls $990	Falls $2,719	Falls $3,709
15–24	MV 3,060	Struck By/Against 974,280	Struck By/Against 974,295	MV $1,303	MV $5,688	MV $6,991
25–44	MV 3,807	Falls 1,264,637	Falls 1,264,848	MV $1,847	MV $8,144	MV $9,991
45–64	MV 2,852	Falls 1,275,607	Falls 1,276,112	Falls $2,289	Falls $6,540	Falls $8,829
65–74	MV 1,245	Falls 493,533	Falls 494,216	Falls $2,058	Falls $1,825	Falls $3,883
75+	Fall 4,914	Falls 1,295,382	Falls 1,300,296	Falls $6,964	Falls $2,428	Falls $9,392

*Includes the following mechanisms: Motor vehicle (*MV*)/other road user, falls, struck by/against, cut/pierce, fire/burn, poisoning, drowning, firearm/gun.
†Includes short- and long-term wage losses and short- and long-term household productivity losses.
‡Approximately 17% of nonfatal struck by/against injuries are intentional.

Other important dimensions of injury not addressed in this chapter include losses in functional and social capacity and reductions in quality of life both for individuals and for their caregivers. An injury episode is not only physical and physiological but is a deeply personal event, occurring in an interpersonal and social context. What determines the ultimate consequences to injured individuals are the quality and extent of medical care received as well as the ability of the individual to attain maximum physical recovery; to survive financially; and to lead secure, productive lives regardless of short-term or permanent functional status.

Despite the extent of the injury problem, much work needs to be done to improve prevention activities and reduce the consequences of injuries. It is critical for epidemiologists to carry out more studies that show which interventions can reduce violence and injuries and their adverse health effects. It is clear that injury prevention practice can be substantially changed by evaluation research that shows significant effects (Doll, Bartenfeld, & Binder, 2003). For example, the installation of smoke detectors and providing fire-injury prevention education grew substantially after it was shown that these programs were highly effective in saving lives and reducing costs of injury (Doll et al., 2003). More specific examples of effective interventions are discussed in later chapters. Even if results do not show an effect on reducing injuries, it is important that these findings are published so that practitioners can direct their resources to other more promising interventions.

Accurate information, collected across the continuum of care, is essential to determining and evaluating which interventions are effective. In addition, as electronic information systems enter the mainstream of injury prevention practice, new opportunities arise to use these data for public health surveillance of injuries. Resolving questions about terminology and classification systems, decisions about linking disparate systems, privacy concerns, and the benefits and costs of new approaches to public health surveillance of injuries are needed.

Finally, the injury practitioner, given limited resources, will often need to decide which specific cause(s) of injury and sector of the population will need to be targeted for prevention. This decision can be problematic given the large burden and demographic disparity by mechanism and intentionality of injury, as noted in this chapter. The local practitioner equipped with the best data available; with the guidance and support of community leaders, stakeholders, and policy makers; and with knowledge obtained from other injury practitioners will need to determine the intervention efforts that have the greatest potential for reducing morbidity and mortality, improving the quality of life, and reducing costs for his or her community. Local insight and effective partnerships and interventions will lead to significant reductions in injury and violence and the adverse health effects resulting from injury.

REFERENCES

AGS Panel on Falls Prevention. (2001). Guideline for the prevention of falls in older persons. *Journal of the American Geriatrics Society, 49*, 664–672.

Caine, D. J., & Maffulli, N. (Eds.). (2005). *Epidemiology of pediatric sports injuries: vol. 48. Individual sports.* Farmington, CT: S. Karger.

Centers for Disease Control and Prevention. (1999). Achievements in public health, 1900–1999 motor-vehicle safety: A 20th century public health achievement. *Morbidity & Mortality Weekly Report, 48*, 369–374.

Centers for Disease Control and Prevention. (2002a). Rapid assessment of injuries among survivors of the terrorist attack on the World Trade Center—New York City, September 2001. *Morbidity & Morality Weekly Report, 51*, 1–5.

Centers for Disease Control and Prevention. (2002b). Psychological and emotional effects of the September 11 attacks on the World Trade Center—Connecticut, New Jersey, and New York, 2001. *Morbidity & Morality Weekly Report, 51*, 784–786.

Centers for Disease Control and Prevention. (2004). Nonfatal and fatal drowning in recreational water settings—United States, 2001–2002. *Morbidity & Mortality Weekly Report, 53*, 447–452.

Centers for Disease Control and Prevention, National Centers for Injury Prevention and Control. (2005). Web-based injury statistics query and reporting system (WISQARS). Retrieved April 19, 2005, from www.cdc.gov/ncipc/wisqars.

Cohen, M. A., & Miller, T. R. (1998). The cost of mental health care for victims of crime. *Journal of Interpersonal Violence, 13* (1), 93–110.

Committee on Trauma, and Committee on Shock, Division of Medical Sciences, National Academy of Sciences/National Research Council (US). (1966). *Accidental death and disability: The neglected disease of modern society.* Washington, DC: National Academy of Sciences.

Committee on Trauma Research, Commission on Life Sciences, National Research Council and the Institute of Medicine. (1985). *Injury in America.* Washington, DC: National Academy Press.

Department of Health and Human Services, Administration on Children, Youth, and Families. (2005). *Child maltreatment 2003.* Washington, DC: U.S. Government Printing Office. Retrieved April 5, 2005, from www.acf.hhs.gov/programs/cb/publications/cm03.pdf.

Doll, L., Bartenfeld, T., & Binder, S. (2003). Evaluation of interventions designed to prevent and control injuries. *Epidemiologic Reviews, 25*, 51–59.

Fife, D. (1987). Injuries and deaths among elderly persons. *American Journal of Epidemiology, 126*, 936–941.

Goldsmith, S. K., Pellmar, T. C, Kleinman, A. M., & Bunney, W. E. (Eds.). Committee on Pathophysiology & Prevention of Adolescent & Adult Suicide, Board on Neuroscience and Behavioral Health. (2002). *Reducing suicide: A national imperative.* Washington, DC: National Academy of Sciences.

Finkelstein, E. A., Corso, P. S., Miller, T. R., & Associates (2006). *Incidence & economic burden of injuries in the United States, 2000.* New York: Oxford University Press.

Haddix, A. C., Teutsch, S. M., & Corso, P. S. (2003). *Prevention effectiveness: A guide to decision analysis and economic evaluation* (2nd ed.). New York: Oxford University Press.

Haddon, W. (1970). On the escape of tigers: An ecologic note. *American Journal of Public Health, 60,* 2229–2234.

Haddon, W., & Baker, S. P. (1981). Injury control. In D. Clark, & B. MacMahon (Eds.), *Preventive and community medicine* (2nd ed., pp. 109–140). Boston: Little, Brown and Company.

Hungerford, D. W., & Pollock, D. A. (Eds.). (2002). *Alcohol problems among emergency department patients: Proceedings of a research conference on identification & intervention.* Atlanta, GA: Centers for Disease Control and Prevention, National Center for Injury Prevention and Control.

Maffulli, N., & Caine, D. J. (Eds.). (2005). *Epidemiology of pediatric sports injuries: vol. 49. Team sports.* Farmington, CT: S. Karger.

Mercy, J. A., & O'Carroll, P. W. (1988). New directions in violence prediction: The public health arena. *Violence & Victims, 3,* 285–301.

National Center for Injury Prevention and Control (NCIPC). (2002). *CDC injury research agenda.* Atlanta, GA: Centers for Disease Control and Prevention.

National Center for Injury Prevention and Control (NCIPC). (2005). *CDC acute injury care research agenda: Guiding research for the future.* Atlanta, GA: Centers for Disease Control and Prevention.

National Highway Traffic Safety Administration. (2005). *Traffic safety facts 2003: A compilation of motor vehicle crash data from the Fatality Analysis Reporting System and the General Estimates System.* (Report No. DOT HS 809-775). Washington, DC: U.S. Department of Transportation.

Paulozzi, L. J., Saltzman, L. E., Thompson, M. P., & Holmgreen, P. (2001). Surveillance for homicide among intimate partners—United States, 1981–1998. *Morbidity & Mortality Weekly Report Surveillance Summaries, 50,* (no. SS-3), 1–15.

Quan, L., & Cummings, P. (2003). Characteristics of drowning by different age groups. *Injury Prevention, 9* (2), 163–168.

Rubenstein, L. Z., & Josephson, K. R. (2002). The epidemiology of falls and syncope. *Clinics in Geriatric Medicine, 18* (2), 141–158.

Sattin, R. W. (1992). Falls among older persons: A public health perspective. *Annual Review of Public Health, 13,* 489–508.

Thompson, R. S., Rivara, F. P., & Thompson, D. C. (1989). A case-control study of the effectiveness of bicycle safety helmets. *New England Journal of Medicine, 320,* 1361–1367.

Tideiksaar, R. (2002). *Falls in older people: Prevention & management.* Baltimore: Health Professionals Press.

Tjaden, P., & Thoennes, N. (2000). *Extent, nature, & consequences of intimate partner violence: Findings from the National Violence against Women Survey* (NCJ 181867). Washington, DC: U.S. Department of Justice, Office of Justice Programs, National Institute of Justice.

Warda, L., Tenenbein, M., & Moffatt, M. E. K. (1999). House fire injury prevention update. Part 1. A review of risk factors for fatal and non-fatal house fire injury. *Injury Prevention, 5,* 145–150.

Youth Violence: A Report of the Surgeon General. Surgeon General's Office, Public Health Service. (2001). Retrieved July 5, 2005, from www.hhs.gov/surgeongeneral/library/youthviolence.

Chapter 2

Injury and Violence Prevention Interventions: An Overview

Lynda S. Doll, Janet R. Saul, and Randy W. Elder

2.1. INTRODUCTION

The traditional goal of research has been to expand the science base in a particular topic area, assuming that sometime in the future others will use that knowledge to address real-world problems. Public health scientists share the goal of increasing knowledge, but their research is also driven by the need to solve public health problems in the near term. This drive for rapid solutions and the demands for research accountability have never been more prominent than now (Office of Management and Budget [OMB], 1993, 2004). Scientists are expected by practitioners and funders to produce findings that can be used in public health practice. Similarly, practitioners are increasingly expected to identify and incorporate interventions with demonstrated effectiveness into their practices.

The fields of injury and violence prevention research are ready for this challenge. There is now a strong and growing scientific basis for injury and violence prevention and control. Injury and violence researchers have followed the public health model to (1) describe the problem, (2) describe risk and protective factors and their causal relationship with injuries, (3) design and evaluate intervention strategies, and (4) ensure widespread use of these strategies. Public health scientists have moved rapidly to the third phase, efficacy and effectiveness intervention trials. The objective of this book is to highlight the results of these trials in unintentional injury and violence prevention. The audience for the book includes both practitioners and researchers. We point out many effective interventions that can be used by practitioners now. Researchers will notice that there are many gaps in what we know. We hope this book will motivate researchers and students to build on this knowledge base to develop and evaluate more effective approaches to preventing unintentional injury and violence.

In this chapter, we provide a brief overview of preventive interventions. We introduce concepts and definitions used throughout the book. We also introduce a framework that describes levels of scientific evidence to use in assessing intervention effectiveness. We end with brief overviews of the history and state of intervention science in unintentional injury and violence prevention.

2.2. PREVENTIVE INTERVENTIONS

In this book we define a *preventive intervention* as a strategy or series of strategies that are implemented with the goal of preventing, reducing, or ameliorating injuries. Measures can include products (e.g., seat belts, smoke alarms, hip protectors, firearm storage boxes), environmental changes (e.g., speed bumps, pool fencing, residential fire sprinklers), behavioral and communications interventions (e.g., individual and group behavior change strategies, parent training, targeted media campaigns), and policy guidelines or laws (e.g., laws preventing persons convicted of intimate partner violence [IPV] to own a firearm, defining permissible blood alcohol levels). Preventive measures can be passive in the sense that the individual need not intentionally behave in a specific way to benefit from the intervention (e.g., childproof cigarette lighters) or can be active as when interventions require specific actions to reduce risk (e.g., buckling a seat belt).

2.3. INTERVENTION CLASSIFICATION SYSTEMS

Different classification systems have been devised to categorize interventions. Preventive interventions have been categorized using terms originally derived from clinical medicine: primary (preventing new cases of disease), secondary (reducing established cases of disease), and tertiary (decreasing the frequency and severity of disability after a disease) (Commission on Chronic Illness, 1957). Using this terminology, this book largely focuses on primary prevention. Gordon (1983) devised a classification system based on population risk levels that is more directly applicable to injury and violence prevention. That system defines three levels of interventions; (1) universal preventive measures targeted to the general population or subpopulations without regard to level of injury risk; (2) selective preventive measures that target populations with increased risk (e.g., those exposed to family violence); and (3) indicated preventive measures that target populations whose behavior or personal history put them at above average risk of future injuries, perpetration, or victimization (e.g., those who use alcohol excessively, elderly persons who have fallen, and perpetrators or victims of sexual violence) (Institute of Medicine [IOM], 1994).

A complementary classification system that describes risk and protective factors was devised by Haddon (1968, 1980) and is used extensively in the unintentional injury control field. The Haddon Matrix is based on epidemiological principles and is used to describe interventions targeted to the host, the agent, and the environment. In injury prevention, the host is the individual and his or her characteristics or behavior (e.g., alcohol-impaired driving, aggressive behavior toward peers); the agent is energy, or the source of energy transfer (e.g., a motor vehicle or weapon); and the environment is the setting or context for the injury, which includes both physical and social environments (e.g., schools, violent neighborhoods).

Another complimentary classification system, sometimes called the social-ecological model (Bronfenbrenner, 1992; Stokols, 1992), defines interventions by the level of risk and protective factors that influence risk and is used extensively in violence prevention. Some work has also progressed applying the social-ecological approach to preventing unintentional injuries (Allegrante, Marks, & Hanson, 2006; Hanson et al., 2005). In this model, interventions can focus on (1) individual risk such as use of medication; (2) risk within dyads or groups, including relationship factors with intimate partners, peers, or families; (3) risks within communities such as high levels of youth violence or poor enforcement of drinking and driving laws; and (4) risks influenced by societal factors such as norms about partner violence.

2.4.   INTERVENTION CHARACTERISTICS

Interventions strategies vary on many different dimensions. In this section, we discuss characteristics that are particularly relevant to public health-oriented preventive interventions for unintentional and violence-related injuries.

2.4.1.   Population-Based Interventions

To distinguish its role from those of medicine, criminal justice, and mental health, the field of public health has traditionally defined its approach to interventions as population based. Such approaches attempt to reach large numbers of individuals by targeting and intervening with groups rather than individuals. Familiar population-based interventions addressing infectious diseases include safe water systems and vaccination programs. Analogous programs in injury and violence include community- and societal-level interventions. As we note later, the field of unintentional injury prevention has taken a course not unlike that of infectious diseases, with much emphasis placed on environmental-, community-, and societal-level interventions. The benefits of individual or social-level interventions are gaining greater acceptance, especially as more behavioral and social scientists enter this field of research (Gielen & Sleet, 2003). The field of violence prevention has in many ways taken a different trajectory. Interventions have long emphasized individual and interpersonal approaches. However, there is growing recognition that there are many community or societal factors that influence individual behavioral choices.

2.4.2.   Behavioral, Social, and Environmental Interventions

Most injury and violence practitioners and researchers now realize that a combination of environmental, behavioral, legislative, and technological solutions is needed to ensure the adoption of safe behaviors (see Chapter 22). But as we noted earlier, this has not always been the case. Environmental, engineering, and legal approaches have been particularly attractive because they have the potential for protecting whole populations. However, even when such interventions are available, they need to be demonstrated to be effective, feasible, and acceptable to communities, which will ultimately decide whether to use them. Similarly, laws and policies that are effective in reducing injury or injury risk must be widely known, adhered to, and enforced to be effective (Shaw & Ogolla, 2006). Proponents of engineering, environmental, or legal interventions often argue against the use of behavioral or educational interventions. Indeed, interventions that provide only information are rarely successful in reducing risk behaviors, although there are some notable exceptions (e.g., Willinger et al., 1998). Well-designed behavioral interventions involve much more than simply providing information. Behavioral interventions that are theory based, focus on risk and protective factors, provide opportunities for skills building, and provide support and reinforcement for behavior change have repeatedly been shown to be effective in changing a variety of health-related risks and behaviors (Fishbein et al., 1992; Halpern, Bates, Beales, & Heathfield, 2004; Schneiderman, Speers, Silva, Tomes, & Gentry, 2001).

2.4.3.   Proximal and Distal Risk

Public health has historically focused on preventive interventions that change proximal or near-term risk (e.g., reducing youth access to drugs and alcohol that is related to violent behaviors, removal of environmental hazards that cause falls among the elderly). It is important to note, however, that preventive interventions also include the promotion of health and well-being by building social and psychological resiliency and mental health and by reducing more distal, long-term social determinants such as poverty, stigma, and racism. The Centers for Disease Control and Prevention's (CDC) work on positive parenting and supervision; promoting prosocial behaviors in children; and building societal norms around healthy, violence-free dating are examples of research that include both risk reduction and health promotion approaches (CDC, 2002).

2.4.4.   Interventions Across Life Stages

It may be tempting to seek brief, one-time interventions that can quickly reduce violence and unintentional injuries. But with few exceptions (Fleming et al., 2002), such interventions are often insufficient, particularly across a lifetime of exposure to risk. For example, parents may be successful in getting young children to wear bicycle helmets, but as these children expand their peer network or mature outside the age limits of helmet laws, they may fail to adhere to this life-saving intervention.

For many behaviors, interventions must be repeated across the life stages and reinforced in different settings with different approaches. For very young children, the most important intervention approach is to enhance parental or caretaker supervision and responsibility for keeping children safe. As children develop their cognitive and motor skills, interventions can be devised to enhance their intrinsic motivation to engage in safe and healthy behaviors. At the same time, communities must also provide tools and environments that reinforce or facilitate safe behaviors (e.g., sidewalks for pedestrians, removing unsafe playgrounds). As these examples suggest, innovation in the design of interventions is essential for meeting the developmental needs of children and adults across the life stages (Mercy, Sleet, & Doll, 2003).

Interventions that prevent youth suicide can provide an example of the changing nature of interventions across the life stages. Universal interventions in the preschool years include those that promote the emotional and physical well-being of the child (e.g., positive parenting, programs building social competence and self-esteem, physical activity programs). School-based, universal interventions can promote prosocial behavior and conflict-resolution skills during the elementary and middle school years. Family interventions can be devised for children who bully or who are bullied by their peers. Screening for depression and counseling referrals are appropriate for high-risk youth. Finally, because youth suicide attempts are often impulsive, preventing access to suicidal means is essential (e.g., providing protective fencing on bridges, removing household poisons and drugs, and storing and locking firearms) (Simon et al., 2001).

2.4.5.   Multilevel, Comprehensive Interventions

Two changes in public health have drawn the fields of unintentional injury and violence toward the support of comprehensive, multilevel interventions, which attempt to intervene at several points of the social-ecological model. The first change came with the recognition that poor health is increasingly a result of risky lifestyle choices or behaviors (e.g., smoking, drinking and driving, unprotected sexual behavior), rather than infectious diseases (CDC, 1999). Such behaviors are usually a result of multiple influences within and across life stages. Evidence increasingly suggests that such risk behaviors are most successfully changed through comprehensive, multilevel approaches (Nation et al., 2003). The second change came with the recognition that public health interventions are not the sole responsibility of public health agencies. Interventions are now conducted in schools, churches, community centers, beauty parlors, and sports stadiums. They are sponsored by health, transportation, and police departments and a variety of community-based organizations, which form community coalitions that together mount simultaneous interventions to address public health problems.

2.4.6.   Effective Interventions

Nation and colleagues (2003) reviewed the scientific literature to identify the principles of effective prevention programs. These principles summarize much of what has been learned in developing and implementing injury and violence-related interventions. Interventions should be comprehensive, use varied teaching methods, deliver a sufficient dosage of the intervention, be theory driven, encourage positive relationships, be appropriately timed, be socioculturally relevant, include an outcome evaluation, and have well-trained staff. Chapters throughout this book describe these and other characteristics of effective interventions in selected topic areas.

2.5.   UNINTENTIONAL INJURY PREVENTIVE INTERVENTIONS

Historically, unintentional injuries have been considered an unavoidable fact of life. Even today, the occurrence of such injuries is commonly attributed to luck or fate. However, the high public health burden resulting from unintentional injuries has prompted epidemiologists and behavioral scientists to study their underlying causal factors in an attempt to develop effective means of prevention. Although there had been isolated efforts to reduce the injury risks from events such as motor-vehicle crashes, it was not until 1949 that unintentional injuries were first comprehensively addressed from a public health perspective (Gordon, 1949), and this approach has been remarkably successful in reducing injury risks (CDC, 2005). Unintentional injury prevention is now a vibrant field in public health and is developing a substantial body of evidence about how to prevent what used to be known as "accidents" (Zaza, Briss, & Harris, 2005).

Despite our progress, unintentional injury remains a major cause of morbidity and mortality. In the United States, unintentional injury is the fifth leading cause of death among people of all ages and the leading cause of death among people aged 1–44 years (CDC, 2005). For every person who dies from unintentional injuries, there are many more who are permanently disabled or who require medical treatment for injuries of varying degrees of severity.

Causal mechanisms, and thus effective prevention activities, generally tend to be unique to the specific type of injury in question, and this is reflected in the organization of this book. One notable exception is the crosscutting role of alcohol consumption as a risk factor for many injuries. Alcohol is an important risk factor for most, if not all of the causes of unintentional injury and many violence-related injuries covered in this book and is described more fully in Chapter 16. The estimated association of alcohol consumption with fatalities from motor-vehicle crashes, fires, drowning, and falls ranges from 38% to 63% (National Highway Traffic and Safety Administration [NHTSA], 2004; Smith, Branas, & Miller, 1999). Thus it is not surprising to find that interventions to reduce excessive drinking, such as the national minimum drinking age (established in 1986), can effectively reduce injuries from multiple causes (see Chapters 4 and 5).

Following in the tradition of the epidemiologic triad and the Haddon Matrix, all the authors in this volume who are concerned with unintentional injury categorize their interventions according to their focus on the person or host (person), the environment, or the agent (energy or sources of energy transfer). In addition to functioning as a useful categorization tool, the perspective that the Haddon Matrix provides on the causal mechanisms underlying injury can guide the development of a comprehensive health promotion approach that addresses multiple causal factors (Gielen & Sleet, 2003; Howat, Sleet, Elder, & Maycock, 2004). This perspective highlights the fact that interventions addressing individual and interpersonal behavioral change are often key components of comprehensive health-promotion efforts aimed at unintentional injury prevention, even when the primary focus is on changing the physical environment. For example, Gilchrist, Saluja, and Marshall (see Chapter 7) discuss a comprehensive approach to changing bicycle helmet use, which includes components such as establishing a coalition, conducting awareness and education campaigns, using incentives (e.g., giveaways, coupons, and rebates), and encouraging legislation mandating helmet use. Similar approaches are necessary to reduce falls among the elderly (see Chapter 3) and drowning (see Chapter 5).

Legislation and regulations are also a particularly important aspect of the broad environment, and they can be important avenues for changing both behavior and the physical environment (Schieber, Gilchrist, & Sleet, 2000; Shaw & Ogolla, 2006). As Warda and Ballesteros point out (see Chapter 6), legislation can also help ensure that effective interventions are widely implemented. These authors note that the public health benefits from highly effective devices for preventing fire-related injuries (e.g., smoke alarms) could be greatly improved if optimal usage of such devices were mandated in building codes. The importance of legislation and regulation to unintentional injury prevention is exemplified by the fact that legislative and regulatory interventions are listed among the most effective interventions for preventing injuries from all of the types of unintentional injury addressed in this volume. Rubenstein, Stevens, and Scott (see Chapter 3) point out that the public health community can play an important role in encouraging legislative action by providing data on costs or costs averted by effective injury prevention intervention (see also Chapter 1).

2.6. VIOLENCE-RELATED PREVENTIVE INTERVENTIONS

Every year, millions of children, women, and men in the United States suffer physical consequences of violence ranging from minor cuts and bruises to death. In 2002, more than 49,000 Americans died as a result of suicide or homicide, and millions more suffered nonfatal injuries due to violence (CDC, 2005).

Perhaps because it is such a widespread problem, many believe that violence is inevitable. Therefore, solutions have traditionally been reactive ones, focusing on what to do with those who commit violent offenses and those who are victimized (i.e., indicated approaches). These solutions are typically carried out by criminal justice, law enforcement, and victim service organizations (Dodge, 2001; World Health Organization [WHO], 2002). Public health, on the other hand, views violence as predictable based on various contributing factors and thus as preventable. This viewpoint evokes solutions that are more proactive, including more focus on universal and selective preventive approaches (WHO, 2002). Mercy and O'Carroll (1988) summarized the history of the emergence of violence as a public health problem. A significant turning point for bringing the public health perspective to violence occurred via the Surgeon General's Workshop on Violence and Public Health in 1985 (Mercy & O'Carroll, 1988). Since then, many people have made the case that violence is a public health problem (IOM, 1999; Mercy, 1999; Mercy, Rosenberg, Powell, Broome, & Roper, 1993; Powell, Mercy, Crosby, Dahlberg, & Simon, 1999; WHO, 2002). In fact, the view of violence as a public health problem is now widely shared globally. The 49th World Health Assembly of WHO declared that violence is a leading public health problem worldwide and thus preventing violence must be a worldwide public health priority (WHO, 2002).

Various authors in this book review the state of prevention science in child maltreatment, youth violence, sexual violence, IPV, suicide, and elder mistreatment. At first glance, these may appear to be disparate problems requiring divergent solutions. On closer examination, however, there are some notable commonalities.

Certainly, some of the fields are farther along in developing and rigorously testing prevention interventions than other fields. Pillemer, Mueller-Johnson, Mock, Suitor, and Lachs (Chapter 13) remind us that elder mistreatment is a very young field and that, as such, there is still a great need for research on modifiable risk and protective factors. Therefore, these authors could not identify any recommended or even promising strategies for elder abuse prevention. Although still at an early stage, the fields of IPV, sexual violence, child maltreatment, and suicide are a bit farther along the evidence-based continuum than elder abuse. Each of these fields has some base of risk factor research, at least one recommended prevention strategy, and multiple promising strategies. On the other end of the continuum is the field of youth violence (Chapter 9) where the authors were able to identify multiple recommended as well as promising strategies.

One note of caution about the observation that some of the violence fields have a more developed research base on risk and protective factors than others: this does not mean that the etiological work in those fields is complete. Whitaker,

Baker, and Arias (Chapter 11) remind us that there are different types of IPV with different risk and protective factors and thus different prevention needs. This is likely to be the situation for other types of violence as well. The four components of the public health model referred to earlier are not meant to be linear but rather iterative. While intervention strategies are designed and tested based on the best available evidence we have about risk and protective factors, the etiological work must continue—there are intricacies in the even more advanced fields that we do not understand. More in-depth work on risk and protective factors (e.g., which factors are more important than others, under what conditions, and for what segments of the population) will help refine, and we hope improve, our current prevention efforts.

Although there are clear differences in the research base for different types of violence, there are similarities as well. First, almost all of the authors in this book point to the critical need for research on comprehensive approaches. As one surmises after reading these reviews, violence in all its forms results from a complex interaction of factors at multiple levels of the social ecology. Because of this complexity, several of the authors assert that focusing on one strategy is highly unlikely to solve the problem at the population level, no matter how strong the scientific evidence is for that strategy (see Chapter 8, 9, 10, and 12). Daro and McCurdy (Chapter 8) point out that in the field of child maltreatment, approaching the problem in a more ecological way would move us "toward a communitywide system of shared responsibility and mutual support" based on a shared moral responsibility to protect children as well as foster their positive growth. Additional support for investigating comprehensive approaches comes from the observation that similar risk factors are mentioned in several of the chapters. A comprehensive approach to violence prevention could perhaps affect shared risk factors and thus affect several types of violence in the same community. Knox (Chapter 10) presents some suggestive evidence that this may, in fact, happen. The comprehensive suicide prevention program implemented by the U.S. Air Force was associated with a decrease not only in suicides but also in severe and moderate cases of family violence and other violent offenses (Knox, Litts, Talcott, Feig, & Caine, 2003).

Pillemer et al. (Chapter 13) and Whitaker et al. (Chapter 11) point out a common lesson that should be kept in mind as we pursue new and better ways of preventing violence in communities: As violence-prevention strategies are developed and tested, both researchers and practitioners must be open to the possibility that their proposed strategies could have the opposite effect from what they intended or hypothesized. The issue of unintended consequences is not unique to violence-prevention research. However, the costs of increasing the likelihood of perpetration or victimization are so dire that vigilant attention to this potential is critical. This argues, of course, for ongoing effectiveness research that tests interventions in real-world settings and for program evaluation that is designed in a way to detect any negative effects as early as possible.

2.7. LEVELS OF EVIDENCE FRAMEWORK

In each chapter of this book, preventive interventions are described with a critical eye toward the question of whether they actually achieve their intended goals. Although practitioners' decisions about which prevention activities to use are almost always made in the context of uncertainty, it is helpful to be aware of the extent to which the available scientific evidence supports the use of different options and of any gaps in the evidence. Armed with this knowledge, practitioners can make more informed decisions about interventions that are both feasible to implement in their local context and likely to result in successful outcomes.

The strongest evidence for effectiveness of interventions comes from systematic reviews of the research literature, such as those presented in the *Guide to Community Preventive Services* (Zaza et al., 2005), and the Cochrane Library (Cochrane Collaboration, 2005). Such reviews have the strong advantage that they consider all of the available literature in a manner designed to minimize bias. Thus they reduce the possibility that results from a single anomalous study—arising from either chance factors or unusual conditions—will provide misleading information. Systematic reviews also provide useful information on the consistency of intervention effects across settings, generalizability issues, and factors that may influence an intervention's effectiveness (Zaza et al., 2001). This information can be valuable both for guiding implementation efforts and for highlighting future research questions. Many of the chapters in this volume describe the results of systematic reviews in various topic areas.

For many interventions, systematic reviews of the evidence have yet to be conducted. In these situations, the results of one or several large and well-designed studies (that are not contradicted by other evidence) may provide a reasonable level of confidence in an intervention's effectiveness, sometimes labeled as "promising interventions." As empirical evidence of effectiveness becomes sparse, theoretical or rational considerations increase in prominence as a means for assessing the likely effectiveness of interventions. These considerations may fall into several categories, including (1) chemical and physical principles as they are applied to product improvements and safety devices, (2) a close analogy between the intervention under consideration and other interventions with demonstrated effectiveness, and (3) a very strong rationale as a solution to a well-documented problem (e.g., use of booster seats to prevent injuries from lap belts). In the absence of evaluation studies, assuming effectiveness based on such considerations is common and generally reasonable. However, evaluation is critical to assess whether the intended effects are achieved and to ensure that there are no unintended negative consequences.

A substantial number of interventions intended to prevent injury and violence do not have a strong evidence base supporting their effectiveness. These should be used only if there are no other feasible and well-supported alternatives or if the primary goal of the intervention is to study its effectiveness. There are situations in which two researchers may interpret similar scientific information on intervention effectiveness in different ways. Some scientists are most comfortable with effectiveness data gathered through a limited set of intervention evaluation methods (e.g., randomized controlled trials), while others are comfortable with a broader set of evaluation methods (see discussions of home visitation interventions in Chapters 8 and 18). In these cases, practitioners must decide the level of evidence they are comfortable with before adopting an intervention. In rare circumstances, there is substantial evidence that interventions are ineffective or even harmful (such as air bags and child passengers). Clearly, such interventions should be avoided. Interventions with each of these levels of effectiveness or ineffectiveness are described in chapters throughout the first two sections of this volume.

2.8.   OVERVIEW OF THE BOOK

This book was written for practitioners and researchers who expressed a need for a volume that synthesized the state of the science in unintentional injury and violence prevention. Part I provides an overview of the epidemiology and costs of injury and violence and the concepts and definitions of preventive interventions. The chapters in Part II, "Effective and Promising Interventions," provide detailed reviews of the scientific literature on unintentional injury and violence prevention interventions, identifying those with strong evidence, those that are promising, and those with little or even negative evidence related to their effectiveness. Part III, "Cross-Cutting Intervention Issues," focuses on interventions and issues that are relevant to both unintentional injury and violence prevention. The science base for some of these areas is just beginning to emerge (see Chapter 19). Part IV, "Interventions in the Field," is oriented toward practitioners who wish to use off-the-shelf curricula or to develop their own interventions. It contains practical information and tools on how to select, develop, implement, and evaluate interventions in the field. Part V, "Dissemination and Adoption of Effective Interventions and Policies," is oriented toward researchers who want to encourage and study the uptake of research findings and practitioners who want to expand the reach of effective interventions to broader audiences and new populations. This volume includes several appendices that provide additional references and resources related to interventions.

REFERENCES

Allegrante, J. A., Marks, R., & Hanson, D. W. (2006). Ecological models for the control and prevention of unintentional injury. In A. Gielen, D. A. Sleet, & R. DiClimente (Eds.), *Injury and violence prevention: Behavior change theories, methods, and applications.* (pp. 105–126). San Francisco, CA: Jossey-Bass.

Bronfenbrenner, U. (1992). Ecological system theory. In R. Vasta (Ed.), *Six theories of child development* (pp. 187–250). London: Jessica Kingsley.

Centers for Disease Control and Prevention. (1999). Achievements in public health, 1900–1999. Motor-vehicle safety: A 20th century public health achievement. *Morbidity & Mortality Weekly Report, 48* (18), 369–374.

Centers for Disease Control and Prevention. (2002). *Injury research agenda.* Atlanta, GA: National Center for Injury Prevention and Control.

Centers for Disease Control and Prevention, National Center for Injury Prevention and Control. (2005). Web-based injury statistics query and reporting system (WISQARS). Retrieved July 10, 2005, from www.cdc.gov/ncipc/wisqars.

Cochrane Collaboration. (2005). The Cochrane Library [On-line]. Retrieved July 10, 2005, from www.cochrane.org.

Commission on Chronic Illness. (1957). *Chronic illness in the United States* (Vol. 1). Cambridge, MA: Harvard University Press.

Dodge, K. A. (2001). The science of youth violence prevention: Progressing from developmental epidemiology to efficacy to effectiveness to public policy. *American Journal of Preventive Medicine, 20* (1S), 63–70.

Fishbein, M., Bandura, A., Triandis, H. C., Kanfer, F. H., Becker, M. H., & Middlestadt, S. (1992). *Factors influencing behavior and behavior change: Final report—theorists' workshop.* Unpublished manuscript, National Institute for Mental Health, Rockville, MD.

Fleming, M. F., Mundt, M. P., French, M. T., Manwell, L. B., Stauffacher, E. A., & Barry, K. L. (2002). Brief physician advice for problem drinkers: Long-term efficacy and benefit-cost analysis. *Alcohol & Clinical Experimental Research, 39,* 548–551.

Gielen, A. C., & Sleet, D. A. (2003). Application of behavior change theories and methods to injury prevention. *Epidemiologic Review, 25,* 65–76.

Gordon, J. E. (1949). The epidemiology of accidents. *American Journal of Public Health, 39,* 504–515.

Gordon, R. (1983). An operational classification of disease prevention. *Public Health Reports, 98,* 107–109.

Haddon, W. (1968). The changing approach to the epidemiology, prevention, and amelioration of trauma: The transition to approaches etiologically rather than descriptively based. *American Journal of Public Health, 58* (8), 1431–1438.

Haddon, W. (1980). Options for the prevention of motor vehicle crash injury. *Israel Journal of Medicine, 16,* 45–68.

Halpern, D., Bates, C., Beales, G., & Heathfield, A. (2004). *Personal responsibility and changing behavior: The state of knowledge and its implications for public policy.* Cabinet Office, Prime Minister's Strategy Unit, Admiralty Arch, The Mall, London. Retrieved May 7, 2005, from www.pm.gov.uk/files/pdf/pr.pdf.

Hanson, D., Hanson, J., Vardon, P., McFarlane, K., Lloyd, J., Muller, R., & Durrheim (2005). The injury iceberg: An ecological approach to planning sustainable community safety interventions. *Health Promotion Journal of Australia, 16,* 5–15.

Howat, P., Sleet, D. A., Elder, R., & Maycock, B. (2004). Preventing alcohol-related traffic injury: Health promotion approach. *Traffic Injury Prevention, 5* (3), 208–219.

Institute of Medicine (1994). *Reducing risks for mental disorders.* Washington, DC: National Academy Press.

Institute of Medicine (1999). *Reducing the burden of injury.* Washington, DC: National Academy Press.

Knox, K. L., Litts, D. A., Talcott, G. W., Feig, J. C., & Caine, E. D. (2003). Risk of suicide and related adverse outcomes after exposure to a suicide prevention programme in the US Air Force: Cohort study. *British Medical Journal, 327,* 376–1380.

Mercy, J. A. (1999). Having new eyes: Viewing child sexual abuse as a public health problem. *Sexual Abuse: A Journal of Research & Treatment, 11* (4), 317–321.

Mercy, J. A., & O'Carroll, P. (1988). New directions in violence prediction: The public health arena. *Violence & Victims, 3* (4), 285–301.

Mercy, J. A., Rosenberg, M. L., Powell, K. E., Broome, C. V., & Roper, W. L. (1993). Public health policy for prevention violence. *Health Affairs, 12* (4), 7–29.

Mercy, J. A., Sleet, D. A., & Doll, L. S. (2003). Applying a developmental approach to injury prevention. *American Journal of Health Behavior, 34* (5), S6–S12.

Nation, M., Crusto, C., Wandersman, A., Kumpfer, K. L., Seybolt, D., Mourissey-Kane, E., & Davino, K. (2003). What works in prevention programs. *American Psychologist, 58,* 6–7, 449–456.

National Highway Traffic Safety Administration. (2004). *Traffic safety facts 2003: A compilation of motor vehicle crash data from the fatality analysis reporting system and the general estimates system* (DOT HS 809-775). Washington, DC: U.S. Department of Transportation, National Highway Traffic Safety Administration, National Center for Statistics and Analysis.

Office of Management and Budget. (1993). *Government Performance and Results Act (GPRA) of 1993.* Retrieved July 25, 2005, from www.whitehouse.gov/omb/mgmt-gpra/gplaw2m.html.

Office of Management and Budget. (2004). *Program assessment rating tool (PART).* Retrieved July 25, 2005, from www.whitehouse.gov/omb/part/index.html.

Powell, K. E., Mercy, J. A., Crosby, A. E., Dahlberg, L. L., & Simon, T. R. (1999). Public health models of violence and violence prevention. In *Encyclopedia of violence, peace, and conflict,* (Vol. 3, pp. 175–187). New York: Academic Press (Elsevier Inc).

Schieber, R. A., Gilchrist, J., & Sleet, D. A. (2000). Legislative and regulatory strategies to reduce childhood unintentional injuries. *Future of Children, 10,* 137–163.

Schneiderman, N., Speers, M. A., Silva, J. M., Tomes, H., & Gentry, J. H. (Eds.). (2001). *Integrating behavioral and social science with public health.* Washington, DC: American Psychological Association.

Shaw, F., & Ogolla, C. P. (2006). Behavior and injury prevention: The role of law and legislation. In A. Gielen, D. A. Sleet, & R. DiClimente (Eds.), *Injury and violence prevention: Behavior change theories, methods, and applications.* (pp. 442–466). San Francisco: Jossey-Bass.

Simon, T. R., Swann A. C., Powell, K. E., Potter, L. B., Kresnow, M., & O'Carroll, P. W. (2001). Characteristics of impulsive suicide attempts and attempters. *Suicide & Life-Threatening Behavior, 32,* 49–59.

Smith, G. S., Branas, C. C., & Miller, T. R. (1999). Fatal nontraffic injuries involving alcohol: A meta-analysis. *Annals of Emergency Medicine, 33,* 659–668.

Stokols, D. (1992). Establishing and maintaining healthy environments: Toward a social ecology of health promotion. *American Psychologist, 47,* 6–22.

Willinger, M., Hoffman, H. J., Wu, K. T., Hou, J. R., Kessler, R. C., Ward, S. L., Keens, T. G., & Corwin, M. J. (1998). Factors associated with the transition to nonprime sleep positions of infants in the United States: The national infant sleep position study. *Journal of the American Medical Association, 280,* 329–335.

World Health Organization. (2002). *World report on violence and health.* Geneva: Author.

Zaza, S., Briss, P. A., & Harris, K. W. (Eds.). (2005). *The guide to community preventive services: What works to promote health?* New York: Oxford University Press.

Zaza, S., Carande-Kulis, V. G., Sleet, D. A., Sosin, D. M., Elder, R. W., Shults, R. A., Bella Dinh-Zarr, T., Nichols, J. L., Thompson, R. S., & the Task Force on Community Preventive Services (2001). Methods for conducting systematic reviews of the evidence of effectiveness and economic efficiency of interventions to reduce injuries to motor vehicle occupants. *American Journal of Preventive Medicine, 21* (4S), 23–30.

Part II

Effective and Promising Interventions

Unintentional Injury

Chapter 3

Interventions to Prevent Falls Among Older Adults

Laurence Z. Rubenstein, Judy A. Stevens, and Vicky Scott

3.1. INTRODUCTION

Falls consistently rank among the most serious problems facing older persons and cause a tremendous amount of morbidity, mortality, and disability (Brown, 1999; Nevitt, 1997; Robbins et al., 1989; Rubenstein, Josephson, & Robbins, 1994; Tinetti, Williams, & Mayewski, 1986). At least a third of community-dwelling people aged 65 years and older fall each year (Centers for Disease Control and Prevention [CDC], 2005; Campbell, Spears, & Borrie, 1990; Rubenstein & Josephson, 2002), and the rates in nursing homes and hospitals are considerably higher (Rubenstein & Josephson, 2002). In 2002 in the United States, falls were responsible for 12,800 deaths and 1.64 million visits to hospital emergency departments (EDs) (CDC, 2005). In addition to physical injury, falls can have major psychological and social consequences. Fear of falling and loss of self-confidence can cause seniors to limit their activities and lead to reduced mobility, decreased physical fitness, and increased fall risk (Brown, 1999; Clark, Lord, & Webster, 1993; Vellas, Wayne, Romero, Baumgartner, & Garry, 1997).

A recent economic analysis of medical payments (rather than billing costs used in earlier calculations) found that in 2000 the direct medical cost of fatal and nonfatal fall injuries was $19.5 billion (Finkelstein, Chen, Miller, Corso, & Stevens, 2005). Of $19.3 billion for nonfatal injuries, 63% ($12.1 billion) were for injuries that required hospitalization, 21% ($4.1 billion) were for injuries treated in EDs, and 16% ($3.1 billion) were for injuries treated in outpatient settings. Overall, falls account for 6% of all medical expenditures for persons aged 65 years and older in the United States (Bernstein & Schur, 1990; Rubenstein, Powers, & MacLean, 2001).

This chapter provides an overview of our current knowledge about fall risk factors, evidence for intervention strategies in various settings, implications for public health practice, and future research needs.

Table 3.1. Fall Risk Factors

Intrinsic/Biological	Behavioral	Environmental	Social/Economic
Advanced age	Multiple medications	Poor building design	Low income
Female gender	Use of:	and/or maintenance	Lack of education
Chronic illness/disability:	Tranquilizers	Inadequate building	Illiteracy/language
Stroke	Antidepressants	codes	barriers
Parkinson disease	Antihypertensives	Poor stair design	Poor living conditions
Heart disease	Excessive alcohol	Lack of:	Unsafe housing
Incontinence/	Risk-taking behaviors	Handrails	Poor social environment
frequency	Lack of exercise	Curb ramps	Living alone
Acute illness	Previous fall/recurrent	Rest areas	Lack of support
Cognitive impairment	falls	Grab bars	networks and social
Gait disorders	Fear of falling	Poor lighting or sharp	interaction
Poor balance	Inappropriate	contrasts	
Postural sway	footwear	Slippery or uneven	
Muscle weakness	Lack, inappropriate	surfaces	
Poor vision	use, or improper use	Obstacles and tripping	
Impaired touch and/or	of mobility aids	hazards	
proprioception	Poor nutrition or		
	hydration		

3.2. RISK FACTORS

Epidemiologic studies have identified numerous fall risk factors. These are frequently classified as either intrinsic (i.e., originating within the body, such as leg weakness, balance disorders, and visual deficits) or extrinsic (i.e., originating outside the body, such as environmental hazards). Some researchers have further expanded this classification to include behavioral and social/economic risk factors (Scott, Dukeshire, Gallagher, & Scanlan, 2001), although the evidence for some factors is indirect (e.g., low income is highly associated with poor health status and disability, which, in turn, are associated with increased fall risk) (Evans, Barer, & Marmor, 1994; Raina, Dukeshire, Chambers, Toivonen, & Lindsay, 1997). Table 3.1 summarizes this broader representation.

Based on a recent literature review, the most important risk factors include muscle weakness, a prior history of falls, difficulties with gait and balance, visual impairment, arthritis, functional limitations, depression, and the use of psychotropic medications (Rubenstein & Josephson, 2002). However, falls rarely have a single cause. Most are the result of an interaction between a number of risk factors, and risk increases with the number of factors present (Nevitt, Cummings, Kidd, & Black, 1989; Robbins et al., 1989; Tinetti et al., 1986; Tinetti, Speechley, & Ginter, 1988). For example, in one survey of community-dwelling older adults, the proportion of people who reported falling increased from 27% for those with no or one risk factor to 78% for those with four or more risk factors (Tinetti et al., 1988).

3.3. FALL PREVENTION INTERVENTIONS

The high incidence of falls among older persons, combined with high susceptibility to injury—the result of age-related physiological changes (e.g., decreased muscle strength and endurance, delayed reaction times, slower reflexes) and a high prevalence of chronic conditions (e.g., osteoporosis, arthritis)—makes even a relatively mild fall potentially dangerous. Unfortunately, older people frequently are not aware of their risk of falling and fail to discuss these issues with their health care providers. Consequently, opportunities to prevent injury and disability are often missed (Cumming, Kelsey, & Nevitt, 1990; Cummings, Nevitt, & Kidd, 1988; Jarrett, Rockwood, Carver, Stolee, & Cosway, 1995).

It is critical that we find ways to prevent falls and fall-related declines in function and independence. Many of the major risk factors are potentially modifiable such as muscle weakness, medication use, vision impairment, and environmental hazards. In 1994, Tinetti and colleagues published a landmark study demonstrating that an intervention addressing multiple risk factors could significantly reduce falls among community-dwelling seniors. During the past two decades, various fall prevention interventions in both community and institutional settings have been tested in randomized controlled trials. The results have provided much useful information about effective interventions. Several meta-analyses have confirmed that some multicomponent interventions were effective, although it was not possible to determine precisely which components contributed most to the outcomes.

3.3.1. What Has Been Studied? What Works?

A number of systematic reviews and meta-analyses (Chang et al., 2004; Gillespie et al., 2003; Rand Corporation, 2003) have assessed the effectiveness of various interventions for preventing falls among older adults living independently and in institutions. These reviews included only randomized controlled trials that reported the number of fallers or falls as outcome measures. The following section describes five types of community-based interventions that studies have shown reduce the risk of falling. Most interventions include multiple components (e.g., physical activity and home modification); some, such as specific exercise programs, consist of a single component.

3.3.1.1. Clinical Assessment and Risk Reduction

The most effective fall prevention intervention used individualized clinical assessment of fall risk factors, performed by a physician, combined with strategies directed toward reducing these risks (Chang et al., 2004; Rand Corporation, 2003). When analyzed as a group, interventions using clinical assessment and risk reduction lowered the risk of falling by 18% and reduced the average number of falls by 43%. For example, one effective intervention included a postfall assessment in an outpatient clinic followed by a home visit by an occupational therapist who provided advice and education about home safety and assisted with some environmental modifications (e.g., removed loose rugs, provided minor equipment) (Close et al., 1999).

3.3.1.2. Exercise

The next most effective interventions used exercises intended to improve balance, strength, flexibility, and/or endurance. Overall, exercise interventions reduced the risk of falls by 12% and the mean number of falls by 19% (Chang et al., 2004; Rand Corporation, 2003). Effective exercise programs included tai chi groups (Wolf, Barnhart, Kutner, McNeely, Coogler, & Xu, 1996), balance and gait training, and strength building (Campbell, Robertson, Gardner, Norton, & Buchner, 1999; Judge, Lundin-Olsson, Nyberg, & Gustafson, 1993; Lord, Caplan, & Ward, 1993). Program approaches have included group classes (Barnett, Smith, Lord, Williams, & Baumand, 2003; Day et al., 2002; Gardner, Buchner, Robertson, & Campbell, 2001; Lord et al., 2003) and individualized in-home programs (Campbell et al., 1999; Robertson, Devlin, Gardner, & Campbell, 2001). Furthermore, exercise was effective in reducing falls when used alone and when included as part of a multi-component intervention.

3.3.1.3. *Medication Management*

Studies have demonstrated that psychoactive medications, specifically benzodiaze-pines, antidepressants, and sedatives/hypnotics, increase fall risk (Cumming, 1998; Ensrud et al., 2003; Leipzig, Cumming, & Tinetti, 1999; Lord et al., 1993). Review-ing and modifying medications reduced fall rates, particularly when included as part of a multicomponent intervention (Campbell et al., 1999). The majority of participants, however, resumed their prior medication use within 6 months after the study ended.

3.3.1.4. *Multicomponent Programs*

Some of the most effective interventions have involved multicomponent programs (Jensen, Lundin-Olsson, Nyberg, & Gustafson, 2002; Tinetti et al., 1994). Such interventions may incorporate a variety of components: risk-factor screening (which may occur in various settings), tailored exercise or physical therapy to improve gait, balance, and strength; environmental modification; medication management; and other elements such as education about fall risk factors, referrals to healthcare providers for treatment of chronic conditions that may contribute to fall risk, and having vision assessed and corrected (Clemson et al., 2004; Close et al., 1999; Day et al., 2002; McMurdo, Miller, & Daly, 2000; Nikolaus & Bach, 2003).

3.3.1.5. *Home Assessment and Modification*

Although studies have not demonstrated that home modification alone will reduce falls, environmental factors do play a part in about half of all home falls (Nevitt et al., 1989). Home assessment and modification may be effective in reducing falls when done by trained professionals such as occupational therapists and when focused on those at high risk. Home modification has been included in a number of effec-tive multicomponent interventions, particularly among individuals with a history of previous falls (Carter, Campbell, Swanson-Fisher, & Redman, 1997; Cumming et al., 1999; Day et al., 2002; Hornbrook et al., 1994; Nikolaus & Bach, 2003).

3.3.2. Health Care Settings

Compared to community interventions, interventions in acute care hospitals and nursing homes have been studied less frequently. Fall prevention in most health care settings involves screening for fall risk at admission and periodically thereafter, combined with interventions to address the identified risks. Several studies have found that successful nursing home programs included fall risk assessment and modification, low-intensity exercise, and staff education.

3.3.2.1. Nursing Homes

While falls are common in the community, they are even more common in nursing homes. It has been estimated that institutionalized elderly persons fall three times more often than elderly persons living in the community (Rubenstein et al., 1994). Between 30% and 50% of all nursing home residents fall each year and of these, 40% fall twice or more each year (Aronow & Ahn, 1997; Kiely, Kiel, Burrows, & Lipsitz, 1998; Nygaard, 1998; Tinetti, 1987). A 1994 analysis estimated that there were about 1.5 falls per bed per year in nursing homes (Rubenstein et al., 1994). A facility with 100 beds, for example, would be expected to have about 150 falls among its residents every year.

Over 10% of falls in nursing homes cause serious injury and about 5% result in fractures (Butler, Norton, Lee-Joe, Cheng, & Campbell, 1996; Thapa, Gideon, Cost, Milam, & Ray, 1998). The risk of sustaining a hip fracture is 10.5 times higher for women who are in nursing homes than for those living in the community; and less than 15% of nursing home residents who sustain a hip fracture regain preinjury functional status (Folman, Gepstein, Assaraf, & Liberty, 1994).

There are a number of reasons why the nursing home residents may be more vulnerable to falling:

- *High level of frailty:* The most dependent and least ambulatory seniors tend to live in institutions.
- *Multiple co-morbidities:* It is common for nursing home residents to suffer from a number of diseases that can increase their risk of falling.
- *Cognitive deficits common:* Alzheimer disease and other dementias as well as other diseases undermine mental competency and make this population more prone to falling. Available evidence points to the effects of neuro-chemical degeneration caused by the dementia process as well as to the medications commonly taken by those with dementia, both of which impair balance, gait, judgment, and reaction time (Oleske, Wilson, Bernard, Evans, & Terman, 1995).
- *Inactivity:* Maintaining muscle strength and physical abilities is difficult in institutional settings that lack the resources to provide physiotherapists or exercise programs.
- *Side effects of medications:* Nursing home residents often take numerous medications that are known to increase fall risk, particularly psychoactive medications.
- *Nurse to patient ratios:* Nursing home residents are highly dependent. Low nurse to patient ratios can mean that aid from nurses may not be available when a frail elderly patient attempts activities that may lead to a fall (for example, getting out of bed on his or her own).
- *Availability of physiotherapists and occupational therapists:* There may be limited availability of professionals who can design fall prevention programs and assess high-risk individuals.

Prevention strategies in health care settings focus on identifying risk factors and implementing individualized interventions. Health professionals use fall risk assessment tools to identify modifiable risk factors among those who are at greatest risk of sustaining a fall or fall-related injury. These instruments typically provide a scoring system, and an individual is ranked for level of risk based on known fall risk factors. There are two general types of risk assessment tools: screening tools and functional mobility assessments (Perell et al., 2001). *Screening tools* typically rank a person's fall risk as high, medium, or low based on responses to a list of questions about fall risk factors (e.g., psychological status, mobility, elimination patterns, acute/chronic illnesses, sensory deficits, medication use, and a history of falling.) The tools also may include physical assessments. Most screening tools are brief, are typically administered by a nurse at admission, and are usually updated regularly or when there is a change in health status. In contrast, *functional mobility assessments* focus on functional limitations in gait, strength, and balance. These are usually administered by physical therapists or physicians and require patients to perform activities that demonstrate functional abilities.

Examples of assessment tools employed in nursing homes include the following:

- Downton Index (Rosendahl et al., 2003)
- Functional Reach (Rockwood, Awalt, Carver, & Macknight, 2000)
- Morse Fall Scale (Morse, Black, Oberle, & Donahue, 1989)
- Mobility Interaction Fall Chart (Lundin-Olsson, Nyberg, Gustafson, 2000; Lundin-Olsson, Jensen, Nyberg, & Gustafson, 2003)
- Timed Up and Go (Rockwood et al., 2000)
- Tinetti Balance Subscale (Thapa, Gideon, Brockman, Fought, & Ray, 1996)

The sensitivity of assessment tools to predict fall risk varies considerably. An example of a tool with good predictive validity in a nursing home setting is the Mobility Interaction Fall Chart, which has a demonstrated sensitivity of 85% (85% of those screened and who fell were correctly predicted to fall) and specificity of 82% (82% of those predicted not to fall, did not fall) (Lundin-Olsson et al., 2000).

Few nursing home interventions have been shown to be effective, although the evidence is strongest for multicomponent interventions. One study showed a 19% decrease in the number of recurrent fallers after implementing a comprehensive risk assessment, with specific safety recommendations targeting suboptimal practices for environmental and personal safety, including transferring and ambulation, wheelchair use, and psychotropic drug use (Ray et al., 1997). A study by Rubenstein, Robbins, Josephson, Schulman, & Osterweil (1990) used medical assessments followed by targeted interventions. Although this study did not show a significant reduction in falls, the intervention group had 25% fewer hospitalizations and 52% fewer hospital days over the 2-year follow-up period. Another study that tested an intervention consisting of staff education, environmental changes, exercise, drug reviews, hip protectors, and postfall problem-solving conferences found 25% fewer falls among the intervention group (Jensen et al., 2002).

Other promising interventions for reducing falls and fall-related injuries include using vitamin D and calcium supplements to enhance bone and muscle strength (Bischoff et al., 2003; Chapuy et al., 1992) and using hip protectors to prevent hip fractures if a fall occurs (Kannus et al., 2000; Lauritzen, Petersen, & Lund, 1993). Exercise as a fall prevention strategy in nursing homes has been linked to improved muscle strength, gait, and endurance but not to a reduction in falls (Schoenfelder, 2000).

3.3.2.2 Acute Care Hospitals

Acute illness and hospitalization may increase the risk of falls (Evans, Hodgkinson, Lambert, Wood, & Kowanko, 1998; Gaebler, 1993; Hill et al., 2004). Among older hospital patients, consequences of falls include an increased risk of complications, a likelihood of developing a fear of falling or lack of confidence, an extended length of stay, added diagnostic procedures and/or surgeries, a potential for litigation, an increased risk for institutionalization, and additional hospital costs (estimated at an extra $4,233 U.S. for each faller compared to nonfallers) (Aditya, Sharma, Allen, & Vassallo, 2003; Bates, Pruess, Souney, & Platt, 1995; Gluck, Wientjes & Rai, 1996; Hendrich, Nyhuis, Kippenbrock, & Soja, 1995).

A review of the literature has identified a number of patient characteristics associated with high rates of falls in the hospital (Evans et al., 1998; Hill et al., 2004). These include prior falls; incontinence or urinary frequency; and acute illness that can cause sudden changes in physical health, abilities, and functions (Tinetti & Speechley, 1989); immobility and extended bedrest, which can diminish coordination and body strength, slow reflexes and mobility, undermine balance and increase body sway, and cause postural hypotension (Deitrick, Whedon, & Shorr, 1948; Greenleaf, 1984; Taylor, Henschel, & Brozek, 1949); and delirium, which occurs in up to 50% of elderly hospital patients and can cause unpredictable behavior (Inouye et al., 1993).

In addition, fall risks are increased by psychoactive medications, such as sleeping pills and antianxiety medications, which are commonly prescribed to hospital patients (Leipzig et al., 1999; Ray et al., 1997) and by staffing shortages that can make it difficult for patients to obtain help getting out of bed and contribute to their reduced mobility.

While there are few rigorous studies of fall prevention in hospital settings, there are some promising interventions that need to be tested in controlled trials (Bakarich, McMillian, & Prosser, 1997; Haines, Bennell, Osborne, & Hill, 2004; Hanger, Ball, & Wood, 1999; Murdock, Goldney, Fisher, Kent, & Walmsley, 1999). These include proactive nursing interventions that focus on patient mobility, toileting, and increased supervision; restraint reduction; medication reviews; and multicomponent strategies.

Interventions also need to be implemented at the institutional level. Such an approach would likely require a facilitywide, multidisciplinary team that was directly responsible for implementing and evaluating fall prevention activities. Logically, it would include programs to educate staff, residents, family members, and visitors; procedures to orient patients to their new surroundings and available services; systems for assessing patients' fall risk at admission and over time; and mechanisms for identifying high-risk individuals (e.g., bracelets, color coding on charts or above beds) (Hill et al., 2004; Scott, Peck, & Kendall, 2004; Tideiksaar, 2002).

To assess the effectiveness of fall interventions, hospitals and nursing homes must be able to identify falls in a systematic way. Current practices for recording falls and fall-related injuries need to be standardized to enable better data collection on the person, place, time, and circumstances of a fall. Being able to compare numbers and fall rates over time and across institutions is critical to evaluating fall prevention strategies in health care settings. This will require designing and/or refining surveillance systems to monitor the frequency, type, severity, and contributing factors for falls; developing procedures to assess the effectiveness of interventions; and incorporating procedures for recognizing and rewarding the efforts of staff and residents for their fall prevention efforts.

3.4.   RECOMMENDATIONS FOR CLINICIANS

An evidence-based clinical practice guideline for fall prevention and management was developed by a joint task force of the American Geriatrics Society, the British Geriatrics Society, and the American Academy of Orthopedic Surgeons (AGS-BGS-AAOS) (Rubenstein, Kenny, Martin, Tinetti, & the AGS-BGS-AAOS Panel on Falls Prevention, 2001). The guideline was intended to help health care professionals assess and manage older persons who had fallen or were at risk of falling. Using standard criteria, the panel identified and synthesized relevant publications and developed evidence-based recommendations based on the strength of evidence and tailored to each individual's risk level.

3.4.1.   Assessment

The panel recommended, as part of routine care, that all older persons should be asked at least annually about falls. If they have fallen previously, information should be collected about the circumstances (including a witness account). For relatively low-risk seniors, a routine primary health care visit should include a brief screening assessment. People who reported having had a single fall should be observed as they stand up from a chair without using their arms, walk several paces, and return (i.e., the Get Up and Go Test) (Mathias, Nayak, & Isaacs, 1986; Podsiadlo & Richardson, 1991). Those who have difficulty or are unsteady when performing this test require further assessment. An assessment would identify the individual's fall risk factors, including chronic conditions, functional status, and environmental risks. Although the risk factors identified may be modifiable (e.g., muscle weakness, medication side effect, hypotension) or nonmodifiable (e.g., hemiplegia, blindness), knowledge of all risk factors is important for planning treatment.

Persons at high risk of falling—such as those presenting after a fall, people who fall repeatedly, nursing home residents, and people who failed the brief fall risk assessment—should receive a more comprehensive and detailed evaluation. This would include a complete history, including fall circumstances, current medications, acute and chronic medical conditions, and mobility problems. The individual should also undergo an examination of vision, gait and balance, and lower extremity joint function as well as of basic neurological function, including mental status; muscle strength; lower extremity peripheral nerves; proprioception; reflexes; and tests of cortical, extrapyramidal, and cerebellar function. An assessment of basic cardiovascular status should include heart rate and rhythm; postural pulse and blood pressure; and if appropriate, heart rate and blood pressure responses to carotid sinus stimulation. Depending on the complexity of the patient's condition and the level of training of the practitioner, a comprehensive assessment could require referral to a specialist such as a geriatrician. In addition, referral to a physical or occupational therapist might also be required for assessment of the need for mobility aids or other equipment and for a home hazard evaluation.

3.4.2.   Interventions

Interventions for community-dwelling seniors should address the results of the individual's risk assessment and likely will use a number of approaches. Such interventions may include gait training, exercise programs that include balance training (especially for people who have fallen repeatedly), review and modification of medications (especially for people taking four or more medications and those taking psychotropic medications), treatment of postural hypotension, treatment of cardiovascular disorders including cardiac arrhythmias, appropriate use of assistive devices, and modification of environmental hazards. An environmental home assessment by an occupational therapist or other trained home-health professional should be considered when older patients who are at high risk of falling are discharged from the hospital.

Interventions designed for individuals in long-term care and assisted-living settings should include staff education programs, gait training, review and modification of medications (especially psychotropic medications), and advice on the appropriate use of assistive devices (including bed alarms, canes, walkers, and hip protectors). Fall-prone individuals should be evaluated by physical and occupational therapists to obtain the correct fit and learn appropriate use of these assistive and/or protective devices. However, without attention to other risk factors, assistive devices alone are not recommended as a fall prevention strategy. More research is needed to determine the role of these devices in preventing falls.

3.5.   ADDITIONAL PROMISING INTERVENTIONS

Several additional fall interventions have been proposed based on limited study experience.

- Strategies to strengthen bones (e.g., hormone-replacement therapy, calcium, vitamin D, antiresorptive agents) have been shown to reduce fracture rates; however, with the possible exception of vitamin D, these agents do not appear to reduce fall rates.
- Falls caused by cardiovascular factors may be amenable to strategies to prevent syncope, such as medication change or cardiac pacing.
- Changes in footwear may improve intermediate outcomes such as balance and sway but have not been shown to reduce falls. However, a recent study found that not wearing shoes (e.g., going barefoot or wearing socks) significantly increased fall risk (Koepsell et al., 2004).
- Hip protectors are a promising strategy for reducing hip fractures if a fall occurs. More research is needed to improve staff compliance and patient adherence and to evaluate the effectiveness of these devices among community-based as well as institutional-based older adults.

3.6.   FUTURE RESEARCH NEEDS

While much is known about fall risk factors and prevention strategies, a national initiative and other large-scale approaches are required to support and expand current fall prevention research and promote widespread use of effective measures. Areas that should be addressed include improving fall injury surveillance and data collection, improving the validity and reliability of fall risk assessment tools for use in all settings, tailoring the most effective fall prevention approaches to specific older adult populations, conducting research about barriers to adopting and sustaining proven interventions, and identifying effective strategies for preventing falls among high-risk seniors in hospital and nursing-home settings. In addition, specific research questions include the following:

General approaches
- What are the core elements of successful fall-intervention approaches?
- How cost-effective are various effective interventions?

Populations
- How do the core intervention elements differ in specific settings, such as hospitals, nursing homes, and assistive housing?
- What specific types of exercises are most effective for different populations?
- How can we develop tailored interventions for populations with differing characteristics (e.g., cognitive impairment) and risk factors (e.g., balance problems)?
- For whom and when is home assessment by an occupational therapist or other home-care specialist effective?

Specific interventions
- What are the key characteristics of exercise programs (such as type, duration, intensity, and frequency)?
- How effective are assistive devices, such as canes and walkers, in preventing falls?
- To what extent does treating and/or correcting visual problems prevent falls?
- What is the safest type of footwear for people at risk of falling?

Dissemination research
- How can we successfully disseminate and sustain effective intervention programs and promote their widespread adoption at the regional and local level?

3.7. IMPLICATIONS FOR PUBLIC HEALTH PRACTICE

To effectively address the problem of falls, we will need national and regional initiatives to provide vision, set priorities, and establish an organizational infrastructure to address issues related to falls and fall-related injuries in our aging society. To accomplish this, fall prevention will need to be integrated into our health care systems. Therefore, actions will need to be taken by organizations at the national, regional, and local levels. Such initiatives will need to focus on the critical areas of legislation, administration, and education. The following sections describe these areas and recommendations.

3.7.1. Legislation

To encourage legislative action, it is essential to assess the cost of health care for fall-related injuries. Specifically, this will require evaluating more precisely the economic impact of falls on Medicare and Medicaid and developing innovative ways to reduce medical costs by expanding coverage for prevention and intervention services. One possible approach is to amend Medicare legislation to provide coverage for a variety of fall prevention activities by health care professionals. For example, Medicare coverage could be expanded to reimburse (1) clinicians for fall

assessments and risk factor reduction for high-risk individuals, (2) physical therapists for providing balance and gait training to seniors to reduce their fall risk, (3)
pharmacists for reviewing seniors' medications and providing counseling about fall
prevention, and (4) occupational therapists for conducting home assessments and
modification for seniors who have sustained falls or fall-related injuries.

3.7.2.   Administration

Government agencies such as the Administration on Aging and the National
Center for Injury Prevention and Control at the Centers for Disease Control and
Prevention can provide national leadership, establish priorities, and oversee
and support national efforts to reduce falls and fall-related injuries. Partnerships
and coalitions of a wide variety of organizations—including regional, state, local,
nonprofit, voluntary, and charitable organizations—will be pivotal in supporting
these efforts.

   An important national objective will be to coordinate regional and state efforts
to disseminate programs that can be implemented at the local level. Regional
and state-level organizations can provide communities with information about
effective, evidence-based fall prevention strategies; provide technical support to
community-based organizations; and encourage expanded roles for local community and service organizations. In addition to state health departments, regional
and state area agencies on aging are well positioned to coordinate state activities, whereas local area agencies on aging, health departments, service providers,
faith-based and volunteer groups, and other local organizations must be engaged
and supported so that they can integrate these programs into existing community-
based services. Another objective will be to provide financial support from a variety
of public and private sources to communities and local organizations to implement effective fall prevention programs. Such support can be used to increase the
availability of balance and strength-training programs for older adults, including
both in-home and community-based settings such as senior centers and retirement
homes, and/or to encourage local communities to develop and implement self-
sustaining fall prevention programs.

   Municipal governments also have an important role to play in the design and
maintenance of safe public environments intended to reduce the risk of falling
among seniors and those with disabilities. The urgency of this issue is reflected
in the changing U.S. demographics, with growing numbers of older people with
chronic health problems and disabilities living longer and choosing to remain in
community settings. Examples of design issues are providing walking routes that
have good lighting and clear signage and are free of obstacles, tripping hazards,
and slippery surfaces. These issues are best addressed through a collaborative
process among municipal officials, community groups, and those with expertise in
environmental design for an aging population.

3.7.3.   Education

A national initiative to reduce falls among older adults will need to include the
development and implementation of effective education strategies. One approach
is to design and conduct national education campaigns to provide fall prevention
information to seniors, family members, employers, caregivers, senior service providers, health care professionals, and others who are involved in providing for the

health and welfare of older adults. Such campaigns, targeting a variety of audiences and implemented at multiple levels (e.g., through continuing-education programs and various print media), will provide information about fall risks and describe effective prevention strategies. Another approach is to develop national education and training guidelines for health care professionals and service providers about fall risk factors and prevention strategies. Such training is essential if fall prevention is to become integrated into our health care and public health systems.

The activities in these three areas are interrelated. Administration and legislation may be handled most appropriately at the national and state levels, while education and prevention programs are implemented most effectively by coalitions of local organizations. In contrast, research involves activities at all levels—for example, government funding of university researchers to conduct community-based studies. The activities of organizations at national, regional, and local levels are all critical to shaping public policy and promoting fall prevention.

3.8.   CURRENT ACTIVITIES

Many communities are implementing activities designed to reduce older adult falls. One of the most extensive fall prevention approaches has been undertaken by California. In 2003, California developed a state-based initiative, *Creating a California Blueprint for Fall Prevention*, to assess current best-practices models and how to best integrate these into new and existing programs in community, hospital, and nursing-home settings (Kramer, Courtright, & Smith, 2004).

Other states provide programs with a range of services (e.g., exercise classes and education) in various settings such as senior centers, retirement homes, and churches. One example is the Florida Injury Prevention for Seniors (FLIPS) program, a program that is supported by the Florida Department of Health. This program is a broad-based collaborative effort between the Departments of Florida Elder Affairs, Health, and Insurance (Fire Marshal's Office); universities; the Florida Student Nurses Association; hospitals, county health departments; and many other local agencies and organizations. However, most programs are limited in scope, with only a small portion of those at risk in each state being exposed to comprehensive fall prevention strategies. Moreover, few programs, regardless of size, have been evaluated for effectiveness or use science-based effective interventions.

Although many states and local communities have been making efforts to address the problem of falls, the full range of U.S. fall programs is unknown. The National Council on the Aging (NCOA), a 3200-member network that is actively promoting fall prevention, recently conducted a survey of current fall prevention programs and services. A total of 63 organizations responded, primarily not-for-profit organizations, trade groups, government agencies, and medical associations that focus on the needs of older adults. These organizations provided information about their fall prevention activities, such as creating and distributing education materials and programs for consumers and professionals, funding research projects on fall prevention, and providing health care services.

In summarizing the results of the survey, NCOA noted that while many programs, products, resources, and services were available, there were some important gaps. First, few educational programs had been developed for minority populations, those with low income, or individuals with limited education. Second, although the non-English-speaking population in the United States is growing rapidly, few materials were available in languages other than English. Third, many organizations provided information through the Internet, which many older adults do not access. Fourth, continuing education for health providers tended to rely on traditional methods such as seminars, conferences, and journal articles. There may be opportunities for establishing collaborative initiatives among professional organizations, including the development and dissemination of clinical guidelines. Finally, it was noted that additional approaches for educating both health care providers and older adults about fall risks and prevention strategies needed to be explored.

In December 2004, NCOA, with support from the Archstone Foundation and the National Safety Council, sponsored the Falls Free Summit, a two-day meeting in Washington, D.C. Small facilitated work groups studied five fall-risk areas (physical mobility, medication management, home safety, environmental safety in the community, and cross-cutting issues) and developed specific goals and recommendations. The outcome of this meeting was a national action plan, a document that describes fall prevention activities that can be used on the local, state, and national level (National Council on Aging Center for Healthy Aging, 2005).

3.9.   CONCLUSIONS

Successful prevention interventions depend on understanding the interaction between the risk factors and the settings where falls take place. In addition, practical interventions must be feasible, sustainable, and cost effective. Research has identified a number of fall prevention interventions. These include

- Clinical assessment and risk reduction.
- Exercise.
- Medication management.
- Vision correction.
- Home modification.

Some interventions are effective by themselves (e.g., clinical assessment, exercise), whereas others are most appropriately used as one part of a multicomponent intervention (e.g., home modification).

To reduce falls and fall injuries, efforts are needed at all levels. Local organizations and health providers can promote effective interventions and encourage seniors to incorporate fall prevention into their daily lives. In addition, national, state, and local organizations will need to act cooperatively. This is going to be challenging because many of these organizations have traditionally operated independently. Cooperation across jurisdictions and disciplines is crucial if we are going to implement effective fall prevention interventions, reduce these debilitating and costly injuries, and improve the health and quality of life for our older citizens.

REFERENCES

Aditya, B. S., Sharma, J. C., Allen, S. C., & Vassallo, M. (2003). Predictors of a nursing home placement from a non-acute geriatric hospital. *Clinical Rehabilitation, 17* (1), 108–113.

Aronow, W. S., & Ahn, C. (1997). Association of postprandial hypotension with incidence of falls, syncope, coronary events, stroke and total mortality at 29-month follow-up in 499 older nursing home residents. *Journal of the American Geriatrics Society, 45* (9), 1051–1053.

Bakarich, A., McMillian, V., & Prosser, R. (1997). The effect of a nursing intervention on the incidence of older patient falls. *Australian Journal of Advanced Nursing, 15*, 26–31.

Barnett, A., Smith, B., Lord, S. R., Williams, M., & Baumand, A. (2003). Community-based group exercise improves balance and reduces falls in at-risk older people: A randomized controlled trial. *Age & Aging, 32*, 407–414.

Bates, D. W., Pruess, K., Souney, P., & Platt, R. (1995). Serious falls in hospitalized patients: Correlates and resource utilization. *American Journal of Medicine, 99* (2), 137–143.

Bernstein, A. B., & Schur, C. L. (1990). Expenditures for unintentional injuries among the elderly. *Journal of Aging Health, 2*, 157–178.

Bischoff, H. A., Stahelin, H. B., Dick, W., Akos, R., Knecht, M., & Salis, C., et al. (2003). Effects of vitamin D and calcium supplementation on falls: A randomized controlled trial. *Journal of Bone & Mineral Research, 18* (2), 343–351.

Brown, A. P. (1999). Reducing falls in elderly people: A review of exercise interventions. *Physiotherapy Theory & Practice, 15*, 59–68.

Butler, M., Norton, R., Lee-Joe, T., Cheng, A., & Campbell, J. (1996). The risks of hip fracture in older people from private homes and institutions. *Age & Ageing, 25*, 381–385.

Campbell, A. J., Robertson, M. C., Gardner, M. M., Norton, R. N., & Buchner, D. M. (1999). Falls prevention over 2 years: A randomized controlled trial in women 80 years and older. *Age & Ageing, 28*, 513–518.

Campbell, A. J., Spears, G. F., & Borrie, M. J. (1990). Examination by logistic regression modelling of the variables which increase the relative risk of elderly women falling compared to elderly men. *Journal of Clinical Epidemiology, 43*, 1415–1420.

Carter, S. E., Campbell, E. M., Swanson-Fisher, R. W., & Redman, S. (1997). Environmental hazards in the homes of older people. *Age & Ageing, 26*, 195–202.

Centers for Disease Control and Prevention, National Centers for Injury Prevention and Control. (2005). Web-based injury statistics query and reporting system (WISQARS). Retrieved on February 8, 2005, from www.cdc.gov/ncipc/wisqars.

Chang, J. T., Morton, S. C., Rubenstein, L. Z., Mojica, W. A., Maglione, M., Suttorp, M. J., Roth, E. A., & Shekelle, P. G. (2004). Interventions for the prevention of falls in older adults: Systematic review and meta-analysis of randomized clinical trials. *British Medical Journal, 328*, 680–687.

Chapuy, M. C., Arlot, M. E., Duboeuf, F., Brun, J., Crouzet, B., Arnaud, S., Delmas, P. D., Meunier, P. J. (1992). Vitamin D3 and calcium to prevent hip fractures in elderly women. *New Engl and Journal of Medicine, 327*, 1637–1642.

Clark, R. D., Lord, S. R., & Webster, I. W. (1993). Clinical parameters associated with falls in an elderly population. *Gerontology, 39*, 117–123.

Clemson, L., Cumming, R. G., Kendig, H., Swann, M., Heard, R., & Taylor, K. (2004). The effectiveness of a community-based program for reducing the incidence of falls in the elderly: A randomized trial. *Journal of the American Geriatrics Society, 52*, 1487–1494.

Close, J., Ellis, M., Hooper, R., Glucksman, E., Jackson, S., & Swift, C. (1999). Prevention of falls in the elderly trial (PROFET): A randomized controlled trial. *Lancet, 353*, 93–97.

Cumming, R. G., Thomas, M., Szonyi, G., Salkeld, G., O'Neill, E., Westbury, C., & Frampton, G. (1999). Home visits by an occupational therapist for assessment and modification of environmental hazards: A randomized trial of falls prevention. *Journal of the American Geriatrics Society, 47*, 1397–1402.

Cumming, R. G. (1998). Epidemiology of medication-related falls and fractures in the elderly. *Drugs & Aging, 12* (1), 43–53.

Cumming, R. G., Kelsey, J. L., & Nevitt, M. C. (1990). Methodologic issues in the study of frequent and recurrent health problems. Falls in the elderly. *Annals of Epidemiology, 1*, 49–56.

Cummings, S. R., Nevitt, M. C., & Kidd, S. (1988). Forgetting falls. The limited accuracy of recall of falls in the elderly. *Journal of the American Geriatric Society, 36*, 613–616.

Day, L., Fildes, B., Gordon, I., Fitzharris, M., Flamer, H., & Lord, S. (2002). Randomised factorial trial of falls prevention among older people living in their own homes. *British Medical Journal, 325* (7356), 128–133.

Deitrick, J. E., Whedon, G. D., & Shorr, E. (1948). Effects of immobilization upon various metabolic and physiological functions of normal men. *American Journal of Medicine, 4*, 3–36.

Ensrud. K. E., Blackwell, T., Mangione, C. M., Bowman, P. J., Bauer, D. C., Schwartz, A., Hanlon, J. T., Nevitt, M. C., & Whooley, M. A. (2003). Central nervous system active medications and risk for fractures in older women. *Archives of Internal Medicine, 163*, 949–957.

Evans, D., Hodgkinson, B., Lambert, L., Wood, J., & Kowanko, I. (1998). *Falls in acute care hospitals: A systematic review.* Adelaide, Australia: Joanna Briggs Institute for Evidence Based Nursing and Midwifery.

Evans, R. G., Barer, M. L., & Marmor, T. R. (1994). *Why are some people healthy and others are not?: The determinants of health of populations.* New York: Aldine.

Finkelstein, E. A., Chen, H., Miller, T. R., Corso, P. S., & Stevens, J. A. (2005). A comparison of the case-control and case-crossover designs for estimating medical costs of non-fatal fall-related injuries among older Americans. *Medical Care, 43,* 1087–1091.

Folman, Y., Gepstein, R., Assaraf, A., & Liberty, S. (1994). Functional recovery after operative treatment of femoral neck fractures in an institutionalized elderly population. *Archives of Physical Medicine & Rehabilitation, 75,* 454–456.

Gaebler, S. (1993). Predicting which patient will fall again . . . and again. *Journal of Advanced Nursing, 18,* 1895–1902.

Gardner, M. M., Buchner, D. M., Robertson, M. C. & Campbell, A. J. (2001). Practical implementation of an exercise-based falls prevention programme. *Age & Ageing, 30* (1), 77–83.

Gillespie, L. D., Gillespie, W. J., Robertson, M. C., Lamb, S. E., Cumming, R. G., & Rowe, B. H. (2003). Interventions for preventing falls in elderly people (Cochrane Database Systematic Review). In: The Cochrane Library, Issue 3, 2003. Chichester, UK: John Wiley & Sons, Ltd.

Gluck, T., Wientjes, H. J., & Rai, G. S. (1996). An evaluation of risk factors for in-patient falls in acute and rehabilitation elderly care wards. *Gerontology, 42* (2), 104–107.

Greenleaf, J. E. (1984). Physiological responses to prolonged bed rest and fluid immersion in humans. *Journal of Applied Physiology, 57,* 619–633.

Haines, T., Bennell, K., Osborne, R., & Hill, K. (2004). Effectiveness of a targeted falls prevention program in a sub-acute hospital setting. *British Medical Journal, 328,* 676.

Hangar, H., Ball, M., & Wood, L. (1999). An analysis of falls in the hospital: Can we do without bedrails? *Journal of the American Geriatrics Society, 47,* 529–531.

Hendrich, A., Nyhuis, A., Kippenbrock, T., & Soja, M. E. (1995). Hospital falls: Development of a predictive model for clinical practice. *Applied Nursing Research, 8* (3), 129–139.

Hill, K., Vrantsidis, F., Haralambous, B., Fearn, M., Smith, R., Murry, K., Sims, J., & Dorevitch, M. (2004). *An analysis of research on preventing falls and falls injury in older people: Community, residential and hospital settings.* Canberra, Australia: National Ageing Research Institute.

Inouye, S. K., Wagner, D. R., Acampora, D., Horowitz, R. I., Cooney, L. M., & Tinetti, M. E. (1993). A controlled trial of a nursing-centred intervention in hospitalized elderly medical patients: The Yale Geriatric Program. *Journal of the American Geriatrics Society, 41* (12), 1353–1360.

Hornbrook, M. C., Stevens, V. J., Wingfield, D. J., Hollis, J. F., Greenlick, M. R., & Ory, M. G. (1994). Preventing falls among community-dwelling older persons: Results from a randomized trial. *The Gerontologist, 34* (1), 16–23.

Jarrett, P. G., Rockwood, K., Carver, D., Stolee, P., & Cosway, S. (1995). Illness presentation in elderly patients. *Archives of Internal Medicine, 155,* 1060–1064.

Jensen, J., Lundin-Olsson, L., Nyberg, L., & Gustafson, Y. (2002). Fall and injury prevention in older people living in residential care facilities. *Annals of Internal Medicine, 136,* 733–741.

Judge, J. O., Lindsey, C., Underwood, M., & Winsemius, D. (1993). Balance improvements in older women: Effects of exercise training. *Physical Therapy, 73* (4), 254–262, 263–265.

Kannus, P., Parkkari, J., Niemi. S., Pasanen, M., Palvanen, M., Jarviven, M., & Vuori, L. (2000). Prevention of hip fracture in elderly people with use of a hip protector. *New England Journal of Medicine, 343,* 1506–1513.

Kiely, D. K., Kiel, D. P., Burrows, A. B., & Lipsitz, L. A. (1998). Identifying nursing home residents at risk for falling. *Journal of the American Geriatrics Society, 46,* 551–555.

Koepsell, T. D., Wolf, M. E., Buchner, D. M., Kukull, W. A., LaCroix, A. Z., Tencer, A. F., et al. (2004). Footwear style and risk of falls in older adults. *Journal of the American Geriatrics Society, 52,* 1495–1501.

Kramer, B. J., Courtright, M. E. K., & Smith, P. (2004). *Creating a California blueprint for fall prevention.* Long Beach, CA: Archstone Foundation.

Lauritzen, J. B., Petersen, M. M., & Lund, B. (1993). Effect of external hip protectors on hip fractures. *Lancet, 341,* 11–13.

Leipzig, R. M., Cumming, R. G., & Tinetti, M. E. (1999). Drugs and falls in older people: A systematic review and meta-analysis: I. Psychotropic drugs. *Journal of the American Geriatrics Society, 47,* 30–39.

Lord, S. R., Caplan, G. A., & Ward, J. A. (1993). Balance, reaction time, and muscle strength in exercising older women: A pilot study. *Archives of Physical & Medical Rehabilitation, 74* (8), 837–839.

Lord, S. R., Castell, S., Corcoran, J., Dayhew, J., Batters, B., Shan, A., & William, P. (2003). The effect of group exercise on physical functioning and falls in frail older people living in retirement villages: A randomized controlled trial. *Journal of the American Geriatrics Society, 51,* 1684–1692.

Lundin-Olsson, L., Nyberg, L., & Gustafson, Y. (2000). The mobility interaction fall chart. *Physiotherapy Research International, 5* (3), 190–201.

Lundin-Olsson, L., Jensen, J., Nyberg, L., & Gustafson, Y. (2003). Predicting falls in residential care by a risk assessment tool, staff judgement, and history of falls. *Aging Clinical Experimental Research, 15* (1), 51–90.

Mathias, S., Nayak, U. S., & Isaacs, B. (1986). Balance in elderly patients: The "get-up and go" test. *Archives of Physical & Medical Rehabilitation, 67,* 387–389.

McMurdo, M. E. T., Millar, A. M., & Daly, F. (2000). A randomized controlled trial of fall prevention strategies in old peoples' homes. *Gerontology, 46,* 83–87.

Morse, J. M., Black, C., Oberle, K., & Donahue, P. (1989). A prospective study to identify the fall-prone patient. *Social Science & Medicine, 28* (1), 81–86.

Murdock, C., Goldney, R., Fisher, L., Kent, P., & Walmsley, S. (1999). A reduction in repeat falls in a private psychiatric hospital. *Australian & New Zealand Journal of Mental Health Nursing, 7,* 111–115.

National Council on the Aging Center for Healthy Aging. (2005). Falls free: Promoting a national falls prevention action plan: National action plan. Retrieved October 20, 2005, from www. healthyagingprograms.org/content.asp?sectionid=69&ElementID=220.

Nevitt, M. C., Cummings, S. R., Kidd, S., & Black, D. (1989). Risk factors for recurrent nonsyncopal falls. A prospective study. *Journal of the American Medical Association, 261,* 2663–2668.

Nevitt, M. C. (1997). Falls in the elderly: Risk factors and prevention. In J. C. Masdeu, L. Sudarsky, & L. Wolfson (Eds.), *Gait disorders of aging: Falls and therapeutic strategies* (pp. 13–36). Philadelphia: Lippincott-Raven.

Nikolaus, T., & Bach, M. (2003). Preventing falls in community-dwelling frail older people using a home intervention team (HIT): Results from the randomized Falls-HIT trial. *Journal of the American Geriatrics Society, 51* (3), 300–305.

Nygaard, H. A. (1998). Falls and psychotropic drug consumption in long-term care residents: Is there an obvious association? *Gerontology, 44* (1), 46–50.

Oleske, D. M., Wilson, R. S., Bernard, B. A., Evans, D. A., & Terman, E. W. (1995). Epidemiology of injury in people with Alzheimer's disease. *Journal of the American Geriatrics Society, 43* (7), 741–746.

Perell, K. L., Nelson, A., Goldman, R. L., Luther, S. L., Prieto-Lewis, N., & Rubenstein, L. Z. (2001). Fall risk assessment measures: An analytic review. *Journal of Gerontology Series A: Biological Sciences & Medical Sciences, 56A* (12), M761–M766.

Podsiadlo, D., & Richardson, S. (1991). The timed "Up & Go": A test of basic functional mobility for frail elderly persons. *Journal of the American Geriatrics Society, 39,* 142–148.

Raina, P., Dukeshire, S., Chambers, L., Toivonen, D., & Lindsay, J. (1997). *Prevalence, risk factors, and health care utilization for injuries among Canadian seniors: An analysis of 1994 National Population Health Survey* (IESOP Research Report No. 15). Hamilton, Ontario, Canada: McMaster University.

Rand Corporation, Southern California Evidence-Based Practice Center. (2003). *Evidence report and evidence-based recommendations: Fall prevention interventions in the Medicare population* (Contract number 500-98-0281). Santa Monica, CA: Author.

Ray, W. A., Taylor, J. A., Meador, K., Thapa, P. B., Brown, A. K., Kajihara, H. K., Davis, C., Gideon, P., et al. (1997). A randomized trial of a consultation service to reduce falls in nursing homes. *Journal of the American Medical Association, 278,* 557–562.

Robbins, A. S., Rubenstein, L. Z., Josephson, K. R., Schulman, B. L., Osterweil, D., & Fine, G. (1989). Predictors of falls among elderly people. Results of two population-based studies. *Archives of Internal Medicine, 149,* 1628–1633.

Robertson, M. C., Devlin, N., Gardner, M. M., & Campbell, A. J. (2001). Effectiveness and economic evaluation of a nurse delivered home exercise programme to prevent falls. I: Randomised controlled trial. *British Medical Journal, 322,* 697–701.

Rockwood, K., Awalt, E., Carver, D., & Macknight, C. (2000). Feasibility and measurement properties of the functional reach and the timed up and go tests in the Canadian Study of Health and Aging. *Journal of Gerontology Series A: Biological Sciences & Medical Sciences, 5,* M70–M73.

Rosendahl, E., Lundin-Olsson, L., Kallin, J., Jensen, Y., Gustafson, & Nyberg, L. (2003). Prediction of falls among older people in residential care facilities by the Downton Index. *Aging Clinical & Experimental Research, 15* (2), 142–147.

Rubenstein, L. Z., Josephson, K. R., & Robbins, A. S. (1994). Falls in the nursing home. *Annals of Internal Medicine, 121,* 442–451.

Rubenstein, L. Z., & Josephson, K. R. (2002). The epidemiology of falls and syncope. *Clinical Geriatric Medicine, 18* (2), 141–158.

Rubenstein, L. Z., Kenny, R. A., Martin, F. C., Tinetti, M. E., & the AGS-BGS-AAOS Panel on Falls Prevention. (2001). Guideline for prevention of falls in older persons. *Journal of the American Geriatrics Society, 49,* 664–772.

Rubenstein, L. Z., Powers, C., & MacLean, C. (2001). Quality indicators for management and prevention of falls and mobility problems in vulnerable older persons. *Annals of Internal Medicine, 135,* 686–693.

Rubenstein, L. Z., Robbins, A. S., Josephson, K. R., Schulman, B. S., & Osterweil, D. (1990). The value of assessing falls in an elderly population: A randomized clinical trial. *Annals of Internal Medicine, 113* (4), 308–316.

Schoenfelder, D. P. (2000). A fall prevention program for elderly individuals. Exercise in long-term care settings. *Journal of Gerontology Nursing, 26,* 43–51.

Scott, V., Dukeshire, S., Gallagher, E., & Scanlan, A. (2001). *An inventory of Canadian programs for the prevention of falls and fall-related injuries among seniors living in the community* (Monograph prepared for the Canadian Federal/Provincial/Territorial Committee of Official for the Ministers Responsible for Seniors): Ottawa, Ontario.

Scott, V., Peck, S., & Kendall, P. (2004). *Prevention of falls and injuries among the elderly: A special report of the Office of the Provincial Health Officer.* Victoria, British Columbia: Ministry of Health Planning.

Taylor, H., Henschel, A., & Brozek, J. (1949). Effects of bed rest on cardiovascular function and work performance. *Journal of Applied Physiology, 2,* 223–239.

Thapa, P. B., Gideon, P., Brockman, K. G., Fought, R. L., & Ray, W. A. (1996). Clinical and biomechanical measures of balance as fall predictors in ambulatory nursing home residents. *Journal of Gerontology: Medical Sciences, 51A* (5), M239–M246.

Thapa, P. B., Gideon, P., Cost, T. W., Milam, A. B., & Ray, W. A. (1998). Antidepressants and the risk of falls among nursing home residents. *New England Journal of Medicine, 339,* 875–882.

Tideiksaar, R. (2002). *Falls in older people: Prevention & management.* Baltimore: Health Professionals Press.

Tinetti, M. E. (1987). Factors associated with serious injury during falls by ambulatory nursing home residents. *Journal of the American Geriatrics Society, 35,* 644–648.

Tinetti, M. E., Baker, D. I., McAvay, G., Claus, E. B., Garrett, P., Gottschalk, M., Koch, M. L., Trainor, K., & Horwitz, R. (1994). A multifactorial intervention to reduce the risk of falling among elderly people living in the community. *New England Journal of Medicine, 331,* 821–827.

Tinetti, M. E., & Speechley, M. (1989). Prevention of falls among the elderly. *New England Journal of Medicine, 320* (16), 1055–1059.

Tinetti, M. E., Speechley, M., & Ginter, S. F. (1988). Risk factors for falls among elderly persons living in the community. *New England Journal of Medicine, 319,* 1701–1707.

Tinetti, M. E., Williams, T. F., & Mayewski, R. (1986). Fall risk index for elderly patients based on number of chronic disabilities. *American Journal of Medicine, 80,* 429–434.

Vellas, B. J., Wayne, S. J., Romero, L. J., Baumgartner, R. N., & Garry, P. J. (1997). Fear of falling and restriction of mobility in elderly fallers. *Age & Ageing, 26,* 189–193.

Wolf, S. L., Barnhart, H. X., Kutner, N. G., McNeely. E., Coogler, C., & Xu, T. (1996). Reducing frailty and falls in older persons: An investigation of tai chi and computerized balance training. Atlanta FICSIT Group. *Journal of the American Geriatrics Society, 44* (5), 489–497.

Chapter **4**

Interventions to Prevent Motor Vehicle Injuries

Ann M. Dellinger, David A. Sleet, Ruth A. Shults, and Caryll F. Rinehart

4.1. MAGNITUDE OF THE PROBLEM

Motor-vehicle-related deaths and injuries take a heavy toll on health in the United States, and motor vehicle crashes result in more than 40,000 deaths and more than three million nonfatal injuries each year. They are the leading cause of death among children, youth, and young adults (Centers for Disease Control and Prevention [CDC], 2005).

Motor-vehicle-related deaths and injuries include those among vehicle occupants, pedestrians, and cyclists. The overall motor vehicle death rate was 15.8 deaths per 100,000 population in 2002, representing 45,579 deaths. Motor-vehicle occupants (drivers and passengers) represent the majority of motor-vehicle-related deaths. Males have occupant death rates twice as high as females (10.0 vs. 4.9 per 100,000). The age distribution of occupant deaths is lowest among children too young to drive, highest in teenagers and young adults aged 15–24 years, and lowest among persons in their 50s. Older adults are particularly vulnerable to death in a motor-vehicle crash given their physical frailty (Evans & Phil, 1988; Li, Braver, & Chen, 2003).

More than 6,000 pedestrians were killed in 2002, including on- and off-road collisions with motor vehicles. Pedestrian death rates are also twice as high for males as females (3.0 vs. 1.3 per 100,000). After age 30, the pedestrian death rate climbs with age, reaching a high of 5.1 per 100,000 among people aged 85 and older. In 2002, 766 cyclists were killed in collisions with motor vehicles. Males had cyclist death rates ten times higher than females (0.50 vs. 0.05). The highest cyclist death rates were among those aged 10–14 and 45–49 years (CDC, 2005).

There are racial and ethnic differences in motor-vehicle-related deaths. Generally, Native American and Alaska Native populations have the highest death rates while Asian and Pacific Islander populations have the lowest; African American and

White populations have similar death rates (CDC, 2005). However, when adjusting for time on the road or vehicle miles traveled, vehicle occupants who are African American or Hispanic have higher death rates than Whites (Baker, Braver, Chen, Pantula, Massie, 1998; Braver, 2003).

It has been estimated that 4.5 million people sought medical care in a hospital emergency department for nonfatal motor-vehicle injury in 2002 (1,553 per 100,000 population). It is interesting that males and females have similar numbers (2.4 million vs. 2.2 million) and rates of injury (1,615 per 100,000 for males vs. 1,503 for females). The highest rates of nonfatal injury were among those aged 15–24 years; the lowest were among children aged 0–4 (CDC, 2005).

4.1.1. Motor-Vehicle Injury Prevention and Public Health

Motor vehicles dominate all other modes of travel in the United States. The motor vehicle accounts for 94% of all transportation-related deaths in the United States (Evans, 1999). This phenomenon is part of a long history of rapid growth in motor-vehicle-related exposure and related mortality and morbidity. In the span of 100 years, the number of registered automobiles in the United States grew from 8,000 in 1900 to 239 million in 2003, and the number of licensed drivers grew to nearly 197 million (National Safety Council [NSC], 2004). The number of annual vehicle miles traveled trap (VMT) has reached 2.9 trillion (National Highway Traffic Safety Administration, 2005a). This remarkable expansion has brought a growing safety problem. But despite the rapid growth in vehicles and vehicle miles traveled, deaths per 100 million VMT have declined since 1925 in the United States (see Figure 4.1).

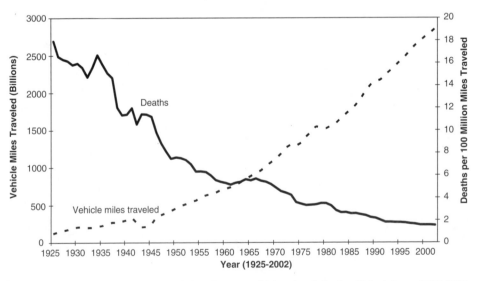

Figure 4.1. Annual vehicle miles traveled and motor-vehicle-related deaths, United States 1925–2002. Data source: National Safety Council, Injury Facts, 2004.

The fundamental role of public health in traffic safety was evident in the appointment of William Haddon, a public health physician who was the first administrator of the National Highway Traffic Safety Administration (NHTSA), U.S. Department of Transportation. He applied the infectious disease conceptual framework of agent, host, and environment to the prevention of motor-vehicle crashes. He also added the dimension of time in three phases, precrash, crash and postcrash. The result was the Haddon Matrix (Haddon, 1968). Given the mandate of regulating vehicles and roadways, the traffic safety community has focused more attention (and made good progress) in the areas of the agent (i.e., vehicle) and environment (i.e., roadways) to prevent injury. Public health has traditionally focused more on the host, or person. Making the host more resistant or separating the host from the energy exchange in a crash is part of the public health approach to injury prevention (Sleet, Egger, & Albany, 1991).

The historic role of public health is the application of knowledge to promote health and prevent disease. The public health sector is the principal architect of programs to influence individual and collective health behavior, to alter environmental conditions protecting health, and to improve health resources and services. Health departments, for example, collectively form a national infrastructure through which to address health problems such as alcohol-impaired driving, safety belt use, or pedestrian injuries. They have the statutory responsibility for public health, provide direct personal health services to a significant part of the population, deliver programs to underserved populations, and are experienced in working with community groups and collaborating with health and social service agencies. As such, public health plays a key role in any plan to promote traffic safety.

4.1.2. Focus of the Chapter

This chapter focuses on interventions that are designed to address person or host factors as the more traditional domain of public health, but includes information on vehicles and roadways where appropriate. The reader can refer to chapter 14 and Elvik and Vaa (2004) for syntheses of interventions related to roads and the built environment. NHTSA (2004a) provides an analysis of the effects of vehicle-related interventions, including vehicle safety standards resulting in improvements in vehicle design. This chapter has a distinctive domestic focus, and interventions implemented in international settings, for the most part, are not addressed. The intent is to provide a practical review of interventions designed to reduce motor-vehicle-related deaths and injuries that can be implemented in the United States by public health practitioners.

This chapter combines interventions into categories by level of effectiveness, starting with interventions with the strongest evidence of effectiveness and ending with interventions that have evidence of unintended harmful effects. Within a topic, interventions related to death and injury prevention are described first, followed by interventions that modify behavior. For example, alcohol-impaired-driving interventions that are effective in reducing mortality and morbidity are followed by interventions related to reducing alcohol-impaired driving or level of intoxication. These sections are followed by a discussion of some of the cross-cutting issues in this area. The chapter includes a summary evidence table (Table 4.1) for many of the interventions described in the text.

(*Continued on page 66*)

Table 4.1. Evidence Table for Selected Motor-Vehicle-Related Public Health Interventions

Intervention (Qualifying Studies)	Level of Evidence[a]	Intervention Description	Key Findings	How Widely Used?	Barriers to Implementation	Other Positive (+) or Negative (−) Effects
Interventions to Reduce Alcohol-Impaired Driving						
Minimum legal drinking age (MLDA) (n = 33)	Strong evidence (maintenance of MLDA of 21 years)	• Specifies an age below which the purchase and/or consumption of alcoholic beverages are not permitted	■ Among 14 studies looking at the effects of raising the MLDA, crash-related outcomes *declined* a median of 16% for the targeted age groups ■ Among 9 studies looking at the effects of lowering the MLDA, crash-related outcomes *increased* by a median of 10% within the targeted age groups ■ Effects were stable over follow-up times ranging from 7 to 108 months	• All 50 states and the District of Columbia have MLDA laws • In many other countries, the drinking age is 18 years • Studies were conducted in the United States, Canada, and Australia	• Some opponents of MLDA laws believe that prohibiting drinking among young adults unjustly punishes them for the irresponsible behavior of the subgroup that drives after drinking	• (+) Several studies reported that the 21 MLDA resulted in decreased alcohol consumption • (+) 9 studies that examined the higher MLDA on crashes involving younger adolescent drivers indicated that raising the MLDA resulted in a median decline of crashes; however, the size of this effect was inconsistent across studies, with several showing no effect • (+) Although some have postulated that the MLDA laws may lead to higher risk of alcohol-impaired driving due to lack of drinking experience at age 21, one study found that if the putative drinking experience effect exists, it does not substantially diminish the benefits of raising the MLDA
Sobriety checkpoints (n = 23)	Strong evidence	• At random breath testing (RBT) checkpoints, all drivers stopped are given breath tests for blood alcohol levels; Such checkpoints are not conducted in the United States • At selective breath testing (SBT) checkpoints, police	■ Crashes thought to involve alcohol dropped a median of 18% (for RBT) and 20% (for SBT) after implementation of sobriety checkpoints ■ Fatal crashes thought to involve alcohol dropped a median of 22% (for RBT) and 23% (for SBT) after implementation of sobriety checkpoints	• Studies were conducted on interventions at the city, county, state, and national levels, and were evaluated in rural areas, urban areas, and mixed rural and urban areas	• Although the U.S. Supreme Court has determined that SBT are permissible, some state courts prohibit them • Where checkpoints are permitted, police concern about low arrest rates can be an important barrier • Informing police officers about the	• (+) Several studies report the arrest of drivers stopped at sobriety checkpoints for other offenses, such as driving with a suspended license or carrying weapons, as an added benefit • (−) Stopping drivers at checkpoints results in inconvenience and intrusion on driver privacy. According to the U.S. Supreme Court, the brief intrusion of a properly conducted sobriety

Table 4.1. *Continued*

Intervention (Qualifying Studies)	Level of Evidence[a]	Intervention Description	Key Findings	How Widely Used?	Barriers to Implementation	Other Positive (+) or Negative (−) Effects
		must have reason to suspect the driver has been drinking before using breath tests. • Media campaigns that publicize the enforcement activity are an important intervention component.	■ Crashes declined regardless of the follow-up time of the study, dropping a median of 18% for follow-up times of less than 1 year and 17% for follow-up times of more that than 1 year		general deterrence benefit of their efforts and providing them with regular feedback that links these efforts to crash prevention may decrease this frustration	checkpoint is justified in the interest of reducing alcohol-impaired driving; some civil libertarian groups have endorsed this position
0.08% blood alcohol concentration (BAC) law (n = 9)	Strong evidence	Lowers the BAC at which it is illegal to drive a motor vehicle from 0.10% to 0.08%	■ 9 studies evaluated 0.08% BAC laws in one or more of the 16 states that implemented the laws before January 1, 1998 ■ Following implementation of the laws, the median decrease in fatal alcohol-related motor-vehicle crashes was 7% ■ Estimates (in 3 studies) of the number of lives that could be saved if all states enacted 0.08% BAC laws ranged from 400 to 600 lives per year	• As of August 1, 2005, all states had 0.08% BAC laws. • Studies analyzed data from statewide police incident reports of fatal crashes in geographically diverse states with varying population densities; thus the evidence of effectiveness should be applicable to all drivers affected by 0.08% BAC laws. Subgroups were not included in the data	• One potential barrier is the view that 0.08% BAC laws discourage "social drinkers" from driving after drinking a small amount of alcohol but do not deter "hard-core" drinking drivers • Results of the systematic review provide some evidence to counter this view • 5 studies measured fatalities involving drivers with BACs of 0.10% or higher and reported post law reductions for most states	• 3 studies measured outcomes other than motor-vehicle crashes, including public knowledge and perception of impaired driving laws, self-reported impaired driving, and impaired driving arrests; information about these potential effects was not summarized in this review
Mass media campaigns (n = 15)	Strong evidence	• Persuade individuals either to avoid drinking and driving or to prevent others from doing so	■ 7 studies found that mass media campaigns were associated with a median decrease of 13% in total alcohol-related crashes (interquartile range, 6% to 14% decrease) ■ 6 studies found that mass media campaigns were associated with a median decrease of 10% in injury-producing alcohol-related crashes (interquartile range, 6% to 14% decrease)	• National, state, community	• According to the "efficacy paradox," the results of poorly implemented programs are of questionable value for making generalizations about the potential utility of such programs • On the other hand, typical resource constraints often make it impossible to implement programs that meet all the requirements for maximal efficacy.	(+) Mass media campaigns likely have indirect effects in addition to those evaluated in this review e.g.,mass media could play an "agenda-setting" role by influencing public perceptions of the importance of social issues. (+) As media coverage increases the perceived importance of a problem, public support for actions to address it may also increase

Table 4.1. *Continued*

Intervention (Qualifying Studies)	Level of Evidence[a]	Intervention Description	Key Findings	How Widely Used?	Barriers to Implementation	Other Positive (+) or Negative (−) Effects
			■ 2 studies found that mass media campaigns were associated with decreases in the proportion of drivers who had consumed alcohol (net decreases of 30% and 158%)		● Before undertaking a campaign, planners should assess whether they have adequate resources and a supportive environment to implement an effective mass media campaign	● (+) Using the mass media to influence social policies may offer much larger benefits than attempting to change individual behavior ● It is suggested that future mass media campaigns should explicitly focus on these broader goals
School-based interventions: instructional (n = 9)	Sufficient evidence for reduction in riding with alcohol-impaired drivers	● School-based instructional programs to reduce riding with alcohol-impaired drivers, alcohol-impaired driving, or alcohol-related crashes	■ Instructional programs varied widely with respect to exposure time, program content, and degree of interaction with students ■ Self-reported drunk driving indicated small and inconsistent benefits (median change: −0.10 standard deviations; range: −0.22 to 0.04) ■ Self-reported riding with a drunk driver indicated small but consistent benefits (median change: −0.18 standard deviations; range: −0.72 to −0.10)			
Lower blood alcohol concentration (BAC) for young and inexperienced drivers (n = 6)	Sufficient evidence	● Establishes a separate, lower illegal BAC (usually ≤0.02%) for drivers targeted by the law ● Studies assessed changes in state laws in the United States and Australia; U.S. laws apply to all drivers under the MLDA; in other countries, laws apply to either newly licensed drivers or	■ 3 studies that examined fatal crash outcomes reported declines of 24%, 17%, and 9% ■ 2 studies that examined injury crash outcomes reported declines of 17% and 4% ■ 1 study that examined crashes in which the investigating police officer believed that the driver had been drinking alcohol reported a decline of 11%	● All U.S. states currently have lower BAC laws for drivers younger than 21 years ● Studies analyzed data from statewide police incident reports of fatal crashes in geographically diverse states with both urban and rural populations (subgroups not included); thus, the evidence of effectiveness should be	● Young people are less likely than adults to drink in bars; therefore, police who target bar neighborhoods are likely to miss underage drinking drivers ● Officers may also be unable to identify underage drinking drivers with low BACs who show no signs of impairment ● Some state laws do not authorize officers to test the BAC of an underage driver	● (−) In some jurisdictions in the United States, it is possible that drivers aged 20 years or younger with BACs above the legal limit for adult drivers would receive the less serious "zero-tolerance" citations instead of being arrested for driving under the influence of alcohol

Table 4.1. *Continued*

Intervention (Qualifying Studies)	Level of Evidence[a]	Intervention Description	Key Findings	How Widely Used?	Barriers to Implementation	Other Positive (+) or Negative (−) Effects
		newly licensed drivers under a specified age		applicable to all drivers affected by these lower BAC laws	without probable cause to believe the driver's BAC is above the legal limit for adults	
Designated driver programs (n = 9)	Insufficient evidence*	• Population-wide promotion campaigns and incentive programs to encourage individuals in drinking establishments to act as designated drivers	Population-wide campaigns: ■ 1 study found a 13% increase in "always" selecting a designated driver but no significant change in self-reported alcohol-impaired driving or riding with an alcohol-impaired driver Incentive programs: ■ 7 studies found a median increase of 0.9 designated drivers per drinking establishment per night (interquartile range, 0.3–3.2 designated drivers per night) ■ 1 study found a 6% decrease (p < 0.01) in self-reported drinking and driving or riding in a car with an intoxicated driver ■ The public health impact of changes unknown due to lack of information regarding their effect on alcohol-impaired driving or alcohol-related crashes			
Interventions to Increase Child Safety Seat Use						
Child safety seat laws (n = 9)	Strong evidence	• Requires children aged 0–5 years traveling in motor vehicles to be restrained in federally approved child safety seat (infant or child safety seats) appropriate for the child's age and size • Specifies children to whom the law applies by age, height, weight, or a combination of factors, which vary by state	■ Laws decreased fatal injuries by a median of 35% ■ Laws decreased fatal and nonfatal injuries combined by a median of 17% ■ Laws increased child safety seat use by a median of 13% ■ Among the studies that evaluated the laws' effects on injury rates, researchers found no differences in the effect size based on the age of children who were required to be in safety seats	• Child safety seat laws have been enacted in all 50 states and the District of Columbia, which were all represented • Evidence of effectiveness should be applicable to the United States • No study adequately described study population in terms of age, gender, race, socioeconomic status, region, etc.	• Experts in child passenger safety may encounter political barriers to strengthening the requirements of laws or to implementing or enhancing enforcement of existing laws, especially in the absence of data on how variations in existing laws are related to outcomes	• None identified • (+) However, a better understanding of these laws will help policymakers in their efforts to strengthen these regulations. In addition, differences in effectiveness based on the variability in state laws might bolster efforts to maintain or strengthen some state laws and to reduce gaps in coverage and protection for some children

Table 4.1. *Continued*

Intervention (Qualifying Studies)	Level of Evidence[a]	Intervention Description	Key Findings	How Widely Used?	Barriers to Implementation	Other Positive (+) or Negative (–) Effects
Distribution and education programs (n = 10)	Strong evidence	• Provide approved child safety seats to parents through loans, low-cost rentals, or giveaways • Include educational components of varying intensity	■ Safety seat distribution and education programs increased both possession of and proper use of safety seats by a median of 23% ■ Distribution programs were effective when implemented in hospitals and clinics, as part of postnatal home visits, and when provided by an auto insurance company ■ Effectiveness of these programs was found among urban, suburban, and rural populations, and among affluent and poor populations	• The same body of evidence was used to evaluate the applicability of these programs in different settings and populations, including hospitals and clinics, and in urban, suburban, and rural populations, and among affluent and poor populations • Studies conducted in United States, Canada, Australia, and Sweden	• Implementing organizations need to consider potential liability; the initial expense for purchasing seats; cleaning and storage of child safety seats; and training of personnel to provide education and to distribute child safety seats • Also, some child safety seats might be incompatible with certain vehicles	• None identified • (–) However, because distribution programs increase number of seats available, they might also increase misuse of safety seats, especially among new users
Community-wide information plus enforcement campaigns (n = 4)	Sufficient evidence	• Use mass media mailings and child safety seat displays in public sites to promote use. • Use special enforcement strategies such as checkpoints, dedicated law-enforcement officials, or alternative penalties to enforce existing child safety seat laws.	■ Child safety seat use increased by a median of 12% ■ Studies involved populations at all socioeconomic levels and settings including cities, suburbs, and states ■ Design and implementation of campaigns involved community organization and government agencies such as public safety and public health groups, schools, advocacy organizations, and parent groups	• Studies were conducted in the United States, Canada, and Australia and involved populations of all socioeconomic levels. • Included parents of children birth to 11 years and likely included urban, suburban, and rural populations	• None identified in the literature but might include the cost of developing and disseminating public information and education material; cost of television and radio announcements; and of enlisting the support and cooperation of the media, police departments, and other community leaders • Training enforcement personnel on the importance of enforcing child-restraint device laws and the additional burden on court systems resulting from increased law enforcement may also	• (+) Communitywide information and enhanced enforcement campaigns can increase public awareness of child safety seat laws and the dangers of unrestrained travel, which might be a predisposing factor for other interventions • (+) Enhanced enforcement might also increase detection and arrest for alcohol-impaired driving and other offenses

Table 4.1. *Continued*

Intervention (Qualifying Studies)	Level of Evidence[a]	Intervention Description	Key Findings	How Widely Used?	Barriers to Implementation	Other Positive (+) or Negative (−) Effects
Incentive plus education programs (n = 4)	Sufficient evidence	• Provide rewards to children and parents for purchasing and correctly using child safety seats • Include educational components of varying intensity	▪ Child safety seat use increased by a median of 10%, measured between 1 and 4.5 months after the programs were conducted; effectiveness of these programs beyond 4.5 months has not been evaluated ▪ Baseline rates of safety seat use were similarly low in all four studies (median = 27%) ▪ Programs were implemented in day-care centers and community-wide among a variety of target populations (children and parents, all socioeconomic groups, urban and rural populations, white and African American populations) with similar positive effects	• Programs were implemented in day-care centers and community-wide among a variety of target populations (children and parents of children 6 months to 12 years, all socioeconomic groups, urban and rural populations, white and African American populations)	be barriers to implementing these programs • None identified in the literature but might include the cost of purchasing incentive reward; maintaining appropriate schedules of reinforcement; training of personnel to provide the education component; and garnering support of schools, day-care centers, and other sites to sponsor incentive and education programs	• None of the identified studies measured safety seat misuse as a result of incentive and education programs in the population, and no other studies of the likelihood of misuse with this intervention were identified in the literature
Education-only programs (n = 6)	Insufficient evidence*	• Provide information and teach skills to parents, children, or professional groups about the use of child safety seats	▪ 3 studies evaluated the effect on parents of perinatal education programs regarding correct use of child safety seats ▪ 1 study evaluated the effect of an education program for preschool children on the correct use of child safety seats ▪ 2 studies evaluated the effect of professional education—1 each for nurses and law-enforcement officers—on implementation of patient education programs or on citation rates, respectively	• Implemented in hospitals, preschools, and work sites • Targeted parents, children, or professional groups • Urban and suburban populations of low, middle, and upper socioeconomic status were represented in some studies • No studies reported racial or ethnic makeup of the study population	• Evidence about barriers was not collected for this intervention because effectiveness was not established	• (+) Educational programs for parents might increase their knowledge about child safety seat laws and the effectiveness of safety seats • (+) Improved knowledge might be a predisposing factor for other interventions • (+) Safety seat misuse and incorrect seat placement can occur when parents who have not previously used safety seats have had inadequate education about the devices • (+) Educational programs might increase children's knowledge about the benefits of using safety seats or safety belts, which might be a predisposing factor for other interventions

Table 4.1. *Continued*

Intervention (Qualifying Studies)	Level of Evidence[a]	Intervention Description	Key Findings	How Widely Used?	Barriers to Implementation	Other Positive (+) or Negative (−) Effects
Interventions to Increase Safety Belt Use						
Safety belt laws (n = 39)	Strong evidence	• Requires the use of safety belt systems by motor-vehicle occupants 6 years of age and older • Specific requirements (e.g., age, seating, position, fines, exceptions) vary by state • Studies assessed laws in the United States and Canada	■ Laws decreased fatal injuries by a median of 9% ■ Laws decreased nonfatal injuries by a median of 2% ■ Laws increased observed safety belt use by a median of 33 percentage points	• Results may be more applicable to adolescent and adult populations because study populations consisted of individuals older than 5 years • 12 studies reported data for those over 16 (i.e., drivers, university students, employees) • 1 study included only those older than 10 and another only older than 11 years. Some studies analyzed subpopulations (e.g., women, older drivers, and adolescents)	• As with many legislative interventions, public opposition is a potential barrier to effective implementation; political climate influences the enactment of laws and level of enforcement • The common argument against early seat belt laws was based on personal freedom • Recent surveys conducted by NHTSA report that 86% of individuals 16 years and older support safety belt laws, with 63% supporting them "strongly" and 23% supporting them "somewhat."	• (+) Adults who do not use safety belts are less likely to buckle up the children they transport; thus laws that increase safety belt use among adults will likely increase use among child passengers • (+) 1 study reported that a law mandating safety belt use in the front seat increased use by children 2–10 years in all positions within the vehicle • (−) Weak laws, laws that do not include all vehicles, exemptions for back seat occupants, high-risk drivers (young men, drinking drivers), and perhaps risk compensation may explain a lower than expected decrease in fatal and nonfatal injuries associated with increased safety belt use
Primary enforcement laws (instead of secondary laws) (n = 13)	Strong evidence	• Primary enforcement law allows a police officer to stop a vehicle solely for an observed belt law violation (without having other reasons for stopping the vehicle) • Secondary enforcement law allows a police officer	■ Of the 13 qualifying studies, 9 compared states with primary laws to those with secondary laws, and 4 evaluated the effect of changing from secondary to primary laws ■ 5 studies looked at changes in the number of fatalities; the median decrease in fatalities was 8% greater in primary law states than in secondary law states	• Primary and secondary safety belt laws in 49 states and Washington, D.C. were evaluated • Although belt use in general is higher among Whites than others, 2 studies showed that with primary enforcement safety belt use increased more	• Perceived public opposition to these laws is a potential barrier to their implementation • Infringement on personal freedom and the potential for differential enforcement are the most frequently voiced concerns • To increase public acceptance, several states have added	• Similar to those of safety laws in general • (+) If primary laws are more effective than secondary laws in increasing usage rates among adults, they may also be more effective in increasing usage among their child passengers • (−) Differential enforcement is a potential concern because African Americans and Hispanics may be

Table 4.1. *Continued*

Intervention (Qualifying Studies)	Level of Evidence[a]	Intervention Description	Key Findings	How Widely Used?	Barriers to Implementation	Other Positive (+) or Negative (−) Effects
		to issue a belt law citation only if the vehicle has been stopped for another violation	■ 5 studies looked at changes in safety belt use; the median increase in primary law states relative to secondary law states was 14 percentage points for observed use	among African Americans and Hispanics than among whites	antiharassment language to their primary safety belt legislation to reduce the potential for differential enforcement • As with safety belt laws in general, public support for primary laws appears to be strong	more likely than whites to be stopped for a safety belt violation; however, studies in several states found either no difference in the rate of white versus nonwhite ticketing, or they found a greater increase in the proportion of whites ticketed after enactment of primary laws
Enhanced enforcement (n = 16)	Strong evidence	• Increased, rather than routine, enforcement at specific locations and times to target violations of safety belt laws • Always includes a publicity component	■ Among 15 qualifying studies, programs reported a median increase in observed safety belt use of 16 percentage points ■ Increases in safety belt use were similar for supplemental patrols and targeted patrols ■ 2 studies reported reductions of 7% and 15% in fatal and nonfatal injuries combined	• Programs conducted in a variety of settings in the United States and Canada, including at city, county, state, provincial, and national levels; involving varying levels of publicity and enforcement climates	• Possible resistance by state policy makers because of perceived public opposition • 2 surveys (California and North Carolina) indicated 70% and 87% favorable responses • Concern by police officers of diversion of enforcement of more serious crimes; 1 study found no increase • Interviews with police and public revealed increasingly positive attitudes toward these programs	• (+) Enhanced enforcement may lead to increased arrests for other crimes, such as possession of weapons or drugs, impaired driving, or license violations (the 1993–94 North Carolina "Click It or Ticket" programs reported arresting 56 fugitives, recovering 46 stolen vehicles, and stopping 2094 alcohol-impaired drivers)

Interventions to Reduce Young Driver Crashes

Intervention (Qualifying Studies)	Level of Evidence[a]	Intervention Description	Key Findings	How Widely Used?	Barriers to Implementation	Other Positive (+) or Negative (−) Effects
Graduated driver licensing systems (n = 13)	Strong evidence	• Drivers licensing system to ensure that novices meet certain minimal requirements deemed necessary to operate a motor vehicle safely in traffic	■ Median decrease in per population overall crash rates during the first year was 31% (range 26–41%)	• 46 North American jurisdictions (40 U.S. states, the District of Columbia, 4 Canadian provinces, and 1 Canadian territory) currently have all three stages, but the systems vary in strength (IIHS 2003)	• Slowness of states to enact full GDL laws • Parental and teen resistance in some states (e.g., Wisconsin)	• (−) There are concerns that enactment of GDL laws would reduce mobility among teens, especially in rural areas

*A determination that evidence is insufficient should not be seen as evidence of ineffectiveness. A determination of insufficient evidence assists in identifying areas of uncertainty regarding effectiveness of an intervention and specific continuing research needs. In contrast, evidence of ineffectiveness leads to a recommendation that the intervention not be used.

4.2.   INTERVENTIONS BY LEVEL OF EVIDENCE

4.2.1.   Strategies with Evidence of Effectiveness

4.2.1.1.   Alcohol-Impaired Driving

In 2002, 41% of all traffic fatalities were alcohol involved—that is, some level of alcohol was present among either a vehicle occupant or nonoccupant such as a pedestrian (NHTSA, 2002a). There are several interventions that have been shown to be effective through rigorous scientific study, such as legislation, law enforcement, mass media campaigns (if in conjunction with other activities), and training.

4.2.1.1.1. Zero-Tolerance Laws.   Zero-tolerance laws make it illegal for people under age 21 to drive after any drinking, but the threshold is usually set at 0.02% BAC. These laws have been associated with declines in alcohol-related deaths (Hingson, Heeren, & Winter, 1994; Shults et al., 2001). Voas, Tippetts, and Fell (2003) found declines of 19–24% in underage drinking drivers in fatal crashes. This is solid evidence that zero-tolerance laws decrease alcohol-impaired driving among drivers under age 21. However, there is also evidence that when zero-tolerance laws are in effect, young drivers who are legally drunk often receive citations for zero tolerance offenses rather than being arrested for drunk driving. Voas, Lange, and Tippetts found that 57% of underage drivers in California who received zero-tolerance citations had BACs above the legal limit of 0.08 g/dL (Voas, Lange, & Tippetts, 1998). This essentially converted about half of the possible arrests for drunk driving among underage drivers to less serious citations. All states have passed zero-tolerance laws for young drivers.

4.2.1.1.2. Minimum Legal Drinking Age Laws.   Minimum legal drinking age (MLDA) laws are effective in reducing alcohol-related crashes and injuries (Shults et al., 2001). This type of law is especially important given the high crash and death rates of young drivers (Voas et al., 2003; Wagenaar, O'Malley, & LaFond, 2001; Wagenaar & Toomey, 2002; Zwerling & Jones, 1999). At the same blood alcohol level, crash risk is higher for young drivers than for older drivers (Zador, Krawchuk, & Voas, 2000). All states have increased their MLDA to 21 years.

4.2.1.1.3. Sobriety Checkpoints.   Alcohol roadside checkpoints, whether randomly or selectively implemented, are an effective law enforcement intervention. Sobriety checkpoints are generally paired with media efforts for publicity, which helps to increase the perceived risk of arrest. Sobriety checkpoints have been shown to decrease fatal and nonfatal injury crashes (Shults et al., 2001).

4.2.1.1.4. Lower Blood Alcohol Concentration.   Blood alcohol concentration (BAC) laws make it illegal "per se" to operate a motor vehicle at or above a specified BAC. Originally set at 0.10 or 0.15, these laws have had their limits lowered over time; 0.08% BAC laws have been found effective in reducing alcohol-impaired driving (Hingson, Heeren, & Winter, 2000; Shults et al., 2001; Wagenaar & Toomey, 2002). As of 2005, all 50 states have 0.08% BAC laws that place the legal BAC limit for driving after drinking for adults below 0.08%.

4.2.1.1.5. Mass Media.   Media campaigns have been a popular method to deter drinking and driving, although only the highest quality campaigns have been found effective. These campaigns were carefully planned, well-executed, high-intensity campaigns that attained adequate target audience exposure. The content commonly included themes related to the fear of arrest, the legal consequences of arrest, fear of harm to self or others, and the social stigmatization of drinking drivers. They were also conducted in conjunction with other alcohol-impaired driving activities, such as enhanced law enforcement. Under similar circumstances, mass media campaigns are effective in reducing alcohol-impaired driving (Elder et al., 2004).

4.2.1.1.6. Ignition Interlocks. Devices that prevent a drinking driver from starting the vehicle have been discussed in the United States since the 1960s. These devices require the driver to provide a breath sample before starting the vehicle. If the breath sample exceeds a specified BAC, the ignition is locked and the vehicle will not start. Systematic reviews have found ignition interlock devices effective in reducing alcohol-impaired driving recidivism while the devices are installed in the vehicle (Coben & Larkin, 1999; Willis, Lybrand, & Bellamy, 2004). Evidence of a lasting effect after removal of the device is lacking.

4.2.1.1.7. School-Based Instruction. School educational programs have been shown effective in deterring riding with a drinking driver. These programs vary widely in their focus; consequently, studies evaluating their effectiveness vary in the factors deemed important for program success—for example, length of exposure to the program, program content, and degree of interaction with students. Although there is sufficient evidence to recommend school-based instructional programs for reducing riding with a drinking driver, there is insufficient evidence to recommend these programs for the reduction of drinking and driving among students (Elder et al., 2005) (See also Section 4.2.3).

4.2.1.1.8. Server Intervention Training. Server intervention and training programs are designed to prevent patron intoxication and alcohol-impaired driving. Although no universally recognized standards exist for these programs, examples of server strategies include offering food with drinks, delaying service to rapid drinkers, and refusing service to intoxicated patrons. Evidence for the effectiveness of server intervention training programs comes from studies of establishments that volunteered to participate; therefore, management support was well established. Results of the literature to date indicate that intensive, high-quality, face-to-face server training, when accompanied by strong management support, is effective in reducing the level of intoxication of patrons (Shults et al., 2001).

4.2.1.2. Occupant Protection

Occupant restraints, including child safety seats (CSS), lap and shoulder belts, booster seats, and air bags, are among the most effective injury prevention interventions available. All states require children to be restrained, although the specifics of coverage vary (Insurance Institute for Highway Safety [IIHS], 2004). CSS are 71% effective in reducing fatalities among infants and 54% effective among toddlers (NHTSA, 2002b). Booster seats are 59% more effective than adult belts alone in reducing injury in age-appropriate children (Durbin, Elliott, & Winston, 2003).

4.2.1.2.1. Child Safety Seats. There is strong evidence for the effectiveness of several types of interventions. CSS use laws require children to be restrained in federally approved safety seats appropriate for the child's age and size. CSS use laws were found to decrease fatal and nonfatal injury and to increase child safety seat use. Distribution plus education programs provide CSS through giveaways, low-cost purchases or rentals, or seat loans. These programs also contain an educational component that varies from providing written materials such as brochures, to active educational and behavioral activities such as discussions, CSS demonstrations, rehearsal, and problem solving. Distribution plus education programs were found to decrease fatal and nonfatal injury, increase CSS use, and increase possession of CSS. Community-wide information plus enhanced enforcement campaigns typically target geographically defined communities and use mass media (e.g., television, radio, newspapers), information and publicity (e.g., direct mailings), CSS displays in public locations, and enhanced enforcement activities such as checkpoints or dedicated law enforcement officials in their programs. In addition, alternative penalties may be used, such as warnings or vouchers instead of citations if a CSS is purchased. These programs were found to increase child safety seat use. Finally, incentive plus education programs include rewards for either parents or children for correctly using CSS. Rewards have varied from inexpensive fast-food coupons to more expensive prizes donated by community merchants. These programs have shown increased CSS use (Grossman & Garcia, 1999; Zaza et al., 2001).

4.2.1.2.2. Booster Seats.   Children who have outgrown their safety seats but are too small to ride safely in adult safety belts should be properly restrained in belt-positioning booster seats. These booster seats are designed to raise a child so that the vehicle lap and shoulder belts fit properly. They are recommended for children who are 4 to 8 years old or who weigh at least 40 pounds and are 4 feet 9 inches tall (NHTSA, 2005b; American Academy of Pediatrics [AAP], 2005). In 2005, the NHTSA estimated that only 10–20% of children aged 4 to 8 years who should be using belt-positioning booster seats were actually using them (NHTSA, 2005b). As of May 2005, a total of 32 states and the District of Columbia had booster seat laws. The specific provisions of the laws vary across states, with half requiring booster seat use only for children up to age 6.

A recently published meta-analysis of interventions to increase booster seat use showed that educational interventions and those that combine education with distribution of booster seats or incentives such as discounted coupons were effective in increasing booster seat use (Ehiri, King, Ejere, & Mouzon, 2006).

4.2.1.2.3. Safety Belts.   The National Occupant Protection Use Survey (NOPUS) conducted in 2003 found belt use to be 79% nationwide. The combination of lap and shoulder belts is 45% effective in reducing fatalities and 50% effective in reducing moderate to critical injury for front seat passenger car occupants. For light truck occupants, belts reduce fatalities by 60% and moderate to critical injury by 65%.

To date, 49 states, the District of Columbia, Puerto Rico, and all U.S. territories have adult safety belt use laws in place; however, coverage varies by state. There are two types of laws: primary enforcement, in which a law-enforcement officer can stop a motorist based on a belt violation alone, and secondary enforcement, in which the officer must have another reason to stop the motorist. Both primary and secondary enforcement laws have been shown to be effective in increasing belt use and reducing fatal and nonfatal injury (Rivara, Thompson, & Cummings, 1999), but primary laws have been shown more effective than secondary laws (Dinh-Zarr et al., 2001).

Enhanced enforcement programs can entail increasing the number of officers on patrol, increasing the number of citations issued for belt violations during regular patrols, safety belt checkpoints, or a combination of these activities. Enhanced enforcement programs are effective in reducing fatal and nonfatal injuries, and increasing belt use (Dinh-Zarr et al., 2001).

4.2.1.2.4. Air Bags. Front air bags are designed as supplemental restraint systems to be used in conjunction with belts, giving added protection in frontal crashes. The overall effectiveness of these air bags for reducing fatalities is 12% (NHTSA, 2002c). Because front air bags were initially designed to protect unbelted adult male occupants, they inflated quickly and with high force. This resulted in deaths and injuries to occupants in crashes that would otherwise be expected to produce minor or no injuries (e.g., low-speed crashes). This was especially true for children. In 1997, the NHTSA permitted a change in vehicle safety testing that resulted in vehicles with depowered air bags successfully meeting safety requirements. Recent research indicates that the change to depowered air bags in model years 1998 and 1999 passenger vehicles (cars, sport utility vehicles [SUVs], and minivans) resulted in an 11% decrease in fatality risk compared to 1997 models, indicating that depowered air bags retained their protective value. However, this improvement was not seen in pickup trucks, which showed an increase in fatalities (Braver, Kyrychenko, & Ferguson, 2005). Passenger-side front air bags remain a risk to children (see Section 4.2.5 for more information).

4.2.1.3. Motorcycle Helmets

Motorcycle helmets are estimated to be 37% effective in preventing fatal injury to motorcyclists (Deutermann, 2004) and 72% effective in reducing head injury (Liu, Ivers, Norton, Blows, & Lo, 2003). Helmet use is especially important given the fact that per vehicle mile, motorcyclists are more than 25 times as likely as passenger car occupants to die in a traffic crash. Motorcycle helmet use laws are effective. In states with mandatory or universal (covers riders of all ages) helmet use laws, nearly 100% of motorcyclists wear them; without a law, helmet use is 50% or lower. In 2003, 20 states required helmet use by all operators and passengers; in an additional 27 states, use was required for riders up to a certain age, generally 18 years old (NHTSA, 2003a). An estimated 71% of motorcyclists wore helmets in 2000, compared to only 58% in 2002 (NHTSA, 2002d).

4.2.1.4. Bicycle Helmets

Bicycle helmets are effective in preventing head injury, brain injury, facial injury and death (Attewell, Glase, & McFadden, 2001; Elvik & Vaa; 2004; Thompson, Rivara, & Thompson, 1999). Interventions designed to increase bicycle helmet use generally target children and adolescents, as does legislation requiring helmet use. Legislation with supporting helmet promotional activities has successfully increased observed helmet use in the United States (Peden et al., 2004; Towner et al., 2002). Community-based interventions that included free helmets and an educational component had the strongest evidence. Interventions in school settings and interventions with subsidized helmets also appeared effective in increasing helmet use (Royal, Kendrick, & Coleman, 2005).

4.2.1.5. Graduated Drivers Licensing Systems

Graduated drivers licensing systems (GDL) address the high risks faced by new drivers by requiring an apprenticeship of planned and supervised practice (learners permit stage), followed by a provisional license that places temporary restrictions on unsupervised driving (Williams & Ferguson, 2002). Two commonly imposed restrictions are limits on nighttime driving and passenger limits. These restrictions are lifted as new drivers gain experience and teenage drivers mature (full licensure). Although the specific requirements for advancing through the three stages of GDL vary across jurisdictions (IIHS, 2003), they provide a protective environment while new drivers become more experienced. GDL has proven effective in reducing new driver crash risk. Evaluations of the effectiveness of GDL in New Zealand, Canada, and the United States have reported reductions in crashes involving new drivers in the range of 9% to 43% (Begg & Stephenson, 2003; Hartling et al., 2005; Shope & Molnar, 2003; Simpson, 2003).

4.2.2.   Promising Strategies

4.2.2.1.   *Rear Seating Position*

The number of children sitting in the front seat is declining; in 2002, the proportion of children riding in the front seat was 15% for infants, 10% for toddlers, and 29% for booster-age children (NHTSA, 2003b). Although the catalyst for moving children to the rear seat was the danger from passenger-side air bags, rear seating position is still the safest place for children whether or not there is a passenger-side air bag present (Berg, Cook, Corneli, Vernon, & Dean, 2000; Braver, Whitfield, & Ferguson, 1998; Durbin et al., 2003; Durbin, Elliott, Arbogast, Anderko, & Winston, 2005). Intervention studies for improving rear seating among children are limited. A systematic review in 1999 (Segui-Gomez, 1999) found only one intervention specifically designed to promote rear seating position. There has been some research since that time (Greenberg-Seth, Hemenway, Gallagher, Ross, & Lissy, 2004), but not a sufficient body of evidence in this area.

4.2.2.2.   *Automated Enforcement*

Automated enforcement, such as speed cameras and red light cameras, have several advantages over conventional enforcement strategies. First, conventional enforcement requires law-enforcement officers to stop drivers and issue citations, a time-consuming activity that requires officers to observe the violation. Second, traffic enforcement may have a lower priority than other types of offenses (e.g., violent crime). In addition, chasing drivers for violations is risky for law-enforcement personnel and for civilians. Finally, the likelihood of being caught speeding is relatively low, so the deterrence effect of conventional enforcement may be short lived.

4.2.2.2.1. Speed Cameras.   Two systematic reviews of the effectiveness of speed cameras have found decreases in both crashes and injuries (Elvik & Vaa, 2004; Pilkington & Kinra, 2005). Speed cameras remain in the promising category because of the marginal quality of some of the research supporting their effectiveness, and because only a limited amount of the research to date has been conducted in the United States.

4.2.2.2.2. Red Light Cameras.   A recent systematic review of three studies found that red light cameras appear to reduce crashes and injuries. However, the body of research is not sufficient to determine effectiveness, and these studies were done outside of the United States (Elvik & Vaa, 2004). One systematic review that included information from the United States (Aeron-Thomas & Hess, 2005), found evidence of effectiveness for total injury crashes but less evidence for all crashes. Other published syntheses (McFadden & McGee, 1999; McGee & Eccles, 2003) found that there was a preponderance of evidence, albeit not conclusive, indicating that red-light-running camera systems improve the overall safety of intersections. However while angle crashes were reduced, rear-end crashes increased. It will be important to determine the net benefit with respect to crashes and injuries.

4.2.3. Strategies with Insufficient Evidence of Effectiveness

4.2.3.1. Education-Only Programs for Child Safety Seat Use

Education only programs for CSS use provide information to parents, children, or professional groups. Although education is an important component of many other types of interventions—for example, distribution or incentive programs— education-only programs do not have sufficient high-quality scientific evidence of effectiveness to support their use apart from other interventions (Zaza et al., 2001).

4.2.3.2. Designated Driver Programs

A designated driver is a person who agrees to either abstain or limit alcoholic consumption and drive others home. Designated driver promotion programs set in restaurants or drinking establishments encourage individuals to act as designated drivers by offering incentives such as free nonalcoholic drinks, free food, or free admission. Despite their widespread use in the United States, relatively few programs have been thoroughly evaluated. A recent systematic review of designated driver programs in drinking establishments found insufficient evidence of their effectiveness in reducing alcohol-impaired driving or alcohol-related crashes (Ditter et al., 2005).

4.2.3.3. School-Based Instructional Programs for Drinking and Driving

School-based instructional programs for drinking and driving among students have recently been reviewed and the evidence was found to be inconsistent. In addition, the results suggested that any initial effects tended to dissipate over time. While there is insufficient evidence of effectiveness among drivers, school-based instructional programs appear effective for reducing *riding* with a drinking driver (as discussed in Section 4.2.1) (Elder et al., 2005).

4.3.3.4. Increasing Pedestrian and Bicyclist Visibility

Several interventions have been tried to increase the visibility of pedestrians and bicyclists on the road by using, for example, fluorescent materials in bright colors during the day and lights and retroreflective materials at night. Results suggest that these interventions can improve drivers' detection and recognition, but there is insufficient evidence of the effect on pedestrian and bicyclist crashes or injuries (Kwan & Mapstone, 2002).

There are also road engineering measures designed to increase the visibility and conspicuity of pedestrians. Studies conducted in the United States include relocating bus stops to discourage pedestrians from entering the roadway in front of a stopped bus and diagonal vehicle parking to encourage scanning traffic before entering the roadway (Retting, Ferguson, & McCartt, 2003). These studies report favorable pedestrian behavior change but are not of sufficient number and rigor to reach a threshold for recommendation.

4.2.4. Strategies with Evidence of Ineffectiveness

4.2.4.1. School-Based Driver Education

The debate over the effectiveness of school-based driver education has been long-standing and contentious and is based on just a few studies that are now quite dated. A review by Vernick et al. (1999) included both randomized controlled trials and ecological studies. The randomized controlled trials included two studies conducted in the late 1970s and early 1980s. The results indicated that driver's education did not reduce violations or crashes among students. A review by Roberts, Kwan, and the Cochrane Injury Group Driver Education Reviews (2001) found similar results; however, only one of the studies was different from those reviewed by Vernick and co-workers. It is unclear how school-based driver education programs implemented today differ from those evaluated above or how any differences might affect violation or crashes among students today. There is also evidence that driver education sometimes leads to early licensure, which itself can be harmful (See next section).

4.2.5. Harmful Strategies

Sometimes safety interventions can have unintended consequences. These can be positive or negative. Negative consequences threaten the success of the intervention and can compromise the health and safety of the target population.

4.2.5.1. Air Bags and Children

Air bags have been shown to be a risk factor for fatal injury to young children. From January 1990 to January 2005, a total of 157 children under age 13 years were killed as passengers in low-speed, otherwise survivable crashes, when the air bag deployed. The explosive force of an air bag's inflation can cause serious injury or even death to children. One recent analysis of NHTSA data (Newgard & Lewis, 2005) on 3,790 children aged 1 month to 18 years who were seated in the right front seat of a vehicle when an airbag deployed, found that children 14 and under were at higher risk for serious injury from air bags, whereas those 15 and over were at lower risk. However, the number of children killed has been decreasing, partially due to more children being placed in the back seat, more restrained children, and depowered air bags starting with 1998 model year vehicles (Durbin et al., 2003). Placing a rear-facing CSS in front of a passenger-side air bag remains risky for infants; thus rear-facing CSSs should never be placed in front of an air bag.

4.2.5.2. Early Licensure for Novice Teenage Drivers

As noted above, school-based driver education training has not been shown to decrease crashes among teenage drivers. Another safety consequence to consider is that driver education often qualifies drivers for early licensure. Studies by Levy (1990), Vernick et al. (1999), and Roberts et al. (2001) consistently indicated that young drivers who take driver education tend to get their licenses earlier. Early licensure leads to earlier novice driving which results in more crashes. Driver education may not have resulted in a decrease in crashes among teenage drivers because any potential safety benefit from the training would be offset by the increased exposure to traffic resulting from early licensure.

4.3. GENERAL ISSUES THAT AFFECT THE SUCCESS OF MOTOR VEHICLE SAFETY INTERVENTIONS

4.3.1. Exposure

There are several issues in motor-vehicle injury prevention that have important effects on the success of interventions. For example, exposure, or the amount of time spent on the road contributes to the risk of a motor-vehicle collision and, therefore, the risk of a motor-vehicle-related death or injury. Most of our exposure occurs as occupants of motor vehicles. From 122 billion miles in 1925 to the 2.9 trillion in 2003, Americans have steadily increased their time on the road. In the period from 1993 to 2003, the number of vehicle miles traveled increased 25% (NSC, 2004). The number of vehicles and the number of drivers have also seen significant growth. The United States has reached a point at which the average number of vehicles in the household exceeds the average number of licensed drivers (Hu & Reuscher, 2004). As an illustration of the potential effect on safety interventions, consider CSS use. Should a family obtain seats for each vehicle in the household, move seats from vehicle to vehicle and increase the chance of improper installation, or restrict travel of children to the vehicle with appropriate restraints?

4.3.2. Rural Crashes

Another issue effecting motor-vehicle safety is the location of a crash. Of the 3.9 million miles of roads in United States, 3.1 million are in rural areas with populations of less than 5000. The majority of fatal crashes that occur in the United States involve rural or small-town residents traveling on rural roads (Blatt & Furman, 1998). In 2002, 39% of travel and 60% of motor-vehicle fatalities occurred in rural areas. The rural fatality rate per 100 million vehicle miles traveled is more than twice the urban fatality rate (2.3 vs. 1.0) (NHTSA, 2003c).

Factors that contribute to the higher fatality rate in rural areas include driver characteristics (e.g., age, nonuse of safety belts, speeding, alcohol-impaired driving), the roadway design (e.g., two-lane highways, narrow or nonexistent shoulders, limited sight distance due to hills and curves), vehicle design (e.g., presence of air bags, roll-over propensity) and medical care delivery after a crash (Blatt & Furman, 1998; General Accounting Office [GAO], 2004). Approaches to reduce fatalities on rural roads include engineering improvements such as paved shoulders, midlane rumble strips, enhanced pavement markings, skid-resistant pavement surfaces, and eliminating shoulder drop-offs (Transportation Research Board [TRB], 2003), small-scale sobriety checkpoints (NHTSA, 2004b), and safety belt campaigns that are tailored to the needs and resources or rural communities (McGinnis & Quick, 2001).

4.3.3. Speed

The historically competing outcomes of mobility and safety are readily apparent in the area of speed. From the driver's perspective, the faster we can get to our destination the better. However, speed affects both the likelihood of a crash and the severity of a crash. Crashes at higher speeds are more severe; therefore, the risk of injury is greater. For vulnerable road users such as pedestrians and cyclists, this is especially problematic. The public perceives speeding to be a low-risk activity, and the majority of drivers admit to doing it. This perception of speeding as a pervasive and harmless activity hinders speed-control efforts such as setting and enforcing speed limits. Reviews of studies that evaluated changes in crashes and injuries in conjunction with changes (or introduction) of speed limits have generally supported the notion that increases in speed limits (without other concurrent changes) are associated with increases in crashes. Conversely, setting or reductions in speed limits are associated with crash and injury reductions (TRB, 1998).

4.3.4. Maintaining Progress after Initial Success

For some interventions, we have made great progress. Child safety seat use is over 90% for children under 5 years. Some form of GDL has been enacted in all 50 states. Safety belt use laws have increased use to nearly 80% in the country as a whole. These successes might leave the impression that the problem of restraint use has been solved. The challenge, then, is to maintain interest and support for safety interventions. For laws with all 50 states on board, the next thing to do is strengthen those laws and reduce the gaps in coverage. For example, CSS laws can be extended through booster seat age, graduated driver licensing laws can be strengthened to encompass all suggested components (e.g., nighttime driving and teenage passenger restrictions), and adult safety belt laws can be strengthened by eliminating exemptions such as back seating position.

4.4. IMPLICATIONS FOR PUBLIC HEALTH PRACTICE

Despite the great success in reducing motor-vehicle-related death rates in the past 40 years, motor vehicle crashes remain the leading cause of injury-related deaths in the United States. Public health practitioners have the opportunity to reduce death and injury using a variety of strategies; interventions can influence behaviors, improve vehicles, or modify roadways. Interventions can reduce exposure to risk, including slowing levels of motorization, selecting alternative travel modes, reducing the volume of unnecessary trips, and efficient and safe land use policy. Interventions can reduce crash occurrences by reducing speed, and drinking and driving, and by promoting stepped-up enforcement. Interventions can also reduce injury severity in a crash by increasing safety belt use, child safety seat use and helmet use, and making roads and vehicles more forgiving to the forces in a crash. Finally, interventions can improve postcrash survival by early detection of crashes and improved emergency medical services and trauma care systems.

4.4.1. What Public Health Can Do

- Include road safety in health-promotion and disease-prevention activities
- Set goals for the reduction of motor-vehicle-related deaths, injuries, and health care costs

- Expand surveillance to better monitor nonfatal injuries, detect new problems, and set priorities
- Strengthen interagency partnerships and collaboration in road safety
- Support research on risk factors and interventions to reduce all forms of motor-vehicle-related trauma
- Implement the most effective programs and policies.

Research still to be done includes demonstrating the effectiveness of promising behavioral and environmental interventions such as the overall safety impact of red light cameras to decrease red-light running, designated-driver programs to reduce alcohol-impaired driving or changes to the built environment to reduce pedestrian exposure. Research is also needed on the recent advances in technology that have enabled computer-assisted communications systems in vehicles and on highways to communicate information to motorists about road and travel conditions and to automatically guide or brake a vehicle to safety. Innovative use of radar and on-board computers may help prevent vehicle collisions. Some early warning devices may even alert drowsy drivers and assist older drivers with slow reaction times. At the individual and community level, we need to carefully and systematically measure, intervention implementation and a variety of intervention outcomes and use both qualitative and quantitative tools to document unintended outcomes.

4.5. CONCLUSIONS

John Last (1980) once noted that we sometimes recognize as public health problems aspects of life that we have taken for granted. As long as the enormous toll of motor-vehicle injuries and death is considered normal and acceptable, we will make little progress in the future. We know injuries related to motor-vehicle crashes are not "accidents," they are predictable and preventable. Many known and effective strategies exist to prevent injuries, if only we would use them. These include:

- legislation and enforcement (recognizing the value of law, applying it appropriately, and strengthening it through enforcement);
- interventions that are community based and participatory, tailored to the problems of local communities (e.g., rural areas);
- interventions that have documented evidence of effectiveness and using scarce resources most efficiently to implement them.

As the United States continues to increase its own motorization, partnerships between public health, vehicle safety, and road engineering communities will be even more urgently needed to prevent the possibility of rising fatalities in the future.

REFERENCES

Aeron-Thomas, A. S., & Hess, S. (2005). Red-light cameras for the prevention of road traffic crashes. *The Cochrane Database of Systematic Reviews* (Issue 2, No. CD003862.pub2.DOI: 10.1002/14651858. CD003862.pub2). Chichester, UK: Wiley.

American Academy of Pediatrics. (2005). Car safety seats: A guide for families 2005. Retrieved June 10, 2005, from www.aap.org/family/carseatguide.htm.

Attewell, R. G., Glase, K., & McFadden, M. (2001). Bicycle helmet efficacy: A meta-analysis. *Accident Analysis & Prevention, 33*, 345–352.

Baker, S. P., Braver, E. R., Chen, L.i-Hui, Pantula, J. F., & Massie, D. (1998). Motor vehicle occupant deaths among Hispanic and black children and teenagers. *Archives of Pediatrics & Adolescent Medicine, 152*, 1209–1212.

Begg, D., & Stephenson, S. (2003). Graduated driver licensing: The New Zealand experience. *Journal of Safety Research, 34* (1), 99–105.

Berg, M. D., Cook, L., Corneli, H. M., Vernon, D. D., & Dean, J. M. (2000). Effect of seating position and restraint use on injuries to children in motor vehicle crashes. *Pediatrics, 105*, 831–835.

Blatt, J., & Furman, S. M. (1998). Residence location of drivers involved in fatal crashes. *Accident Analysis & Prevention, 30* (6), 705–711.

Braver, E. R. (2003). Race, Hispanic origin, and socioeconomic status in relation to motor vehicle occupant death rates and risk factors among adults. *Accident Analysis & Prevention, 35* (3), 295–309.

Braver, E. R., Kyrychenko, S. Y., & Ferguson, S. A. (2005). Driver mortality in frontal crashes: Comparison of newer and older airbag designs. *Traffic Injury Prevention, 6*, 1–7.

Braver, E. R., Whitfield, R., & Ferguson, S. A. (1998). Seating positions and children's risk of dying in motor vehicle crashes. *Injury Prevention, 4*, 181–187.

Centers for Disease Control and Prevention, National Center for Injury Prevention and Control. (2005). Web-based injury statistics query and reporting system (WISQARS). Retrieved February 8, 2005, from www.cdc.gov/ncipc/wisqars.

Coben, J. H., & Larkin, G. L. (1999). Effectiveness of ignition interlock devices in reducing drunk driving recidivism. *American Journal of Preventive Medicine, 16* (1S), 81–87.

Deutermann, W. (2004). *Motorcycle helmet effectiveness revisited* (Report No. DOT HS 809-715). Washington, DC: U.S. Department of Transportation, National Highway Traffic Safety Administration.

Dinh-Zarr, B., Sleet, D. A., Shults, R. A., Zaza, S., Elder, R. W., Nichols, J. L., Thompson, R. S., Sosin, D. M., & the Task Force on Community Preventive Services. (2001). Reviews of evidence regarding interventions to increase the use of safety belts. *American Journal of Preventive Medicine, 21* (4S), 48–66.

Ditter, S. M., Elder, R. W., Shults, R. A., Sleet, D. A, Compton, R., Nichols, J. L., & the Task Force on Community Preventive Services. (2005). Effectiveness of designated driver programs for reducing alcohol-impaired driving: A systematic review. *American Journal of Preventive Medicine, 28* (5S), 280–287.

Durbin, D. R., Elliott, M., Arbogast, K. B., Anderko, R. L., & Winston, F. K. (2005). The effect of seating position on risk of injury for children in side impact collisions. *Pediatrics, 115* (3), e305–e309.

Durbin, D. R., Elliott, M. R., & Winston, F. K. (2003). Belt-positioning booster seats and reduction in risk of injury among children in vehicle crashes. *Journal of the American Medical Association, 289* (21), 2835–2840.

Durbin, D. R., Kallan, M., Elliott, M., Cornejo, R. A., Arbogast, K. B., & Winston, F. K. (2003). Risk of injury to restrained children from passenger air bags. *Traffic Injury Prevention, 4*, 58–63.

Ehiri, J. E., King, B., Ejere, H. O. D., Mouzon, P. (2006). Effects of interventions to increase use of booster seats in motor vehicles for 4–8 year olds. Washington, DC: AAA Foundation for Traffic Safety.

Elder, R. W., Nichols, J. L., Shults, R. A., Sleet, D. A., Barrios, L. C., Compton, R., & the Task Force on Community Preventive Services. (2005). Effectiveness of school-based programs for reducing drinking and driving and riding with drinking drivers: a systematic review. *American Journal of Preventive Medicine, 28* (5S), 288–304.

Elder, R. W., Shults, R. A., Sleet, D. A., Nichols, J. L., Thompson, R. S., Rajab, W., & the Task Force on Community Preventive Services. (2004). Effectiveness of mass media campaigns for reducing drinking and driving and alcohol-involved crashes. *American Journal of Preventive Medicine, 27* (1), 57–65.

Elvik, R., & Vaa, T. (Eds.) (2004). *The handbook of road safety measures*. Amsterdam: Elsevier.

Evans, L. (1999). Transportation safety. In R. W. Hall (Ed.), *Handbook of transportation science*. Boston: Kluwer Academic.

Evans, L., & Phil, D. (1988). Risk of fatality from physical trauma versus sex and age. *Journal of Trauma, 28* (3), 368–378.

General Accounting Office. (2004). Highway safety: Federal and state efforts to address rural road safety challenges (Report No. GA04-663). Washington, DC: Author.

Greenberg-Seth, S., Hemenway, D., Gallagher, S. S., Ross, J. B., & Lissy, K. S. (2004). Evaluation of a community-based intervention to promote rear seating for children. *American Journal of Public Health, 94* (6), 1009–1013.

Grossman, D. C., & Garcia, C. C. (1999). Effectiveness of health promotion programs to increase motor vehicle occupant restraint use among young children. *American Journal of Preventive Medicine, 16* (1S), 12–22.

Haddon, W. (1968). The changing approach to the epidemiology, prevention, and amelioration of trauma: The transition to approaches etiologically rather than descriptively based. *Amercan Journal of Public Health, 58* (8), 231–235. (Reprinted in 1999: *Injury Prevention, 5* (3), 231–235).

Hartling, L., Wiebe, N., Russell, K., Petruk, J., Spinola, C., & Klassen, T. P. (2005). Graduated driver licensing for reducing motor vehicle crashes among young drivers. *The Cochrane Database of Systematic Reviews* (Issue 2. Art. No.: CD003300.pub2.DOI: 10.1002/14651858.CD003300.pub2). Chichester, UK: Wiley.

Hingson, R., Heeren, T., & Winter, M. (1994). Lower legal blood alcohol limits for young drivers. *Public Health Reports, 109,* 738–744.

Hingson, R., Heeren, T., & Winter, M. (2000). Effects of recent 0.08% legal blood alcohol limits on fatal crash involvement. *Injury Prevention, 6,* 109–114.

Hu, P. S., & Reuscher, T. R. (2004). *Summary of travel trends 2001 national household travel survey.* Washington, DC: U.S. Department of Transportation, Federal Highway Administration.

Insurance Institute for Highway Safety. (2004). State laws: Child restraint, belt laws as of July 2004. Retrieved February 8, 2005, from www.hwysafety.org/safety_facts/state_laws/restrain.htm.

Insurance Institute for Highway Safety. (2003). U.S. licensing systems for young drivers. Retrieved February 8, 2005, from www.highwaysafety.org/safety_facts/state_laws/grad_license.htm.

Kwan, I., & Mapstone, J. (2002). Interventions for increasing pedestrian and cyclist visibility for the prevention of death and injuries. *The Cochrane Database of Systematic Reviews* (Issue 2. Art. No.: CD003438. DOI: 10.1002/14651858.CD003438). Chichester, UK: Wiley.

Last, J. (1980). *Public health and human ecology.* New York: Prentice Hall.

Levy, D. T. (1990). Youth and traffic safety: The effects of driving age, experience, and education. *Accident Analysis & Prevention, 22* (4), 327–334.

Li, G., Braver, E. R., & Chen, L. (2003). Fragility versus excessive crash involvement as determinants of high death rates per vehicle-mile of travel among older drivers. *Accident Analysis & Prevention, 35,* 227–235.

Liu, B., Ivers, R., Norton, R., Blows, S., & Lo, S. K. (2003). Helmets for preventing injury in motorcycle riders. *The Cochrane Database of Systematic Reviews* (Issue 4. Art. No.: CD004333.pub2.DOI: 10.1002/14651858.CD004333.pub2). Chichester, UK: Wiley.

McFadden, J. F., & McGee, H. W. (1999). *Synthesis and evaluation of red light running automated enforcement programs in the United States* (Report No. FHWA-A-IF-00-0040). Washington, DC: U.S. Department of Transportation, Federal Highway Administration.

McGee, H. W., & Eccles, K. A. (2003). *Impact of red light camera enforcement on crash experience* (HCHRP Synthesis 310). Washington, DC: Transportation Research Board.

McGinnis, P., & Quick, R. L. (2001). *Partners for Rural Traffic Safety Action Kit* (Report No. DOT HS 809-299). Washington, DC: U.S. Department of Transportation.

National Highway Traffic Safety Administration. (2002a). *Alcohol. Traffic Safety Facts* (Report No. DOT HS 809-606). Washington, DC: U.S. Department of Transportation.

National Highway Traffic Safety Administration. (2002b). *Children. Traffic Safety Facts* (Report No. DOT HS 809-607). Washington, DC: U.S. Department of Transportation.

National Highway Traffic Safety Administration. (2002c). *Occupant Protection. Traffic Safety Facts* (Report No. DOT HS 809-610). Washington, DC: U.S. Department of Transportation.

National Highway Traffic Safety Administration. (2002d). *Safety Belt and Helmet Use in 2002—Overall Results* (Technical Report No. DOT HS 809-500). Washington, DC: U.S. Department of Transportation.

National Highway Traffic Safety Administration. (2003a). *Motorcycles. Traffic Safety Facts* (Report No. DOT HS 809-764). Washington, DC: U.S. Department of Transportation.

National Highway Traffic Safety Administration. (2003b). *Child restraint use in 2002: Results from the 2002 NOPUS controlled intersection study.* Retrieved on February 8, 2005, from www-nrd.nhtsa.dot.gov/pdf/nrd-30/NCSA/Rpts/2003/ChildRestraints.pdf.

National Highway Traffic Safety Administration. (2003c). *Rural/urban comparison. Traffic Safety Facts* (Report No. DOT HS 809-739). Washington, DC: U.S. Department of Transportation.

National Highway Traffic Safety Administration. (2004a). *Lives saved by the federal motor vehicle safety standards & other vehicle safety technologies, 1960–2002.* Washington, DC: U.S. Department of Transportation.

National Highway Traffic Safety Administration. (2004b). *You drink & drive. You lose. National crackdown law enforcement action planner.* Retrieved February 8, 2005, from www.nhtsa.dot.gov/people/injury/alcohol/StopImpaired/1298%20YDDYL%20Labor%20Day/pages/SmallScaleSB.htm.

National Highway Traffic Safety Administration. (2005a). *Traffic Safety facts 2003: A compilation of motor vehicle crash data from the Fatality Analysis Reporting System and the General Estimates System* (Report No. DOT HS 809-775). Washington, DC: U.S. Department of Transportation.

National Highway Traffic Safety Administration. (2005b). *National child passenger safety week. CPS/ Valentine's mini-planner, facts sheet & talking points.* Retrieved February 8, 2005, from www.nhtsa.dot. gov/CPS/promote/intro.htm.

National Safety Council. (2004). *Injury Facts. 2004 Edition.* Itasca, IL: National Safety Council Press.

Newgard, C. D., & Lewis, R. J. (2005). Effects of child age and body size on serious injury from passenger air-bag presence in motor vehicle crashes. *Pediatrics, 115* (6), 1579–1585.

Peden, M., Scurfield, R., Sleet, D. A., Mohan, D., Hyder, A., Jarawan, E., & Mathers, C. (Eds.). (2004). *World report on road traffic injury prevention.* Geneva: World Health Organization.

Pilkington, P. K., & Kinra, S. (2005). Effectiveness of speed cameras in preventing road traffic collisions and related casualties systematic review. *British Medical Journal, 330,* 331–334.

Retting, R. A., Ferguson, S. A., & McCartt, A. T. (2003). A review of evidence-based traffic engineering measures designed to reduce pedestrian-motor vehicle crashes. *American Journal of Public Health, 93* (9), 1456–1463.

Rivara, F. P., Thompson, C. O., & Cummings, P. (1999). Effectiveness of primary and secondary enforced seat belt laws. *American Journal of Preventive Medicine, 16* (Supplement 1), 30–39.

Roberts, I., Kwan, I., the Cochrane Injuries Group Driver Education Reviews. (2001). School based driver education for the prevention of traffic crashes. *The Cochrane Database of Systematic Reviews* (Issue 3. Art. No.: CD003201.DOI: 10.1002/14651858.CD003201). Chichester, UK: Wiley.

Royal, S. T., Kendrick, D. & Coleman, T. (2005). Non-legislative interventions for the promotion of cycle helmet wearing by children (Review). *The Cochrane Database of Systematic Reviews* (Issue 2. Art. No.: CD003985.pub2.DOI: 10.1002/14651858.CD003985.pub2). Chichester, UK: Wiley.

Segui-Gomez, M. (1999). Evaluating interventions that promote the use of rear seats for children. *American Journal of Preventive Medicine, 18* (4S), 11–22.

Shope, J. T., & Molnar, L. J. (2003). Graduated driver licensing in the United States: Evaluation results from the early programs. *Journal of Safety Research, 34,* 63–69.

Simpson, H. M. (2003). The evolution and effectiveness of graduated licensing. *Journal of Safety Research, 34,* 25–34.

Shults, R. A., Elder, R. W., Sleet, D. A., Nichols, J. L., Alao, M. O., Carande-Kulis, V. G., Zaza, S., Sosin, D. M., Thompson, R. S., & the Task Force on Community Preventive Services. (2001). Reviews of evidence regarding interventions to reduce alcohol-impaired driving. *American Journal of Preventive Medicine, 21* (4S), 66–88.

Sleet, D. A., Egger, G., & Albany, P. (1991). Injury as a public health problem. *Health Promotion Journal of Australia, 1* (2), 4–9.

Thompson, D. C., Rivara, F. P., & Thompson, R. (1999). Helmets for preventing head and facial injuries in bicyclists. *The Cochrane Database of Systematic Reviews* (Issue 4. Art. No.: CD001855.DOI: 10.1002/14651858.CD0031855). Chichester, UK: Wiley.

Towner E., Dowswell, T., Burked, M., Dickinson, H., Towner, J., & Hayes, M. (2002). Bicycle helmets: Review of effectiveness (No. 30). London: Department for Transport.

Transportation Research Board. (2003). Guidance for implementation of the AASHTO Strategic Highway Safety Plan. Retrieved February 8, 2005, from gulliver.trb.org/publications/nchrp/nchrp_rpt_500v6.pdf.

Transportation Research Board. (1998). *Managing speed: Review of current practice for setting and enforcing speed limits* (Special Report 254). Washington, DC: National Academy Press.

Vernick, J. S., Li, G., Ogaitis, S., MacKenzie, E. J., Baker, S. P., & Gielen, A. C. (1999). Effects of high school driver education on motor vehicle crashes, violations, and licensure. *American Journal of Preventive Medicine, 16* (1S), 40–60.

Voas, R. B., Lange, J. E., & Tippetts, A. S. (1998). *Enforcement of the zero tolerance law in California: A missed opportunity?* Paper presented at the 42nd meeting of the Association for the Advancement of Automotive Medicine, Charlottesville, VA.

Voas, R. B., Tippetts, A. S., & Fell, J. C. (2003). Assessing the effectiveness of minimum legal drinking age and zero tolerance laws in the United States. *Accident Analysis & Prevention, 35,* 579–587.

Wagenaar, A. C., and Toomey, T. L. (2002). Effect of minimum drinking age laws: Review and analyses of the literature from 1960 to 2000. *Journal of Studies on Alcohol,* (Supplement) *14,* 206–225.

Wagenaar, A. C., O'Malley, P. M., & LaFond, C. (2001). Lowered legal blood alcohol limits for young drivers: Effects on drinking, driving, and driving-after-drinking behaviors in 30 states. *American Journal of Public Health, 91,* 801–804.

Williams, A. F., & Ferguson, S. A. (2002). Rationale for graduated licensing and the risks it should address. *Injury Prevention, 8* (Supplement 2), 9–14.

Willis, C., Lybrand, S., & Bellamy, N. (2004). Alcohol ignition interlock programmes for reducing drink driving recidivism. *The Cochrane Database of Systematic Reviews* (Issue 3. Art. No.: CD004168.pub2. DOI: 10.1002/14651858.CD004168.pub2). Chichester, UK: Wiley.

Zador, P. L., Krawchuk, S. A., & Voas, R. B. (2000). Alcohol-related relative risk of driver fatalities and driver involvement in fatal crashes in relation to driver age and gender: An update using 1996 data. *Journal of Studies on Alcohol, 61*, 387–395.

Zaza, S., Sleet, D. A., Thompson, R. S., Sosin, D. M., Bolen, J. C., & the Task Force on Community Preventive Services. (2001). Reviews of evidence regarding interventions to increase use of child safety seats. *American Journal of Preventive Medicine, 21* (4S), 31–47.

Zwerling, C., & Jones, M. P. (1999). Evaluation of the effectiveness of low blood alcohol concentration laws for younger drivers. *American Journal of Preventive Medicine, 16* (1S), 76–80.

Chapter 5

Interventions to Prevent Drowning

Linda Quan, Elizabeth E. Bennett,
and Christine M. Branche

5.1. EPIDEMIOLOGY

Drowning refers to an event in which a person's airway is immersed in a liquid medium leading to respiratory difficulty (Idris et al., 2003). This may result in a drowning death or survival.

Drowning is a multifaceted injury, involving multiple patterns that vary by age group, body of water (bath, swimming pool, and open water), and activity. However, the patterns vary consistently wherever studied. In many countries, drowning is among the top three leading causes of injury death. Drowning death rates are highest in preschoolers, aged 1–4 years, and second highest in older adolescents and young adults (15–24 years). Most preschoolers in North America drown after falling into swimming pools while by the water; older children and adults are primarily in or on the water, boating or swimming, when they drown. The highest case fatality rates are in adults. Males predominate. Among older teenagers and young adults who drown, the male to female ratio may be as high as 6:1.

Other risk factors for drowning include race, seizures, and alcohol use. Overall, U.S. drowning death rates for African Americans are 1.4 times those of white Americans and even higher among youths (Branche, Dellinger, Sleet, Gilchrist, & Olson, 2004). Unintentional drowning rates are also higher for American Indians and Asian Americans (Brenner, Trumble, Smith, Kesslers, & Overpeck, 2001; Washington State Department of Health, 2004; Quan & Cummings, 2003).

For persons with seizures, drowning is the most common cause of unintentional injury death. Persons with seizures represent 5–7% of drowning deaths in all age groups studied (Quan & Cummings, 2003). The bathtub is the site of highest drowning risk, certainly related to high exposure and lengthy periods of being unattended (Diekema, Quan, & Holt, 1993). Compared to those without seizures, children with seizures also have a higher risk of drowning in a swimming pool.

Children with autism may also be at increased risk of drowning (Shavelle, Strauss, & Pickett, 2001; Sibert et al., 2002).

Alcohol is a clear risk factor for drowning. The likelihood of drowning death increases with increasing blood alcohol levels (Smith et al., 2001). Alcohol has physiological as well as psychological effects that increase drowning risk and bad outcome. Among adult drowning deaths, 50% have positive blood alcohol levels.

In addition, socioeconomic and geographical factors contribute to risk. Drowning rates are high in rural settings and in warm climates in industrialized countries where swimming pools are common (Children's Safety Network, 2005).

5.2. HISTORY OF DROWNING PREVENTION EFFORTS

Drowning prevention efforts have narrowly focused on specific age groups and specific activities. The U.S. Coast Guard (USCG) has led the need for drowning prevention in boating activities and promoting the availability and use of personal flotation devices (PFDs), also called life jackets, by boat operators and passengers. For years, a national PFD law has required all recreational boats to have readily available an appropriately fitting, USCG-approved PFD in good condition for each person in the boat. In 2002, a federal law requires children to wear PFDs in boats. State PFD laws vary by age of child, length or type of boat, whether the boat must be under way and whether the child is above or below deck. While boat-related drowning rates have decreased, nationally, PFD use remains low (14%) among adolescents and adults, the groups at highest risk for boat-related drowning (U.S. Coast Guard [USCG], 2004).

Drowning prevention for nonboating settings has focused on swimming pools, after Australian and U.S. reports of almost overwhelming experience with young drowned patients. Led by Australia and New Zealand, legislation requiring complete pool isolation with four-sided fencing has been the major intervention for preschooler swimming pool drownings. In the United States, legislation for isolation pool fencing remains at the county level, although statewide legislation exists in a few states, such as Florida.

Open-water drownings outnumber swimming pool drownings, because open water is the major drowning site for schoolage children, adolescents, and adults. Despite this, there has failed to be a comprehensive approach to prevention of open-water drownings. Several phenomena impeded easy recognition of the scope of the problem. Before 1998, external causes of injury codes (E-codes) allowed identification of boat-related drownings but not other open-water drownings in hospital and death records. Thus it was difficult to assess these drownings epidemiologically. Moreover, the medical community has not faced the devastation of these drownings because most open-water drowning victims are rescued too late, declared dead at the scene, and do not enter hospitals.

As personal watercraft (PWC) use has increased, so have the injuries associated with them. Most of the injuries associated with this form of water recreation occur among people older than age 16 years (Branche, Conn, & Annest, 1997). Most injuries occur when PWC collide with other vessels, with other PWCs, or with fixed objects such as docks or tree stumps. Injuries range in severity from lacerations and bruises to death, usually from blunt trauma. Thus the prevention strategies are those that have been used for other types of trauma as well as for drowning; for instance, the American Academy of Pediatrics (AAP) (2000) has recommended that no child younger than 16 years should operate a PWC and that helmets should be worn.

5.3. INTERVENTIONS

5.3.1. Products

5.3.1.1. *Isolation Fencing of Swimming Pools*

In high-income countries, drowning in swimming pools is a leading cause of unintentional injury death among children under age 6 years. Evidence from case-control studies suggests that isolation pool fencing for swimming pools (also known as four-sided pool fencing) is an effective intervention for preventing fatal and nonfatal drowning among children from birth to 5 years (Thompson & Rivara, 2000). The odds ratio for drowning risk in a fenced pool compared to an unfenced pool was 0.27 (95% confidence interval [CI]: 0.16–0.47). Isolation fencing, which isolates the pool from the house, was superior to perimeter fencing (three-sided fencing), in which the house forms the fourth side of the fence, allowing the child in the house easy access to the pool. The odds ratio for pools with isolation fencing compared to three-sided fencing was 0.17 (95% CI: 0.07–0.44). When combined with a self-closing and self-latching gate, such fencing provides a passive intervention that prevents unintended access to the swimming pool by small children (U.S. Consumer Product Safety Commission [CPSC], 2005a).

5.3.1.2. *Personal Flotation Devices (PFDs)*

Observational studies by the USCG and the Canadian Coast Guard, repeatedly show that 80–96% of those who drowned while boating were not wearing personal flotation devices PFDs (Penttila & Pikkarainen, 1990, USCG, 2004). Despite the lack of proof of efficacy, most agencies such as the USCG, the AAP, and National Safe Boating Council recommend PFD use. For two centuries, PFDs have been the basic technological intervention used to keep people afloat, allowing them to keep their airway above water and thereby prevent drowning. In Canada and the United States, efforts are under way to evaluate the potential for all-ages PFD legislation. Universal agreement for such legislation does not exist, however, even among the boating safety community.

In contrast, most states require operators and passengers of personal watercraft to wear a PFD. No study has evaluated the effect of PFD wear on drowning in this group.

5.3.1.3. *Door Alarms*

In residential pool drownings, children usually access the pool from the house. Pool alarms are audible devices designed to alert adults when the door leading directly to the swimming pool area has been opened. CPSC (2005b) recommends an alarm on the door to the yard although their effectiveness has not been examined.

5.3.1.4. Pool Alarms

Various technologies use sensors in, above, or around the pool to detect movement in, into, or near the water that set off alarms. These devices have not been carefully evaluated.

5.3.1.5. Pool Covers

In theory, pool covers provide a layer of protection from unintended access to the swimming pool inside the pool area. However, drowning deaths have occurred with flexible solar pool covers in place; pool covers often trapped the child or hid the child from view, thereby delaying rescue. (Sulkes & van der Jagt, 1990) The CPSC (2005) presently recommends use of powered pool covers that are heavier and more rigid although these devices have not been evaluated for effectiveness.

5.3.1.6. Poolside Equipment

Poolside equipment that enables quick retrieval of the drowning victim and summons for trained help with resuscitation might improve survival and neurological outcome. A host of rescue equipment placed at poolside, from reach poles to a telephone, has been recommended but their effectiveness in drowning prevention has not been evaluated.

5.3.1.7. Signage

The use of signs at water recreation sites for drowning prevention has not been evaluated. Studies have identified factors that increase public attention to signage and messages, including reinforcement by personnel. However, specific drowning prevention signage has not been tested for comprehension, for its effect on behaviors, or for its ability to decrease drownings. Consideration should be given to developing signage with internationally recognized symbols warning of specific hazards such as undertow, currents, dangerous swimming or boating, or beach drop off. These would need to be tested for comprehension before effectiveness can be assessed. Signage to reinforce key messages and promote specific behaviors such as wearing a PFD has not been evaluated.

5.3.1.8. Bathtub Seats/Rings

Several small-case studies document drownings of infants left unattended in a bathtub seat or ring (Byard & Donald, 2004; Rauchschwalbe, Benner, & Smith, 1997). Occasionally, the product itself may have contributed to the drowning, but more than 90% of the drownings occurred because of a lapse in supervision. Focus group interviews suggested that the real hazard of bathtub seats is their effect on risk perception; many parents felt more comfortable leaving their young child unattended in the bathtub when using this device (Rauchschwalbe et al., 1997). Thus most experts agree that bathtub seats are not drowning prevention interventions; when used, the infant still requires attentive, at-hand supervision.

5.3.2. Environmental

5.3.2.1. Restricting Access to Unsafe Swim Areas

In many regions, hazardous waters are known to local emergency medical systems or health departments. Some communities have restricted access to hazardous water sites by banning patrons from using the waters or requiring extra precautions. This intervention has not been evaluated.

5.3.3.   Behavioral: Individual/Social

5.3.3.1.   Physician Counseling

The Injury Prevention Program (TIPP) is an educational program developed by the AAP (2005) for parents of children through 12 years of age to help prevent common injuries, including drowning. The program provides primary-care providers a counseling framework based on child development and scheduled office encounters and includes educational handouts to parents. The effectiveness of the program is predicated on studies showing educational counseling by primary-care providers decreased specific injuries. However, TIPP has not been specifically evaluated. Moreover, despite its availability, pediatricians in high-risk drowning regions do not routinely counsel their families/patients on drowning hazards (Barkin & Gelberg, 1999). No studies have evaluated ways to increase use of this intervention by primary-care providers.

5.3.3.2.   Drowning Awareness Education

Though drowning is the second leading cause of injury-related death for children ages 1–14, approximately 55% of parents reported that they do not worry very much or at all about their child drowning (Cody, Quraishi, Dastur, & Mickalide, 2004). Many organizations distribute education materials to families directly or through health care providers, child-care providers, USCG Auxiliary or community groups such as the YMCA. Their effectiveness is unclear.

Risk Watch is a comprehensive injury prevention curriculum for kindergarten to eighth grade, which includes sections on water safety for each age group. While not specific to drowning, an evaluation of the program showed significant changes in student knowledge (National Fire Protection Association [NFPA], 2001).

5.3.3.3.   Boating Education

USCG, U.S. Power Squadrons, and state and local boating programs have both classroom and online education programs for boaters (Perkins, 1995). The USCG reported that in 2001 a total of 6419 recreational boating accidents resulted in 681 fatalities, of which 80% occurred on boats operated by individuals who had not completed a boating safety education course (Rosenker, 2003). The majority of states have some requirement for boater education. However, no studies to date have assessed the direct relationship between people who have taken boating safety courses and those who have been involved in boating accidents.

5.3.3.4.   Lifeguards

One drowning prevention strategy is to provide lifeguards in public areas where people are known to swim and to encourage people to swim in such protected areas. Data from the U.S. Lifesaving Association (USLA) suggest that during 1988–1997 more than three quarters of drownings at USLA sites occurred at times when beaches were unguarded. The chance of drowning at a beach protected by lifeguards may be less than 1 in 18 million (Branche & Stewart, 2001) Observational data show the success of life-saving resuscitations (Fenner, Harrison, Williamson, & Williamson, 1995). In addition, lifeguards may deter behaviors that could put swimmers at risk for drowning, such as horseplay or venturing into rough or deep water. It is generally accepted that the presence of lifeguards increases the likelihood of a favorable outcome during water recreation. Therefore, the AAP recommends that when choosing natural bodies of water for recreation, parents and caregivers of young children select locations that are designated swim areas with lifeguards present.

Local circumstances can and should determine whether or not a community will insist on lifeguard services, regardless of the evidence, or lack thereof, of lifeguard effectiveness (Branche & Stewart, 2001). Local evidence, public attitudes, and the legal environment are key to the approach for increasing public safety in water recreation settings. Providing a safe water recreation environment and instituting programs, such as lifeguards, to prevent water-related injury or death may offer significant economic savings.

5.3.3.5.   Water (or Child) Watchers

To improve supervision, recommendations call for designating an adult responsible for supervising children around water. To ensure quality supervision, the designated water watcher is to avoid alcohol intake and be dedicated to watching the child or children around the water. Qualifications usually do not address ability to perform a rescue of a drowning child. The concept lacks an educational component of water hazards, hazardous behaviors, recognition of a drowning event, and what to do. The efficacy of this supervisory role, however, has not been evaluated.

5.3.3.6.   Swimming Lessons

The role of swimming lessons for young children as a drowning intervention remains controversial. Children 2–5 years given one-on-one swimming instruction can acquire specific motor skill components needed for swimming (Erbaugh, 1986). A randomized study showed that the behavior of 2-year-old children around swimming pools was safer after swimming classes (Asher, Rivara, Felix, Vance, & Dunne, 1995). In Canada and Europe, swimming lessons focus on water survival versus learning specific strokes. However, no study of a young child's swimming ability or performance after an "accidental" fall into a body of water has been performed. No data show clearly that swimming lessons actually decrease the risk of drowning.

Swimming lessons could potentially be harmful because of risk compensation. In New Zealand where the incidence of preschooler swimming drowning is high, compared to other parents, parents of 2- to 5-year-old children who had swimming lessons reported being more confident in their child's swimming ability and thought their child could be less supervised after taking swimming lessons (K.M. Moran, personal communication, February 2005).

Given the lack of adequate data on effectiveness, the AAP has not recommended swimming lessons for very young children as a means of drowning prevention because generally children are not developmentally ready for formal swimming lessons until age 4 or older. The AAP has cautioned, furthermore, that among older children, knowing how to swim well in one type of body of water (e.g., a swimming pool) does not always make a child safe in another body of water (e.g., a natural body of water like the ocean) (Brenner, 2003) Swimming lessons, usually conducted in a swimming pool, need to address this key difference.

5.3.4. Legislation

5.3.4.1. Swimming Pool Fencing Legislation

Legislation requiring isolation pool fencing for all private, public, and semipublic swimming pools has been recommended, but also with enforcement provisions to enhance the effectiveness of this intervention. Legislation has been effective in decreasing drownings and some drowning rates but not as much as was anticipated (Fergusson, Horwood, & Shannon, 1983; Logan, Branche, Stacks, Ryan, & Peddicord, 1998).

   This is attributed to factors other than the legislation. Failure to adequately educate and enforce laws, even in determined countries like New Zealand, account for failure of the legislation to affect drowning rates (Morrison, Chalmers, Langley, Alsop, & McBean, 1999). Strong behavioral issues explain why education and enforcement are needed; surveyed pool owners believe that supervision is the key to drowning prevention. Pool owners primarily want the aesthetic value of the pool uninterrupted by an intervening barrier. Product design that is sensitive to this issue may well be part of the solution.

5.3.4.2. Personal Flotation Device Availability Legislation

U.S. law requires that boats have a wearable and accessible personal flotation device (PFD) that fits each person on board. USCG and marine patrols conducted vessel checks and found that PFDs may be tucked under decks or benches and not easy to access in an emergency. Thus when passengers fall off boats or boats capsize suddenly they do not have the time and the wherewithal to find and put on the PFD. There is no evidence to show that this law leads to compliance or is effective in preventing drowning.

5.3.4.3. Personal Flotation Device Use Legislation

The age of children mandated to wear PFDs in a boat varies by state, ranging from 5 to 12 years. The federal requirement that is used by states without legislation requires children 12 and under to wear PFDs while the boat is under way. No study of the effect of these laws has been conducted. A major methodologic challenge is PFD use in children before such laws. In Washington State, before a state law requiring children 13 years old and younger to wear PFDs, 63% of those under 15 years were already wearing PFDs in small boats; after the law, 77% were wearing them, an insignificant increase (Quan, Bennett, Cummings, Williams, & Moldrem, 2000). For the past few years, USCG observational studies report that 90% of young children in boats in the United States wear PFDs. In addition, passage of such laws often requires several years of public education for support of such laws and consensus building. Thus, by the time laws are passed, before and after studies may not be able to prove an effect because usage may already be high.

5.3.4.4. Decreasing Alcohol Consumption at Water Activities

Limiting alcohol consumption, a well-demonstrated risk factor for drowning, would make sense as an intervention. Although studies have demonstrated decreasing drowning mortality rates in association with a decrease in rates of alcohol use, no study has demonstrated that decreasing alcohol use would decrease drownings (Cummings & Quan, 1999) All 50 states in the United States prohibit boating under the influence of alcohol and allow issuing "boating under the influence" tickets, some of which append to the boater's motor-vehicle license. Other laws ban the use of alcohol in some parks.

The barrier to changing alcohol consumption during water activities is significant as these activities are strongly linked in the recreational culture, especially the boating culture. Use of alcoholic beverages while boating or going to the beach is portrayed daily in advertisements for alcoholic beverages. These unsafe activities are portrayed even in movies for juvenile audiences (Pelletier et al., 2000) However, the success of the traffic safety community in decreasing drinking and driving may provide important lessons for how normative behavior can be changed among boaters who drink.

5.3.4.5. Alcohol Limit Legislation

One evaluation showed state laws establishing minimum age drinking laws and lowering the alcohol level were not associated with any change in unintentional drowning rates among 18- to 21-year-olds (Howland, Birckmayer, Hemenway, & Cote, 1998). A better outcome measure might be an evaluation of the rates of positive blood alcohol levels among drowning victims. This study did not adjust for an overall downward trend of drowning rates that has been seen nationally (Lunetta, Penttila, & Sarna, 1998).

5.3.5. Multilevel: Drowning Prevention Campaigns

The Handbook on Drowning: Prevention, Rescue, and Treatment (Bierens, 2006) profiles a number of community campaigns in the United States, Canada, Australia, New Zealand, and Europe. The programs were based on data and strategically focused. They used multiple strategies such as media, publicity, public and provider education, policies, environmental change, coalitions, and PFDs loans or sales. Evaluations, primarily through telephone or written surveys, indicated changes in knowledge and awareness of water safety messages and behavioral intentions. Some programs, such as in Canada, include drowning surveillance. However, the authors did not use rigorous evaluation strategies to their confirm findings.

One campaign in King County, Washington, was evaluated by two studies (Bennett, Cummings, Quan, & Lewis, 1999; Treser, Trusty, & Yang, 1997). This campaign had a clear objective and outcome measures: to increase PFD use. It included a community coalition; educational materials and messages using multimedia, including news, radio, and television, billboards, bus advertising; and increasing availability by coupon distribution, PFD loan programs, and working with a PFD manufacturer. A before and after telephone survey indicated a significant increase in PFD use and ownership among children whose parents were aware of the campaign. An observational survey of PFD use by boaters in small boats before, during, and after the campaign, showed a significant increase in PFD use among adults only. A study of an Australian drowning awareness campaign using drowning events as an outcome measure was unable to demonstrate a decrease in drowning deaths (Nixon, Pearn, Wilkey, & Corcoran, 1986).

5.4. IMPLICATIONS FOR PUBLIC HEALTH

Drowning is an important public health problem. The ability to accurately estimate the number of deaths and nonfatal events in all bodies of water and to describe the key factors that contributed to the submersion will improve understanding of the magnitude and complexity of the drowning problem both in the United States and abroad. Compared with other unintentional injuries, drowning prevention has fewer epidemiological and behavioral studies and in general is not as mature scientifically (Branche et al., 2004) While addressing the need for improved data collection, drowning prevention researchers and practitioners will need to think more creatively and draw from the lessons learned from other unintentional injury interventions.

Effective public health is usually less about the dramatic issues and more about addressing everyday threats. Several public health strategies may reduce the risk for drowning, including public education regarding the need for supervision, elimination of hazards, use of PFDs, and environmental changes. Properly draining bathtubs and buckets, fencing backyard pools to separate the pool from the yard and house, and fencing the yard to limit access to natural water hazards such as ditches or ponds can be effective means of preventing drowning among small children. The challenge is the active nature of the multiple interventions required.

Encompassing a complex set of scenarios, drowning prevention requires multiple approaches, depending on age, location, and circumstances. Ideally, people of all ages on or near recreational bodies of water need to be where adequate supervision and rescue can be provided. The message is challenging because the level and type of supervision needed depend on age and ability. Small children need constant at arm's-length supervision; older individuals and those with disabilities need caregivers who are also near and vigilant. Public health can provide the impetus for lifeguard use within the community.

Public health can promote the use of effective prevention technologies. The consistent use of PFDs for children and adults, in and on and around the water, should become a part of every person's water recreation habits. Increasing the availability and cultural acceptance and decreasing the economic burden of this simple piece of portable technology need to be public health mandates.

5.5. RESEARCH GAPS

5.5.1. Products

5.5.1.1. Pool Fencing

Failure of pool fencing laws to achieve expected decreases in swimming pool drownings has been attributed to failure of enforcement. Researchers must explore the effect of enforcing these laws, ways to address the user knowledge gap, methods of assessing attitudes toward use of newer fencing technologies, and the effect of homeowner insurance policies.

5.5.1.2. *Personal Flotation Devices (PFDs)*

To increase PFD use, needed interventions include increasing their availability, ownership, and wearing. To increase availability, PFD loaner programs have been situated across the United States at beaches and boat ramps, usually at no charge. Loaner programs resulted in six documented saves in Washington State and led to increased PFD use in Alaskan communities (State of Alaska Department of Health and Social Services [Alaska], Mar. 2003). To increase ownership, discount coupons have been used as an integral part of successful injury prevention campaigns.

To change the culture around wearing PFDs, marketing of the devices needs to change. Currently, PFD use and marketing is targeted only for use with boats, even though USCG-approved swim belts have been created. Age and perception of swimming ability affect use. PFD use for swimming or playing in or near open water is not well accepted.

5.5.2. Behavioral

5.5.2.1. *Risk Reduction Among Teens*

Although adolescent risk-reduction programs regarding topics such as drugs and alcohol and driving have been developed and evaluated, the equivalent has not been done related to drowning risk reduction.

Using a conceptual framework for adolescent risk behavior, adolescent drowning prevention must consider both risks and protective factors that take into account a combination of biology/genetics, social environment, perceived environment, and personality and behavior (Jessor, 1991). Developmental assets should be considered in designing adolescent drowning prevention interventions. The framework acknowledges the research-based associations of 40 qualities, attitudes, and behaviors—called "development assets"—with success and safety among young people (Scales & Leffert, 2004). Categorized into two groups, external assets identify important roles that families and communities play in promoting healthy development. These might include adult role models who demonstrate positive responsible behavior, positive peer influence, or youth programs such as teen swimming lessons. Internal assets identify characteristics and behaviors that reflect positive internal growth and development of young people, enabling them to make thoughtful and positive choices in challenging situations. Internal assets directly applicable to drowning risk and prevention might include developing responsibility for choices, planning, and decision making and teaching resistance skills.

5.5.2.2. *Bathing vs. Showering*

Drowning in a bathtub is a lethal risk faced by people of all ages with seizures (Quan & Cummings, 2003). An easy risk reduction in this specific population, to avoid bathing in a bathtub and to shower instead, is espoused in the United States and United Kingdom (EpilepsyInfo.co.uk, 2005). Showers are probably safer than a bathtub because drowning in a shower after loss of consciousness, though described, is difficult to achieve. However, the effectiveness of showering as a drowning intervention has not been studied. Moreover, behavioral changes would be required at a family level for children with seizures. Ways to accomplish a change to less-risky bathing behaviors in all age groups need to be studied.

5.5.2.3.   Increased Identification of High-Risk Individuals

High-risk groups—such as those with seizures, autism, and some physical/mental disabilities—may also include people with social risk. Child fatality reviews in several states identified that a disproportionate percent of families who had a child drowning death also had a history of involvement with child protective services (Washington State Department of Health [WSDH], 2004) Families involved with child protective services may well represent a specific population to be targeted for drowning prevention, with a need for specific interventions that would focus on behavioral approaches, the use of safety products, and environmental modifications made in and around the home to reduce risk.

5.5.2.4.   Improve Adult Supervision

For young children, close supervision around any water is a critical strategy for prevention. Inevitable lapses in supervision make supervision alone an insufficient intervention. Recently, what qualifies as adequate supervision for drowning prevention has been defined but not evaluated (Saluja et al., 2004). The kind of rescue ability needed among supervisors and what types of skills are necessary to interpret a potentially dangerous situation need to be defined and assessed.

5.5.3.   Environment and Systems

Altering water recreation environments to decrease drowning risk needs to be better evaluated. Removal of attractive nuisances such as buoys that tempt teens to swim out too far, grading swimming beaches to remove dropoffs, or marking unlifeguarded swimming areas to be no more than 5 feet deep should be considered. Given the difficulties in achieving behavior change, there is a clear need to assess the potential for more passive changes such as beach alterations.

5.5.4.   Audience Focus

5.5.4.1.   Broad Audience Focus

The general public still is unaware of drowning risks to children and young adults. Even in regions where drowning risk is highest, where outdoor swimming pools are ubiquitous, awareness is still either unrecognized or refuted (Brenner, Saluja, & Smith, 2003; Nixon, Pearn, & Dugdale, 1979) The failure to convey the message in a meaningful way that results in action, such as installation of isolation fencing, is the challenge for injury prevention.

5.5.4.2.   Personal Flotation Device (PFD) Use

Broad audiences need to be targeted regarding PFD use. Promotion of PFD use has focused too narrowly on the boating population only and it has failed; only 13% of Washington State motor boaters were observed to wear PFDs, and adult use has stayed relatively constant. Promotion of PFDs has focused on a narrowly defined group of boaters. While PFDs can be purchased in sporting goods and variety stores, knowledgeable staff and a selection of stylish jackets can generally be found only in marine supply or outdoor specialty stores. People who do not own a boat, those who use small watercraft (such as fishermen), and those who use rafts and inflatables do not see themselves as boaters and thus are not reached by the boating community's efforts to promote the need for PFDs. PFD use is low in motor boats, rowboats, and rafts (Quan, Bennett, Cummings, Trusty, & Treser, 1998). In addition, PFD use has focused on the young pediatric age group, despite the data showing that the largest proportion of open-water drownings involve adult males. The need for cross-generational use of PFDs is further underscored by the observation that children in small boats are more likely to be wearing PFDs if adults in the boat also wear them (Quan et al., 1998). In addition, PFD legislation has been fractionated at the state level and does not include the groups at highest risk: teens and adults.

5.5.4.3.   *Alcoholic Beverage Consumers*

The general public may be unaware of the relationship between increasing alcohol consumption and drowning. The effective techniques that have led to societal acceptance of the message "Don't drink and drive" need now to be used for the message that "Water and alcohol don't mix."

5.5.4.4.   *Young Children*

For children younger than 5 years, swimming lessons to decrease their drowning risk is of unclear effectiveness. Instead, effective interventions are those that have primarily focused on implementing more passive interventions such as pool fencing. Families with young children who own or frequent swimming pools and swimming beaches need to be identified. For instance, they could be targeted when buying a swimming pool, when visiting a beach, or when visiting their health provider. Specifically targeting families to inform them of the hazard and provide them with prevention information is done for many products and hazards. Creative ideas include requiring the following groups of people to sign a disclosure regarding water safety: individuals purchasing a single or multiunit property with a swimming pool, tenants signing a lease for an apartment with a swimming pool, an individual applying for a permit to build a swimming pool, or anyone purchasing an above-ground swimming pool (D. Henes, March 2005, personal communication).

5.5.4.5.   *People with Seizure Disorders*

Children and adults of all ages with seizure disorders are a group at high risk for drowning (Quan & Cummings, 2003). It is unclear if they or their health care providers recognize their increased risk. Ways to decrease their risk in swimming pools or around other water activities have not been explored. No interventions have specifically addressed this group.

5.5.4.6.   *Racial and Ethnic Populations*

Recent data have begun to elucidate the increased risk of drowning among diverse racial and ethnic populations in the United States. No studies have sought to explain the differences and no studies have addressed interventions for specific ethnic or cultural groups. Thus, although different groups must be targeted for prevention, the specific, culturally adapted, interventions for each group need to be defined.

Table 5.1. Studies of Interventions for Drowning Prevention

Element	Effective	Promising	Insufficient Evidence	Not Effective	Harmful
Products					
Solar pool covers					Sulkes & van der Jagt (1990)
Isolation pool fencing	Nixon et al. (1986), Present (1987), Thompson & Rivara (2000)				
Environment					
Lifeguards		Branche & Stewart (2001)			
Behavior					
Pool fencing legislation			Milliner Pearn, Guard (1980), Morgenstern Bingham, Reza (2000), Pitt & Balanda (1998)		
Boating education			Perkins (1995)		
Swimming lessons			Asher et al. (1995)		
Drinking laws				Howland et al. (1998), Lunetta et al. (1998)	

5.5.4.7.   Adolescents and Young Adults

It is unclear if the older adolescents and young adults who drown are risk takers, a group defined in the adolescent literature as those who invoke many risk-taking behaviors, such as unprotected sex, smoking, and driving under the influence of alcohol. Specific and different approaches would be needed for this group.

5.5.4.8.   Groups Involved with Other Water Activities

Specific groups of people who spend time near or on the water need to be identified and targeted for drowning prevention. Two examples are fishermen and duck hunters, who do not see themselves as boaters or swimmers and have little exposure to PFD use. Their perceptions, attitudes, and approachability for drowning prevention need to be examined.

Drowning is an injury for which omnipresent risk is in the home for certain age groups and at water recreational sites for all people. Interventions that probably work involve active interventions such as good supervision by lifeguards and caretakers and the use of a simple but not well accepted technological intervention, the PFD.

5.6. CONCLUSION

The only well-researched effective intervention is isolation fencing of swimming pools (Table 5.1). Full commitment to drowning prevention would require broad legislative mandates with enforcement for PFD use by all boaters, boating under the influence of alcohol, and installation of isolation fencing. To achieve changes in education and behaviors, social marketing and awareness campaigns targeting specific groups must be integrated into efforts. Given these challenges, drowning prevention research needs to focus on education and behavioral interventions at the individual level and major changes in societal perceptions of drowning and water-related risk.

REFERENCES

American Academy of Pediatrics. 2005. Age-related safety sheets. Retrieved December 5, 2005, from aap.org/family/tippmain.htm.

American Academy of Pediatrics. Committee on Injury and Poison Prevention. (2000). Personal water-craft use by children and adolescents. *Pediatrics, 105* (2), 452–453.

Asher, K. N., Rivara, F. P., Felix, D., Vance, L., & Dunne, R. (1995). Water safety training as a potential means of reducing risk of young children's drowning. *Injury Prevention, 1* (4), 228–233.

Barkin, S., & Gelberg, L. (1999). Sink or swim—Clinicians don't often counsel on drowning prevention. *Pediatrics, 104* (5, Part 2), 1217–1219.

Bennett, E., Cummings, P., Quan, L., & Lewis, F. M. (1999). Evaluation of a drowning prevention campaign in King County, Washington. *Injury Prevention, 5* (2), 109–113.

Bierens, Joost, J. L. M. (ed) (2006). *Handbook on drowning: Prevention, rescue, and treatment.* Heidelberg, Germany: Springer-Verlag.

Branche, C. M., Conn, J. M., & Annest, J. L. (1997). Personal watercraft-related injuries. A growing public health concern. *Journal of the American Medical Association, 278* (8), 663–665.

Branche, C. M., Dellinger, A. M., Sleet, D. A., Gilchrist, J., & Olson, S. J. (2004). *Unintentional injuries: The burden, risks and preventive srategies to address diversity* (2nd ed.). Westport, CT: Praeger.

Branche, C., & Stewart, S., (Eds.). (2001). *Lifeguard effectiveness: A report of the working group* (Report). Atlanta, GA: Centers for Disease Control and Prevention, National Center for Injury Prevention and Control.

Branche, C., & van Beeck, E. (Eds.). (2006). The epidemiology of drowning. In Bierens J.J.L.M. (ed). *Handbook on drowning: Prevention, rescue and treatment.* Heidelberg, Germany: Springer-Verlag.

Brenner, R. A. (2003). Prevention of drowning in infants, children, and adolescents. *Pediatrics, 112* (2), 440–445.

Brenner, R. A., Saluja, G., & Smith, G. S. (2003). Swimming lessons, swimming ability, and the risk of drowning. *Injury Control & Safety Promotion, 10* (4), 211–216.

Brenner, R. A., Trumble, A. C., Smith, G. S., Kesslers, E. P., & Overpeck, M. D. (2001). Where children drown, United States, 1995. *Pediatrics, 108* (1), 85–89.

Byard, R. W., & Donald, T. (2004). Infant bath seats, drowning and near-drowning. *Journal of Pediatrics & Child Health, 40* (5–6), 305–307.

Children's Safety Network National Center for Rural and Agricultural Health and Safety. (2005). Rural youth drowning: fact sheet: Drowning Prevention Professional Resource Packet, 1991. Retrieved December 6, 2005, from http://notes.edc.org/HHD/CSN/csnpubs.nsf/cb5858598bf707d5852568 6d005ec222?Open View.

Cody, B., Quraishi, A., Dastur, M., & Mickalide, A. (2004). *Clear danger: A national study of childhood drowning and related attitudes and behaviors.* Washington, DC: National SAFE KIDS Campaign.

Cummings, P., & Quan, L. (1999). Trends in unintentional drowning: The role of alcohol and medical care. *Journal of the American Medical Association, 281* (23), 2198–2202.

Diekema, D. S., Quan, L., & Holt, V. L. (1993). Epilepsy as a risk factor for submersion injury in children. *Pediatrics, 91* (3), 612–616.

EpilepsyInfo.co.uk. (2005). Safety and first aid. Retrieved December 2, 2005, from www.efa.org/answerplace/quickstart/forparents/qsprrisks.cfm.

Erbaugh, S. J. (1986). Effects of aquatic training on swimming skill development of preschool children. *Perceptual & Motor Skills, 62* (2), 439–446.

Fenner, P. J., Harrison, S. L., Williamson, J. A., & Williamson, B. D. (1995). Success of surf lifesaving resuscitations in Queensland, 1973–1992. *Medical Journal of Australia, 163* (11–12), 580–583.

Fergusson, D. M., Horwood, L. J., & Shannon, F. T. (1983). The safety standards of domestic swimming pools 1980–1982. *New Zealand Medical Journal, 96* (725), 93–95.

Howland, J., Birckmayer, J., Hemenway, D., & Cote, J. (1998). Did changes in minimum age drinking laws affect adolescent drowning (1970–90)? *Injury Prevention, 4* (4), 288–291.

Idris, A. H., Berg, R. A., Bierens, J., Bossaert, L., Branche, C. M., Gabrielli, A., Graves, S. A., Handley, A. J., Hoelle, R., Morley, P. T., Papa, L., Pepe, P. E., Quan, L., Szpilman, D., Wigginton, J. G., Modell, J. H., & American Heart Association. (2003). Recommended guidelines for uniform reporting of data from a drowning: The "Utstein style." *Resuscitation, 59* (1), 45–57.

Jessor, R. (1991). Risk behavior in adolescence: A psychosocial framework for understanding and action. *Journal of Adolescent Health, 12* (8), 597–605.

Logan, P., Branche, C. M., Sacks, J. J., Ryan, G., & Peddicord, J. (1988). Childhood drowning and fencing of outdoor pools in the United States, 1994. *Pediatrics, 101* (6), E3.

Lunetta, P., Penttila, A., & Sarna, S. (1998). Water traffic accidents, drowning and alcohol in Finland, 1969–1995. *International Journal of Epidemiology, 27* (6), 1038–1043.

Milliner, N., Pearn, J., Guard, R. (1980). Will fenced pools save lives? A 10-year study from Mulgrave Shire, Queensland. *Medical Journal of Australia, 2* (9), 510–511.

Morgenstern, H., Bingham, T., Reza, A. (2000). Effects of pool-fencing ordinances and other factors on childhood drowning in Los Angeles County, 1990–1995. *American Journal of Public Health, 90* (4), 595–601.

Morrison, L., Chalmers, D. J., Langley, J. D., Alsop, J. C., & McBean, C. (1999). Achieving compliance with pool fencing legislation in New Zealand: A survey of regulatory authorities. *Injury Prevention, 5* (2), 114–118.

National Fire Protection Association. (2001). Final report of the three year evaluation of Risk Watch. Retrieved March 11, 2005, from www.nfpa.org/riskwatch/pefs/3yrfinalevaluation.pdf.

Nixon, J., Pearn, J., Wilkey, I., & Corcoran, A. (1986). 15 years of child drowning. A 1967–81 analysis of all fatal cases from the Brisbane Drowning Study and an 11 year study of consecutive near-drowning cases. *Accident Analysis & Prevention, 18*, 199–203.

Nixon, J. W., Pearn, J. H., & Dugdale, A. E. (1979). Swimming ability of children: A survey of 4000 Queensland children in a high drowning region. *Medical Journal of Australia, 2* (5), 271–272.

Pelletier, A. R., Quinlan, K. P., Sacks, J. J., Van Gilder, T. J., Gilchrist, J., & Ahluwalia, H. K. (2000). Injury prevention practices as depicted in G-rated and PG-rated movies. *Archives of Pediatrics & Adolescent Medicine, 154* (3), 283–286.

Penttila, A., & Pikkarainen, J. (1990). Accidents with fatal outcome in Finnish leisure boating 1986–1988. *Beitrage zur Gerichtlichen Medizin, 48*, 185–191.

Perkins, R. (1995). Evaluation of an Alaskan marine safety training program. *Public Health Reports, 110* (6), 701–702.

Pitt, W. R., & Balanda, K. P. (1998). Toddler drownings in domestic swimming pools in Queensland since uniform fencing requirements. *Medical Journal of Australia, 169* (10), 557–558.

Present, P. (1987). *Child drowning study: A report of the epidemiology of drownings in residential pools to children.* Washington, DC: U.S. Consumer Product Safety Commission.

Quan, L., Bennett, E., Cummings, P., Trusty, M. N., & Treser, C. D. (1998). Are life vests worn? A multiregional observational study of personal flotation device use in small boats. *Injury Prevention, 4* (3), 203–205.

Quan, L., Bennett, E., Cummings, P., Williams, K., & Moldrem, C. (2000). *Washington State drowning prevention project PFD observation results.* Seattle: Children's Hospital and Regional Medical Center; Retrieved December 4, 2005, from www.seattlechildrens.org/DP/data.htm.

Quan, L., & Cummings, P. (2003). Characteristics of drowning by different age groups. *Injury Prevention, 9* (2), 163–168.

Rauchschwalbe, R., Brenner, R. A., & Smith, G. S. (1997). The role of bathtub seats and rings in infant drowning deaths. *Pediatrics, 100* (4), E1.

Rosenker, M. V., Vice Chairman, National Transportation Safety Board Before The United States Marine Safety Association, Las Vegas, Nevada, Retrieved September 18, 2003, from www.ntsb.gov/speeches/rosenker/mvr030918.htm.

Saluja, G., Brenner, R., Morrongiello, B. A., Haynie, D., Rivera, M., & Cheng, T. L. (2004). Role of supervision in child injury risk: Definition, conceptual and measurement issues. *Injury Control & Safety Promotion, 11,* 17–22.

Scales, P. C., & Leffert, N. (2004). *Developmental assets: A synthesis of the scientific research on adolescent development.* (2nd ed.). Minneapolis: Search Insitutue.

Shavelle, R. M., Strauss, D. J., & Pickett, J. (2001). Causes of death in autism. *Journal of Autism & Developmental Disorders, 31* (6), 569–576.

Sibert, J. R., Lyons, R. A., Smith, B. A., Cornall, P., Sumner, V., Craven, M. A., & Kemp A. M. (2002). Preventing deaths by drowning in children in the United Kingdom: Have we made progress in 10 years? Population based incidence study. *British Medical Journal, 324* (7345), 1070–1071.

Smith, G. S., Keyl, P. M., Hadley, J. A., Bartley, C. L., Foss, R. D., Tolbert, W. G., McKnight, J. (2001). Drinking and recreational boating fatalities: A population-based case-control study. *Journal of the American Medical Association, 286* (23), 2974–2980.

State of Alaska Department of Health and Social Services. (2003). Promising Practices—Injury prevention programs in Alaska. Retrieved March 11, 2005, from www.hss.state.ak.us/dph/chems/injury_prevention/Assets/EducationMaterials/Best%20Practices.pdf.

Sulkes, S. B., & van der Jagt, E. W. (1990). Solar pool blankets: Another water hazard. *Pediatrics, 85* (6), 1114–1117.

Thompson, D. C., & Rivara, F. P. (2000). Pool fencing for preventing drowning in children (CD001047). *Cochrane Database of Systematic Reviews* (2).

Treser, C. D., Trusty, M. N., & Yang, P. P. (1997). Personal flotation device usage: Do educational efforts have an impact? *Journal of Public Health Policy, 18* (3), 346–356.

United States Consumer Product Safety Commission. (2005a). CPSC warns: Pools are not the only drowning danger at home for kids. Data show other hazards cause more than 100 residential child drowning deaths annually. Retrieved December 2, 2005, from cpsc.gov/CPSCPUB/PREREL/prhtml102/02169.html.

United States Consumer Product Safety Commission. (2005b). *Safety Barrier Guidelines for Home Pools.* Retrieved December 2, 2005, from www.cpsc.gov/cpscpub/puls/pool.pdf.

United States Coast Guard. (2004). Boating Statistics 2003, You're in command boat safety. Retrieved December 2, 2005, from www.uscgboating.org/statistics/Boating_Statistics_2003.pdf.

Washington State Department of Health. (2004). *Child death review state committee recommendations on child drowning prevention.* Olympia: Washington State Department of Health, Community and Family Health.

Chapter 6

Interventions to Prevent Residential Fire Injury

Lynne J. Warda and Michael F. Ballesteros

6.1. EPIDEMIOLOGY OF RESIDENTIAL FIRES IN THE UNITED STATES

The National Fire Protection Association (NFPA) reported 402,000 residential fires in 2003, resulting in 3,165 deaths and incurring $6,074,000,000 in property damage (Karter, 2004). This represented an increase of 17.4% in residential fire deaths compared to 2002, although the overall number of fires and property losses did not increase. Residential fire deaths have been declining steadily since the late 1970s, with a relative plateau since the early 1990s. Smoking materials are the leading cause of fatal residential fires (20%), with 40% of smoking-related fire victims being older than 65 years of age (Hall, 2004). Cooking is the leading cause of residential fires and nonfatal injuries (Hall, 2005). Despite 96% smoke alarm prevalence for U.S. homes with a telephone in 2004, 40% of residential fires still occur in homes without a smoke alarm, and among homes with alarms, 25% are not functioning at the time of the fire. In 1999–2001, an average of 70% of residential fire deaths resulted from fires in homes with either no smoke alarms or in which no smoke alarm sounded (Ahrens, 2004). Nearly every high-risk group for residential fire fatality is less likely to install smoke alarms, including the poor, seniors, heavy drinkers, households with less than high school education, and those in rural areas and in the Southern United States (Ahrens, 2004; Hall, 1985; Hall, 1994).

In 2002, for all ages combined, fires and burns were the 6th leading cause of unintentional injury mortality, and the 14th leading cause of nonfatal injury (Centers for Disease Control and Prevention [CDC], 2005). Approximately 6% of people with residential fire-related injuries are hospitalized, with slightly more than half being admitted for carbon monoxide poisoning and the remainder for burns (CDC, 2003). Children and older adults have the highest rates of fire-related mortality and hospitalization (DiGuiseppi, Edwards, Godward, Roberts, & Wade, 2000). Fires and burns are the 5th leading cause of injury mortality among children younger than 15 years of age and the 10th leading cause of injury-related emergency department visits, with a ratio of 198 emergency department visits for every death (Ballesteros, Schieber, Gilchrist, Holmgreen, & Annest, 2003). For children 1–4 years of age, fires and burns are the 6th leading cause of death and result in almost 63,000 emergency department visits (CDC, 2005). Fatal fire injuries among children are often (30–60%) due to playing with fire, and playing with fire is the leading cause of fatal residential fire injuries for preschool children (Hall, 2003; Istre, McCoy, Carlin, & McClain, 2002; Shai & Lupinacci, 2003).

A number of other risk factors for fatal residential fires have been identified. Mortality rates are significantly higher for American Indian/Alaskan Native and black/African American populations (2.1 and 3.0 per 100,000 in 1998 vs. 1.2 per 100,000 for the total population) (U.S. Department of Health and Human Services [DHHS], 2000). Other risk factors include personal and household factors, such as income, educational level, rural residence, physical and mental disability, smoking, impairment by drugs or alcohol, and male gender, and housing-related factors, such as home ownership, lack of a telephone, housing age, and housing type (e.g., mobile/manufactured home) (Warda, Tenenbein, & Moffatt, 1999a).

6.2. HISTORY OF PREVENTION EFFORTS

Heat detectors for use in residential structures were introduced in 1921 and represented the first available technology for the early notification of fire. Underwriters Laboratories (UL) approved a single-station residential smoke detector in the 1960s, which was followed in 1970 by the now widespread single-station battery-powered smoke alarm. Early recommendations demanded installation of both smoke and heat detectors, at substantial expense to the homeowner. By 1974, research supported the effectiveness of smoke detectors in isolation, and the NFPA eliminated the requirement for an additional heat detecting system (Hall, 1985).

Fire prevention efforts at the national level have a lengthy history. In May 1947, the President's Fire Prevention Conference brought together 2000 leaders including President Harry Truman and representatives from industry, government, the military, higher education, and the fire service. Reports of this event detail an approach not unlike the current one, with a call for multilevel multisectoral interventions, including education, enforcement, and engineering measures (Federal Works Agency, 1947). Further evidence of an organized approach to burn prevention was apparent in the late 1960s and early 1970s. The American Burn Association was founded in 1967 and initially focused on patient care, teaching, and research. In 1972, the association expanded its activities to include public education and added *Prevention* to its name. The U.S. Fire Administration was established in 1974, when Congress passed the Federal Fire Prevention and Control Act, with the mandate to reduce deaths and property loss due to fire through surveillance, education, research, and training (Silverstein & Lack, 1987).

Fire prevention has been acknowledged as a public health priority for several decades. The 1990 health promotion objectives for the nation relating to injury prevention included increasing functioning smoke alarm prevalence to 75% for residential units from baseline rates of 50% in 1980 and 67% in 1982. Subsequently, *Healthy People 2010* injury prevention objectives included two objectives related to residential fire injuries: (1) reduce residential fire deaths to a target level of 0.2 deaths per 100,000 population in 2010 from a 1998 baseline of 1.2 per 100,000 and (2) increase functioning residential smoke alarms from a 1998 baseline of 87% of residences having a functioning smoke alarm on every floor to 100% in 2010 (USDHHS, 2000).

The U.S. Fire Administration, Consumer Product Safety Commission (CPSC), Centers for Disease Control and Prevention (CDC), and other organizations have recently established the goal of eliminating residential fire deaths by 2020 (CDC, 2003). As part of this effort, the CDC has funded smoke alarm installation programs and fire safety education programs in high-risk communities since 1998 and has targeted residential fires as a research priority. The CDC Injury Research Agenda includes the following priorities related to the prevention of residential fire injuries: evaluation of strategies to increase smoke alarm and sprinkler use; identification of behavioral factors that influence safe escape from fires; identification of strategies that improve the ability of high-risk individuals to detect and escape fires; and developing an interdisciplinary research program pertaining to evacuation in mass trauma events, including environmental and human factors, human reaction to fire, and fire risk perception (CDC, 2002).

6.3. CHAPTER ORGANIZATION

This chapter summarizes interventions of relevance to the prevention of fires and fire-related injuries. Three broad groups of interventions are summarized: products (e.g., smoke alarms, sprinklers), environmental interventions (residential design and household equipment factors that reduce the risk of fire injury), and behavioral interventions (strategies to increase smoke alarm use and function). Behavioral strategies are divided into three levels according to the group targeted for behavior change: the individual (e.g., education in clinical settings, schools, and the community), the community (e.g., smoke alarm legislation), and multilevel interventions. Risk factors and interventions are then summarized by vulnerable population. For each intervention type, the level of evidence is noted (effective, promising, insufficient evidence, no evidence, harmful).

6.4. REVIEW OF INTERVENTIONS BY LEVEL OF EVIDENCE

6.4.1. Intervention Types

6.4.1.1. Products

6.4.1.1.1. Smoke Alarms (Effective Strategy).   There are three types of smoke alarms: ionization alarms, photoelectric alarms, and combination types. Photoelectric alarms respond more rapidly than ionization types, have fewer nuisance alarms, and therefore lower disconnection rates. Despite this, ionization alarms remain the most popular ones in U.S. homes (90%). In 1993 most smoke alarms were battery powered (72%), with the remainder being hard-wired to the home's electrical system (23%), portable units powered by an electrical outlet (2%), and hard-wired with battery backup (2%). Hard-wired systems are much more common in new construction, apartments, and manufactured homes, reflecting current fire and building codes and legislation. Although field testing has not confirmed greater effectiveness of hard-wired systems, these systems do not depend on batteries and are statistically much less prone to power source interruptions; therefore, hard-wired interconnected alarms are recommended over battery-powered systems and are now required in many jurisdictions for new construction. Wireless technology is being explored as a means to interconnect existing single-station battery-powered smoke alarms, thereby sounding all alarms if one is activated (Ahrens, 2004).

Current recommendations for smoke alarm placement and number are based on sleeping location and home design; there should be one detector on each level of the home and close to each sleeping area. Detectors should be installed, maintained, and tested according to the manufacturer's instructions and should be replaced at least every 10 years. Batteries should be replaced at least annually (Ahrens, 2004; Reisinger, 1980).

The National Fire Incident Reporting System (NFIRS) has been used to estimate the effectiveness of smoke alarms. Residential fire mortality rates in homes with smoke alarms are 40–50% lower than those in homes not equipped with functioning detectors; this estimate has been consistent since it was first calculated using 1979 NFIRS data (Hall, 1985; Hall, 1994). A recent National Institute of Standards and Technology (NIST) Fire Research Division study reports extensive testing of current residential smoke alarm technologies in a controlled laboratory setting and in a series of real-scale tests conducted in two residential structures. These studies affirmed that both ionization and photoelectric smoke alarms consistently provide time for occupants to escape from most residential fires. Consistent with prior findings, ionization-type alarms provided somewhat better responses to flaming fires than photoelectric alarms, and photoelectric alarms provided considerably faster response to smoldering fires than ionization type alarms. Notably, the escape times documented in these studies (3 minutes) were considerably shorter than those reported in previous similar studies (17 minutes). The addition of a smoke alarm in the bedroom increased escape times significantly, particularly for smoldering fires (Bukowski et al., 2004).

The National Smoke Detector Project Survey conducted in 1993 found that up to 20% of installed smoke alarms are nonoperational. A number of studies have evaluated the performance of smoke alarms in real fires. The most common reason for nonoperational alarms are malfunctions, dead batteries, removed batteries, and disconnection, commonly due to frequent false alarms. In a 1983 study, in fires that produced enough smoke to cause activation, smoke alarms did not properly sound due to dead or missing batteries and other power source problems (69%), incorrect installation (12%), and incorrect location (11%) (Hall, 1994). Disconnection is a significant issue and has contributed to numerous fatal fires. Disabling of alarms occurs frequently in response to nuisance alarms, largely related to cooking. Despite educational efforts and research to reduce nuisance alarms, the current disconnection rate remains high. The National Smoke Detector Project recommended measures to reduce nuisance alarms, including adjusting the installation location, switching to the photoelectric type of detector, and decreasing sensitivity through routine maintenance and replacement after 10 years. Sensitivity drift due to age may increase nuisance alarms or decrease the detection of real fires (Hall, 1994).

Extended-life lithium batteries have been promoted in recent years to address the issue of battery replacement. These batteries are typically advertised as lasting 10 years. Numerous complaints have been documented regarding these batteries, due to premature low battery chirping. The CPSC investigated these complaints and determined that a grease sealing process used during a limited time period in 1998–1999 allowed moisture into the batteries. This problem appears to have been resolved; however, there are no data documenting improved effectiveness over standard batteries (Ahrens, 2004; Lee, 2002). In a randomized controlled trial examining which type of smoke alarm is most likely to remain functional in inner city housing, alarms with lithium batteries were significantly more likely to be functional at follow-up; however, a significant portion were not working after 15 months (Rowland et al., 2002).

The CPSC recently conducted a literature review concerning the audibility of smoke alarm signals to older adults and sleeping children. The authors concluded that current smoke alarms do not reliably wake children younger than 16 years of age or seniors who are hearing impaired. Interconnected alarms could enhance audibility, particularly for units installed in bedrooms. Further research is recommended regarding potential technical solutions, such as alternative audible or visible (strobe light) cues, and/or training and education to improve waking responses (Lee, Midgett, & White, 2004).

6.4.1.1.2. Child Resistant Lighters (Effective Strategy).

In 1994, the CPSC introduced a safety standard for cigarette lighters (16 CFR Part 1210) that requires disposable or novelty lighters to have a child-resistant mechanism that makes them difficult for children younger than 5 years to operate. This standard does not pertain to "multipurpose lighters" used for barbeques and fireplaces because they are covered by a different standard. Lighter manufacturers are required to test their products using panels of children between 42 and 51 months of age, and 85% of these children must not be able to operate them within a defined time limit (Smith, Greene, & Singh, 2002).

The effectiveness of the CPSC standard was estimated by comparing the incidence of fires caused by children younger than 5 years playing with lighters for 1997–1999 (poststandard) to similar data for 1985–1987 (prestandard). There was a 58% reduction in these fires after the introduction of the standard (Odds ratio [OR]: 0.42; 95% confidence interval [CI]: 0.23–0.62). It was estimated that the child-resistant standard prevented 3300 fires, 100 deaths, 660 injuries, and $52.5 million in property losses in 1998 (Smith et al., 2002).

As part of another study, two groups of children 40–60 months of age were given conventional and child-resistant lighters. The children were given 5 minutes to attempt to operate the lighter; if the child could not ignite it, the administrator showed them how to use it and allowed another 5 minutes. Researchers found that 62% were unable to operate the conventional lighter after the second 5 minutes compared to 95% that were still unable to operate the child-resistant one. The child-resistant feature lowered caregivers' risk perceptions related to the lighter and reduced precautionary behaviors; however, the authors concluded that these effects would not significantly affect the effectiveness of the child-resistant feature in terms of fire-related injuries (Viscusi & Cavallo, 1994).

6.4.1.1.3. Residential Sprinklers (Insufficient Evidence).

Residential sprinkler systems are designed to automatically discharge to extinguish fires, giving the occupant time to escape. Sprinkler systems have been available for more than 100 years, but residential systems were not practical until 1978 when technical advancements made them five times faster in response to fires (American Medical Association Council on Scientific Affairs, 1987). More quick-response heads that are now available react as quickly as 35 seconds. Industrial or commercial sprinkler systems have been evaluated by full-scale fire tests and have increased survivor rates, reduced multiple losses, and significantly reduced property losses (one fifth compared to unsprinklered buildings). It has been estimated that while smoke detectors reduce home fire fatalities by about 50%, a residential sprinkler system could reduce home fire fatalities by an additional 30% (Rohr, 2003). In 1999, only 3.4% of fires in one- and two-family dwellings occurred in homes with sprinkler systems (Rohr, 2003). One of the major deterrents to installation of sprinkler systems is the cost, estimated at greater than 20 times that of a smoke alarm system (Hall, 1985). A number of demonstration projects have been conducted to reduce installation costs, simplify installation, and investigate infrastructure and code alternatives and incentives for installation of these systems.

6.4.1.1.4. Fire-Safe Cigarette (Promising Strategy). "Fire-safe" cigarettes are designed to demonstrate a reduced propensity for igniting household materials such as furniture and mattresses and self-extinguish when they are not being smoked. Burn rates of cigarettes are determined by multiple factors, including the circumference of the cigarette, packing density of the tobacco, porosity of the paper, and presence of a filter. Other factors that play a major role are the addition of accelerants such as citrate and phosphate that maintain continuous burning when the cigarette is not inhaled (Botkin, 1988; Chapman & Balmain, 2004).

Legislative efforts to develop fire-safe cigarettes began in the 1920s, as a method to prevent forest fires (Barillo, Brigham, Kayden, Heck, & McManus, 2000). In 1979, the American Burn Association endorsed the first national campaign for fire-safe cigarettes. The 1984 Cigarette Safety Act (PL98-567) established a technical study group to examine the feasibility of the development of fire-safe cigarettes. In 1987 this group released their report, which stated that it was technically feasible to produce a cigarette with low propensity for ignition of other items. Subsequently, a Fire-Safe Cigarette Act was passed in 1990, which mandated the development of a test method and other studies. The final report of these activities was presented to Congress in 1993, and in February 1994, the late Congressman Joseph Moakley sponsored a bill that would have required the CPSC to issue a safety standard for cigarettes. This bill did not pass; however, legislative efforts continue. American Society for Testing and Materials (ASTM) recently introduced a test method for measuring cigarette ignition, and fire-safe cigarette legislation was recently passed in New York State and Canada, requiring manufacturers to publicize or limit ignition strength (Chapman & Balmain, 2004; Hall, 2004); but presently, not enough time has elapsed since the passage of these laws to determine if they have been effective. Preliminary results from the state of New York appear promising.

6.4.1.1.5. Ignition-Resistant Household Materials (Promising Strategy). Mattresses, bedding, and upholstered furniture are the items most commonly ignited in smoking-related home fires and in fires resulting from children playing with fire (Hall, 2003, 2004). Mattresses sold in the United States after 1971 are required to be resistant to ignition by a dropped cigarette (Clarke & Birky, 1981). It has been suggested that continued investigation regarding the ignition resistance and burning properties of household materials could further reduce the risk of injury and death for these types of fires, particularly for smoking-related fires (Hall, 2004).

6.4.1.1.6. Environmental Interventions (Insufficient Evidence). Building design, construction materials and quality, and household furnishings and equipment can contribute to residential fire risk and injury. Hard-wired interconnected smoke alarms, sprinkler systems, and well-planned routes for egress can reduce the risk of a fatal fire, while exposed heating sources, faulty wiring, poorly maintained appliances and fixtures, and substandard cooking facilities are potential fire hazards (Krieger & Higgins, 2002; Neutra & McFarland, 1972).

Heating equipment is the second leading cause of residential fires (Ahrens, 2003). Home heating equipment includes central heating units, portable and fixed space heaters, fireplaces, chimneys, and hot-water heaters. These fires typically involve poorly installed, poorly maintained, or misused heating equipment. Electrical distribution equipment fires are the leading cause of property damage (Ahrens, 2003). This equipment includes wiring; transformers; meters or meter boxes; switches, receptacles, and outlets; light fixtures; cords and plugs; and lamps and light bulbs. "Open flame, ember or torch" is the second leading cause of home fire injuries (Ahrens, 2003). This category includes cutting, welding, or other torches; matches, lighters, and candles not associated with intentional or child-play fires; open fires; and embers. Candles were the leading cause in this category of home fires for 1999. While these household equipment and other home environment fire risks are well characterized, prevention strategies have not been well evaluated. A Cochrane review of modification of the home environment to reduce injuries concluded that there is insufficient evidence to determine the effectiveness of these types of interventions (Lyons et al., 2003). However, fire-prevention education materials and campaigns often cite the need to modify environments to reduce these hazards, yet evidence is insufficient to determine if this works. The effectiveness of educational and behavioral change strategies are discussed in the next section.

6.4.1.2. Behavioral Interventions

Behavioral aspects of residential fire injury and its prevention are not well documented in current research literature. Some of these behaviors relate to routine practices, such as safe cooking behaviors and space heater placement, and are considered primary prevention, which can avert a fire. Other behaviors are considered secondary prevention and reflect decision making or action taken during a fire, which can eliminate or reduce fire-related injuries. Other characteristics of a human behavior approach to fire safety deal with principles of applied behavioral analysis, evacuation modeling, factors affecting perception of fire risk, visual access, residential design concepts, and human performance criteria needed for fire safety engineering (University of Ulster, 2001, 2004).

An understanding of health behavior theory may contribute to new or improved interventions, such as smoke alarm distribution and maintenance campaigns, and fire escape planning and practice (Thompson, Waterman, & Sleet, 2004). A set of key factors to predict and explain behavior change affecting many health problems has been determined, including three that are considered necessary and sufficient—intentions, environmental barriers, and skills—and five that can influence strength and direction of intentions or act directly to influence behavior—outcome expectancies, social norms, self-standards, emotional reactions, and self-efficacy (Fishbein et al., 2001). These eight factors can be applied to the behavior of testing the functionality of a residential smoke alarm.

As described by Gielen and Sleet (2003), if a home owner forms a strong positive intention (i.e., a commitment to test the smoke alarm every month), encounters no environmental barriers to accessing the smoke alarm (i.e., the alarm is reachable by household ladder), and has the skills necessary to successfully test the alarm, then we would expect routine alarm maintenance. Maintenance would be even more likely if the home owner believes that it is useful to do the testing, understands that it is the right thing to do in the neighborhood, expects that conducting smoke alarm maintenance is part of being a responsible home owner, overall feels positively about doing the testing (i.e., the satisfaction of knowing the smoke alarm is operational outweighs the time and effort involved in the testing), and finds it feasible to conduct the testing activities under conditions that could include other competing household or family demands. The more that is known from theory about factors influencing specific fire-related behavior and behavior change, the more likely it is that behavioral-intervention programs will succeed (Thompson et al., 2004). To date, few injury prevention programs have used health behavior theory as a framework for prevention (Trifiletti, Gielen, Sleet, & Hopkins, 2005).

6.4.1.2.1. Individual Education and Counseling (Insufficient Evidence).

A systematic review of controlled trials of interventions to promote smoke alarms estimates that counseling and educational interventions had nonsignificant effects on the likelihood of owning an alarm (OR: 1.26; 95% CI: 0.87–1.81) or having a functioning alarm (OR: 1.19; 95% CI: 0.85–1.66) (DiGuiseppi & Higgins, 2000). Providing smoke alarm counseling as part of routine well-child care had more significant effects on smoke alarm ownership (OR: 1.93; 95% CI: 1.04–3.58) but not functionality (OR: 1.72; 95% CI: 0.78–3.78). However, these published interventions were not based on behavioral theory and did not study the interventions' effects on fire-related injuries. Educational interventions in other settings were not as effective, demonstrating no effect or modest positive, statistically nonsignificant effects on smoke alarm ownership and function; these included education in prenatal classes, discharge teaching for children hospitalized in a burn unit, and mass media and community-based injury prevention education. A more recent study documented significantly higher working smoke alarm rates in households receiving a health visitor delivered safety consultation based on evidence-based educational principles and including free safety devices fitted for the family free of charge (OR: 1.83; 95% CI: 1.33–2.52 at 12 months; OR: 1.67; 95% CI: 1.21–2.32 at 24 months). These and other improved safety practices were not associated with a reduction in injury rates (Watson et al., 2005).

6.4.1.2.2. Community/Societal Interventions, Including Legislation (Promising Strategy).

The effectiveness of smoke alarm legislation was examined in a study of smoke alarm use in a county with a retrofit law requiring a smoke alarm in all homes regardless of age, compared to a county with legislation applying only to new construction. Just 5 years after the retrofit law was introduced, homes in the county with the retrofit law were less likely to have no operational alarms (17% vs. 30%) or to have no detector (6% vs. 16%) when compared to the control county. Fatal fires and fire deaths decreased to a greater extent in the retrofit county than the control county for the 6-year periods before and after the law was introduced (McLoughlin, Marchone, Hanger, German, & Baker, 1985).

Smoke alarm requirements differ considerably by state. By 1999, seven states did not have smoke alarm legislation, and the remainder of states had varying requirements; the dwellings affected include all residences in some states and in others, various combinations of one- and two-family dwellings, multiple-occupancy dwellings, mobile homes, and rental properties (ISCAIP Smoke Detector Legislation Collaborators, 1999). The type and number of detectors required range considerably, as well as the referenced codes (e.g., NFPA 72—the National Fire Alarm Code, Uniform Building Code).

6.4.1.3.   Multilevel

6.4.1.3.1. Community-Based Campaigns (Insufficient Evidence). A recent Cochrane review examined community-based interventions for the prevention of burns and scalds in children 0–14 years of age (Turner, Spinks, McClure, & Nixon, 2004). Eligible interventions were coordinated, multi-strategy initiatives, and controlled community trials were included that reported changes in medically attended injuries. Of 32 studies, 3 met criteria for inclusion (Guyer et al., 1989; MacKay & Rothman, 1982; Ytterstad, Smith, & Coggan, 1998; Ytterstad & Sogaard, 1995). Project Burn Prevention was an educational campaign delivered through mass media, schools, and community organizations and was implemented in two Boston communities from October 1977 to May 1978 (MacKay & Rothman, 1982). The Massachusetts Statewide Childhood Injury Prevention Program (SCIPP) was an injury prevention educational intervention, with burn prevention being one of five target project areas; it was implemented in nine cities between September 1980 and June 1982. SCIPP implemented the Project Burn Prevention curricula through schools, libraries, police and fire authorities, and day-care facilities (Guyer et al., 1989). The Harstad Injury Prevention Study used the Safe Communities method and targeted burns and scalds in children younger than 5 years of age. Multiple community agencies and businesses delivered burn-prevention education using a variety of methods, ranging from individual counseling to local media involvement (Ytterstad & Sogaard, 1995).

Burn injury rates decreased in the Harstad study; however, in this study residential fires was not a focus of the intervention, but rather scalds and contact burns (Ytterstad & Sogaard, 1995). Neither of the other two studies documented significant reductions in burn injuries. Project Burn Prevention may have been limited by its short duration (8 months) (MacKay & Rothman, 1982). The SCIPP program may have been limited by the lack of penetration of its burn-prevention component (Guyer et al., 1989).

6.4.1.3.2. Smoke Alarm Installation (Effective Strategy) and Distribution (Promising Strategy). Another Cochrane review examined interventions for promoting smoke alarm ownership and function (DiGuiseppi & Higgins, 2000, 2001). This review included four published nonrandomized trials with multilevel components (Guyer et al., 1989; MacKay & Rothman, 1982; Mallonee et al., 1996; Schwarz, Grisso, Miles, Holmes, & Sutton, 1993). Two of these studies were described earlier. The Oklahoma City Smoke Alarm Project targeted households in an area with the highest rate of residential fires in the city, and distributed free smoke alarms and related information to residents. By 6 years after the project was implemented, fire-related injury rates had decreased 81% in the target area and only 7% in the remainder of the city. Part of this reduction may have been due to regression to the mean, as the target area had the highest rate at baseline. At 48 months, 46% of the alarms were still installed and functioning (Mallonee, 2000). A subsequent cost-effectiveness analysis documented that the program was cost effective both from a societal and a health care system perspective (Haddix, Mallonee, Waxweiler, & Douglas, 2001). Another smoke alarm giveaway program targetted urban African American households; this campaign increased functional smoke alarm use among the intervention group (96% vs. 77%) and also demonstrated a significant reduction in fire-related injuries in the intervention but not the control group (Schwarz et al., 1993). A more recent cluster randomized controlled trial targeting rental housing in a poor urban population did not reduce fires, hospitalizations, deaths, or alarm installation rates. Few of the alarms had been installed or maintained, suggesting that some distribution campaigns require installation assistance to ensure compliance (DiGuiseppi et al., 2002; Harvey et al., 2004).

Comparisons of the effectiveness of different distribution methods have been reported by several studies. For the Oklahoma City Smoke Alarm Project, the authors describe a comparison of smoke alarm distribution methods and document that direct distribution to homes was the most effective and cost-efficient method, compared to notification by mail, flyer, or public notices alerting residents that fire alarms were available at local fire stations. Contamination of the distribution groups limits this analysis because the distribution methods were assigned by ZIP code, and promotional materials were distributed widely through schools, the media, and community groups (Douglas, Mallonee, & Istre, 1998).

Another study examined two methods—direct distribution/installation and vouchers for free smoke alarms—in high-risk households in five states. Within each state, geographic areas were identified (areas, cities, counties), and comparable areas were randomly assigned to the two methods. All homes were canvassed, and households without any smoke alarms were eligible for randomization. Follow-up home visits at 6–12 months documented 89.8% in the installation group had functioning alarms compared to 65% in the voucher group (OR: 4.82; 95% CI: 3.97–5.85; $p < .0001$). Almost half of the voucher group did not redeem the voucher (Harvey et al., 2004). Another study revealed a positive economy of scale: as the number of smoke alarms installed went up, the costs per alarm went down; for every 1% increase in, smoke alarm installation, the cost per alarm decreased by $1.36 (Parmer, Corso, & Ballesteros, 2005).

One study evaluated the long-term functional status of smoke alarms distributed to high-risk households (Shults et al., 1998). Households were randomly selected for home visits to assess smoke alarms that were distributed 3–4 years earlier, for three different smoke alarm giveaway programs (Minnesota, North Carolina, Oklahoma). The proportion of homes with at least one functioning alarm ranged from 58% to 73%, with the majority (76%) of nonfunctioning alarms due to missing batteries or disconnection. In a more recent randomized controlled trial, almost half of the distributed alarms were not functioning at 15 months (Rowland et al., 2002).

6.4.2. Target Populations

Most smoke alarm distribution studies have targeted "high-risk" households, variably defined as communities or households with at least one risk factor, including increased rates of residential fires or fire-related injury/death or low prevalence of smoke alarm use, households with at least one young child or older adult, low-income areas, and high proportion of rental units. These studies are summarized above, as are other studies that specifically target children and their families. Data regarding other vulnerable populations are presented in this section.

6.4.2.1.   Rural Communities

Rural homes are more likely to lack smoke alarms, and often have multiple risk factors for smoke alarm nonuse and residential fire death (Ahrens, 2004; Forjuoh, Coben, Dearwater, & Weiss, 1997). Although smoke alarm distribution initiatives in rural communities are described in the literature, their effectiveness in terms of reductions in fires, injuries, and deaths are not known. Uncontrolled follow-up studies of targetted smoke alarm distribution campaigns have demonstrated significant increases in functioning smoke alarms. One such study documented an increase from 58.6% to 89.9% at 1-year follow-up. In this study, dead or missing batteries and disabled alarms accounted for approximately 50% of nonfunctioning alarms and could be addressed by installation of alarms with long-life batteries (Jones, Thompson, & Davis, 2001).

Fazzini, Perkins, & Grossman (2000) studied the problem of nuisance alarms in a cohort study conducted in four small villages in Alaska. They compared the false alarm rate between households with ionization and photoelectric types of detectors. Both groups were similar with respect to square footage, household income, family size, and alarm location (distance from cooking source). At 6 months after the detectors were installed, surveys were conducted to determine false alarm and detector disconnection rates. Significant rates of false alarms were documented for ionization detectors (92% vs. 11% for photoelectric) and high rates of disconnection were found in the same group (19% vs. 4%). Of note, these homes were small, and the nuisance alarms were predominantly related to frying foods. The authors conclude that photoelectric alarms may result in higher long-term functioning smoke alarm rates for small homes (<1000 square feet) or those with high rates of nuisance alarms. However, in a subsequent study, ionization alarms were significantly more likely to be functional at follow-up (Rowland et al., 2002).

6.4.2.2.   Homebound and Older Adults

Between 1997 and 2001, a total of 11 "sentinel events" were reported to the Joint Commission on Accreditation of Healthcare Organizations related to home-care patients who were seriously (4) or fatally (7) injured in residential fires (Joint Commission on Accreditation of Healthcare Organizations [JCAHO], 2001). Risk factors identified in these cases included living alone, lack of a functional smoke alarm, cognitive impairment, a history of smoking while using oxygen, and flammable clothing. These cases were analyzed for root causes that contributed to these fires, which included patient care processes, caregivers, the environment of care, and communication factors. Risk-reduction strategies arising from these analyses include development of home safety assessment processes, including obtaining and testing smoke alarms; providing smoking-cessation information and terminating home-care services for noncompliance; and staff training with respect to care of smokers and home-care fire safety. In-depth fire safety assessments of geriatric home-care clients have documented significant personal and environmental risk factors for fire injury (physical impairment, poor fire safety knowledge and equipment, apathy) (Stiles, Bratcher, Ramsbottom-Lucier, & Hunter, 2001). A home safety checklist for homebound adults has been developed for home visitors and other caregivers, but has not been evaluated (Weese, 1995); home safety risk-assessment tools have been developed for home-care professionals but have not been validated (Stiles et al., 2001; Tanner, 2003).

6.4.2.3. Persons with Disabilities and Older Adults

Individuals with disabilities, including many older adults, are at an increased risk of fire-related death; this may be related to limited mobility; sensory or cognitive impairment that prevents awareness of a fire or an alarm; or inability to develop, alter, or complete an escape plan (Gaebler-Spira & Thornton, 2002). In an analysis of victims and survivors of the same residential fires, persons with physical or cognitive disabilities had a 4-fold increased risk of death (OR: 4.18; 95% CI: 1.33–13.11) (Marshall et al., 1998). In this study, the presence of a potential rescuer (unimpaired adult) reduced the risk of death by half, and the presence of a smoke alarm reduced the risk of death by 60%. The risk of death for persons with disabilities (vision, hearing, mobility, mental status) was documented as a 2.5-fold increase compared to nondisabled persons in a previous case-control study by the same authors (OR: 2.5; 95% CI: 1.5–4.4) (Runyan, Bangdiwala, Linzer, Sacks, & Butts, 1992).

Several studies of mildly to profoundly mentally disabled children and adults have documented mastery of safe exit in individual or small group training sessions using behavior-modification techniques (Haney & Jones, 1982; Holburn & Dougher, 1985; Jones & Thornton, 1987; Katz & Singh, 1986; Rae & Roll, 1985; Rowe & Kedesdy, 1988). Maintenance of skills was variable, with good retention at 3–8 months. These studies consistently document the importance of follow-up testing and reinforcement. Two studies examined cognitive-behavioral training to teach blind, mildly mentally disabled adolescents the necessary fire evacuation skills to escape a nighttime fire in their dormitory. In the first study, individuals were trained to respond to four different scenarios. In the second study, group training was used with a single scenario. Both individual and group training were effective in teaching the correct sequence of behaviors (100% mastery), with high levels of maintenance of these skills at 3–4 months (Jones, Sisson, & Van Hasselt, 1984; Jones, Van Hasselt, & Sisson, 1984).

6.4.2.4. Children

Studies that evaluate the effectiveness of fire safety education and smoke alarm counseling in various settings (e.g., primary care, prenatal classes, parenting classes, injured children, community-based programs) and targeted caregivers of young children are summarized in the above sections. Studies that evaluate interventions targeting children themselves include educational programs and fire-response training at schools and day cares and are summarized in detail elsewhere (Warda, Tenenbein, & Moffatt, 1999b). Some of these educational programs documented modest increases in fire safety knowledge but most were limited by short-term outcome evaluation and lack of rigorous evaluation methods. Of note, the single published study of the Learn Not to Burn (LNTB) curriculum documented that pretest and posttest scores among grade 3 and 4 students did not differ between LNTB schools and schools with other fire safety programs or no fire safety program (Grant, Turney, Bartlett, Winbon, & Peterson, 1992). One large school-based program implemented by the New Zealand Fire Service documented a significant increase in correct behavioral responses to two of three simulated fire situations (Dunn & Renwick, 1995). Several small randomized controlled trials have evaluated small group and one-on-one intensive training in fire response behaviors using simulated bedrooms or actual sleeping areas. Several groups of grade 2–4 students successfully mastered these skills; however, loss of skills over time was considerable (Jones & Haney, 1983; Jones, Ollendick, McLaughlin & Williams, 1989; Jones, Kazdin, & Haney, 1981; Hillman, Jones, & Farmer, 1986).

Infants and children generally require more sleep, have longer stages of deep sleep, and are more difficult to arouse from sleep than adults. There has been growing concern regarding the extent to which children will awaken to a smoke detector alarm in the standard hallway location. In response to this concern, a study was conducted using 20 individuals 6–17 years old and 16 adults 30–59 years old (Bruck, 1999). A smoke alarm stand was placed such that the decibel reading at the pillow of each participants was $60\,dBA \pm 3\,dBA$. It was found that 85% of the children slept through the 3-minute alarm, whereas 100% of the adults reliably awoke. Based on these findings, the author recommends that interconnected detectors and alarms be installed in residential settings so that adults can be awoken if a fire occurs in or near children's bedrooms.

Inadequate supervision is a significant risk factor for injury death among children, including residential fire death (Rimsza, Schackner, Bowen, & Marshall, 2002; Landen, Bauer, & Kohn, 2003) Families with previous involvement with child protection services are at higher risk of injury death and hospitalization, including burn injuries. In a retrospective burn center study, 17.6% of admissions were related to abuse or neglect, 36% had been investigated for abuse or neglect, and 12% had lost custody of other children (Hultman et al., 1998). In a similar study of 507 consecutive admissions to a pediatric burn unit, 14% of families were referred to child protection services with suspected or confirmed child abuse or neglect (Andronicus, Oates, Peat, Spalding, & Martin, 1998) A 12-month study of patients treated in a pediatric emergency department documented 431 patients with burn injuries, of which 84 (19.5%) were suspected of being abused or neglected (Rosenberg & Marino, 1989). These case series are primarily scalds and contact burns; however, caregiver neglect has also been documented for residential fire injuries and flame injuries related to playing with lighters and matches; for flame injuries, cases of neglect include children left alone and children supervised by intoxicated adults. Prevention program staff might benefit from communicating with child protection services, to further understand families at risk and to ensure that fire safety and education regarding active supervision are incorporated in home visiting and other early intervention programs.

6.5.   DISCUSSION: IMPLICATIONS FOR PREVENTION

The causes of residential fires and key effective countermeasures (smoke alarms, fire-safe cigarettes) have been well described, with the remaining prevention gaps being widespread implementation of these measures. As with other injury issues, legislation could be instrumental in addressing these gaps. Such legislation could include mandatory compliance with NFPA's Life Safety Code for single- and two-family dwellings, lodging homes, and apartments; the current code requires functioning smoke alarms on every floor and outside every sleeping area, as well as inside bedrooms (excludes apartments). For new construction, interconnected hard-wired alarms are required, and for multistory dwellings greater than four floors, sprinkler systems are also required. As the proportion of nonfunctioning alarms remains significantly high, future efforts must address disconnection and power source (battery) issues; programs that facilitate routine battery replacement and installation of long-life battery alarms or hard-wired systems are potential prevention measures, and careful selection and placement of alarms can reduce false alarm rates and disconnection. Given the new information regarding short escape times afforded by current smoke alarm technology, smoke alarms should be installed inside the bedroom, as well on every level of the home, and interconnected systems should be encouraged. Smoke alarm distribution programs should encourage compliance with these recommendations and should provide education and install alarm units in a manner that reduces false alarm rates.

Federal-level fire-safe cigarette legislation and smoking cessation programs could also contribute significantly to a reduction in fatal residential fires. As the population ages, fires in the home-care setting may increase; the health care system should begin to integrate fire safety precautions in routine standards of care for home-care patients and should also monitor the frequency and patterns of fires in home-care systems.

6.6. RESEARCH GAPS

6.6.1. Intervention Type

A number of research gaps remain with respect to smoke alarm technology, including relative effectiveness and cost-effectiveness of long-life battery-powered alarms systems and hard-wired systems, smoke alarm audibility for children and older adults, relative effectiveness of interconnected alarm systems, and effective and efficient methods to increase functional smoke alarm prevalence in the highest-risk households. Finally, if new technology develops an acceptable smoke, heat, and carbon monoxide combination detector, consumer acceptance and nuisance alarm potential will all have to be carefully evaluated. Residential sprinkler effectiveness in real fires has not been demonstrated, and cost and installation barriers deserve exploration.

6.6.2. Target Audience

American Indian and Alaskan Native communities have significantly elevated residential fire mortality rates and have unique cultural, infrastructure, housing, and equipment (e.g., heating and cooking systems) challenges; effective prevention programs for these communities have not been established. Programs addressing the unique needs of older adults, particularly the frail and homebound elderly in home-care systems, have not been developed or evaluated. The potential for integration of fire-prevention countermeasures with health- and home-care services, such as home visitors, has not been explored. While intensive training methods for fire evacuation responses have been shown to be effective for individuals and small groups with mental and physical disabilities, these methods have not been adopted for more widespread training efforts, and the potential for application of these techniques to teach very young children fire evacuation responses could be further examined.

6.6.3.   Methodological Problems in Existing Research

Smoke alarm promotion interventions in clinical and community settings should evaluate fire-related injury outcomes using more rigorous designs (e.g., randomized controlled trials, where feasible), ensuring adequate allocation concealment, blind outcome assessment, and adequate follow-up (DiGuiseppi & Higgins, 2000). Where different interventions are compared with one another, theory should be used to inform and guide the most promising ones. When a single intervention has produced null results, it doesn't mean all interventions in that class should be abandoned. The search for more useful methods of delivering interventions and methods for disseminating results of effective ones remain important research goals.

Cost-effectiveness and cost utility analyses of these interventions are also needed. The validity of self-report measures has been documented; telephone surveys may overestimate the presence of functioning smoke alarms by more than 20%, and should be interpreted with caution or validated with on-site measurements or verification by testing during a phone interview (Chen, Gielen, & McDonald, 2003; Douglas, Mallonee, & Istre, 1999).

6.7.   CONCLUSIONS

The current research evidence regarding the prevention of residential fire injuries emphasizes the widespread adoption of effective measures, including long-life smoke alarms, child-resistant lighters, and smoke alarm installation programs. The best protection currently available is for interconnected hard-wired smoke alarm systems with detection units on every level, outside of every sleeping area, and in each bedroom. Further research regarding behavioral and engineering interventions to improve compliance with current prevention recommendations is warranted, as well as important research on improving fire escape planning, practice and evacuation behaviors. Coordination and integration of these efforts with other public health, social, and educational services, especially among vulnerable populations, may contribute to cost-effective and efficient implementation of these interventions and long-term maintenance of safer behaviors.

REFERENCES

Ahrens, M. (2003). *The U.S. fire problem overview report: Leading causes and other patterns and trends.* Quincy, MA: National Fire Protection Association.

Ahrens, M. (2004). *U.S. experience with smoke alarms and other fire detection/alarm equipment.* Quincy, MA: National Fire Protection Association.

American Medical Association Council on Scientific Affairs. (1987). Preventing death and injury from fires with automatic sprinklers and smoke detectors. *Connecticut Medicine, 51* (12), 811–814.

Andronicus, M., Oates, R. K., Peat, J., Spalding, S., & Martin, H. (1998). Non-accidental burns in children. *Burns, 24* (6), 552–558.

Ballesteros, M. F., Schieber, R. A., Gilchrist, J., Holmgreen, P., & Annest, J. L. (2003). Differential ranking of causes of fatal versus non-fatal injuries among U.S. children. *Injury Prevention, 9* (2), 173–176.

Barillo, D. J., Brigham, P. A., Kayden, D. A., Heck, R. T., & McManus, A. T. (2000). The fire-safe cigarette: A burn prevention tool. *Journal of Burn Care of Rehabilitation, 21* (2), 162–164.

Botkin, J. R. (1988). The fire-safe cigarette. *Journal of the American Medical Association, 260* (2), 226–229.

Bukowski, R. W., Peacock, R. D., Averill, J. D., Cleary, T. G., Bryner, N. P., Walton, W. D., Reneke, P. A., & Kuligowski, E. D. (2004). *Performance of home smoke alarms. Analysis of the response of several available technologies in residential fire settings* (NIST Technical Note 1455). Washington, DC: National Institute of Standards and Technology.

Bruck, D. (1999). Non-awakening in children in response to a smoke detector alarm. *Fire Safety Journal, 32,* 369–376.

Centers for Disease Control and Prevention. (2002). *CDC injury research agenda.* Atlanta, GA: National Center for Injury Prevention and Control.

Centers for Disease Control and Prevention. (2003). Nonfatal residential fire-related injuries treated in emergency departments—United States, 2001. *Morbidity & Mortality Weekly Report, 52* (38), 906–908.

Centers for Disease Control and Prevention, National Centers for Injury Prevention and Control. (2005). Web-based injury statistics query and reporting system (WISQARS). Retrieved April 18, 2005, from www.cdc.gov/ncipc/wisqars.

Chapman, S., & Balmain, A. (2004). Time to legislate for fire-safe cigarettes in Australia. *Medical Journal of Australia, 181* (6), 292–293.

Chen, L. H., Gielen, A. C., & McDonald, E. M. (2003). Validity of self reported home safety practices. *Injury Prevention, 9* (1), 73–75.

Clarke, F. B., & Birky, M. M. (1981). Fire safety in dwellings and public buildings. *Bulletin of the New York Academy of Medicine, 57* (10), 1047–1060.

DiGuiseppi, C., Edwards, P., Godward, C., Roberts, I., & Wade, A. (2000). Urban residential fire and flame injuries: A population based study. *Injury Prevention, 6* (4), 250–254.

DiGuiseppi, C., & Higgins, J. P. (2000). Systematic review of controlled trials of interventions to promote smoke alarms. *Archives of Disease in Childhood, 82* (5), 341–348.

DiGuiseppi, C., & Higgins, J. P. (2001). Interventions for promoting smoke alarm ownership and function (CD002246). *Cochrane Database of Systematic Reviews, 2* (2), 1–39.

DiGuiseppi, C., Roberts, I., Wade, A., Sculpher, M., Edwards, P., Godward, C., Pan, H., Slater, S. (2002). Incidence of fires and related injuries after giving out free smoke alarms: Cluster randomised controlled trial. *British Medical Journal, 325* (7371), 995.

Douglas, M. R., Mallonee, S., & Istre, G. R. (1998). Comparison of community based smoke detector distribution methods in an urban community. *Injury Prevention, 4* (1), 28–32.

Douglas, M. R., Mallonee, S., & Istre, G. R. (1999). Estimating the proportion of homes with functioning smoke alarms: a comparison of telephone survey and household survey results. *American Journal of Public Health, 89* (7), 1112–1114.

Dunn, K., & Renwick, M. (1995). *Children's knowledge of fire safety stage 2: What standard 2 children know about fire safety and where they got that information from.* Wellington, New Zealand: New Zealand Council for Educational Research.

Fazzini, T. M., Perkins, R., & Grossman, D. (2000). Ionization and photoelectric smoke alarms in rural Alaskan homes. *Western Journal of Medicine, 173* (2), 89–92.

Federal Works Agency. (1947). *A guide to community organization for fire safety. President's Conference on Fire Prevention.* Washington, DC: Author.

Fishbein, M., Triandis, H., Kanfer, F. H., Becker, M., Middlestat, S. E., & Eichler, A. (2001). Factors influencing behavior and behavior change. In A. Baum, T. A. Tevenson, & J. E. Singer (Eds.), *Handbook of health psychology* (pp. 3–16). Mahwah, NJ: Erlbaum Associates.

Forjuoh, S. N., Coben, J. H., Dearwater, S. R., & Weiss, H. B. (1997). Identifying homes with inadequate smoke detector protection from residential fires in Pennsylvania. *Journal of Burn Care & Rehabilitation, 18* (1, Part 1), 86–91.

Gaebler-Spira, D., & Thornton, L. S. (2002). Injury prevention for children with disabilities. *Physical Medicine & Rehabilitation Clinics of North America, 13* (4), 891–906.

Gielen, A. C., & Sleet, D. (2003). Application of behavior-change theories and methods to injury prevention. *Epidemiologic Reviews, 25,* 65–76.

Grant, E., Turney, E., Bartlett, M., Winbon, C., & Peterson, H. D. (1992). Evaluation of a burn prevention program in a public school system. *Journal of Burn Care & Rehabilitation, 13,* 703–707.

Guyer, B., Gallagher, S. S., Chang, B. H., Azzara, C. V., Cupples, L. A., & Colton, T. (1989). Prevention of childhood injuries: Evaluation of the Statewide Childhood Injury Prevention Program (SCIPP). *American Journal of Public Health, 79* (11), 1521–1527.

Haddix, A. C., Mallonee, S., Waxweiler, R., & Douglas, M. R. (2001). Cost effectiveness analysis of a smoke alarm giveaway program in Oklahoma City, Oklahoma. *Injury Prevention, 7* (4), 276–281.

Hall, J. R. (1985). A decade of detectors: Measuring the effect. *Fire Journal* (September), *79,* 37–43, 78.

Hall, J. R. (2003). *Children playing with fire*. Quincy, MA: National Fire Protection Association.

Hall, J. R. (2004). *The smoking-material fire problem*. Quincy, MA: National Fire Protection Association.

Hall, J. R. (2005). *Home cooking fire patterns and trends*. Quincy, MA: National Fire Protection Association.

Hall, J. R. (1994). The U.S. experience with smoke detectors: Who has them? How well do they work? When don't they work? *National Fire Protection Association Journal, 88* (5), 36–46.

Haney, J., & Jones, R. (1982). Programming maintenance as a major component of a community-centered preventive effort: Escape from fire. *Behavior Therapy, 13*, 47–62.

Harvey, P. A., Aitken, M., Ryan, G. W., Demeter, L. A., Givens, J., Sundararaman, R., Goviette, S. (2004). Strategies to increase smoke alarm use in high-risk households. *Journal of Community Health, 29* (5), 375–385.

Hillman H., Jones R., & Farmer L. (1986). The acquisition and maintenance of fire emergency skills: Effects of rationale and behavioral practice. *Journal of Pediatric Psychology, 11*, 247–258.

Holburn, C., & Dougher, M. (1985). The fire-alarm game: Exit training using negative and positive reinforcement under varied stimulus conditions. *Journal of Visual Impairment & Blindness, 79*, 401–403.

Hultman, C. S., Priolo, D., Cairns, B. A., Grant, E. J., Peterson, H. D., & Meyer, A. A. (1998). Return to jeopardy: The fate of pediatric burn patients who are victims of abuse and neglect. *Journal of Burn Care & Rehabilitation, 19* (4), 367–376.

ISCAIP Smoke Detector Legislation Collaborators. (1999). International smoke detector legislation. *Injury Prevention, 5* (4), 254–255.

Istre, G. R., McCoy, M., Carlin, D. K., & McClain, J. (2002). Residential fire related deaths and injuries among children: Fireplay, smoke alarms, and prevention. *Injury Prevention, 8* (2), 128–132.

Joint Commission on Accreditation of Healthcare Organizations. (2001). Lessons learned: Fires in the home care setting. *Sentinel Event Alert, 17*, 1–3.

Jones, A. R., Thompson, C. J., & Davis, M. K. (2001). Smoke alarm ownership and installation: A comparison of a rural and a suburban community in Georgia. *Journal of Community Health, 26* (5), 307–329.

Jones, R. & Haney, J. (1983). *Refinement of a primary preventive approach to fire emergencies: A comparison of external and self-instruction strategies for training and maintaining fire emergency responding*. Pittsburgh, PA: University of Pittsburgh.

Jones, R., Kazdin, A., & Haney, J. (1981). Social validation and training of emergency fire safety skills for potential injury prevention and life saving. *Journal of Applied Behavior Analysis, 14*, 249–260.

Jones, R., Ollendick, T., McLaughlin, K., & Williams, C. E. (1989). Elaborative and behavioral rehearsal in the acquisition of fire emergency skills and the reduction of fear of fire. *Behavior Therapy, 20*, 93–101.

Jones, R., & Thornton, J. (1987). The acquisition and maintenance of emergency evacuation skills with mildly to moderately retarded adults in a community living arrangement. *Journal of Community Psychology, 15*, 205–215.

Jones, R. T., Sisson, L. A., & Van Hasselt, V. B. (1984). Emergency fire-safety skills for blind children and adolescents. Group training and generalization. *Behavior Modification, 8* (2), 267–286.

Jones, R. T., Van Hasselt, V. B., & Sisson, L. A. (1984). Emergency fire-safety skills. A study with blind adolescents. *Behavior Modification, 8* (1), 59–78.

Karter, M. J. (2004). *Fire loss in the United States during 2003*. Quincy, MA: National Fire Protection Association.

Katz, R. C., & Singh, N. N. (1986). Comprehensive fire-safety training for adult mentally retarded persons. *Journal of Mental Deficiency Research, 30* (part 1), 59–69.

Krieger, J., & Higgins, D. L. (2002). Housing and health: Time again for public health action. *American Journal of Public Health, 92* (5), 758–768.

Landen, M. G., Bauer, U., & Kohn, M. (2003). Inadequate supervision as a cause of injury deaths among young children in Alaska and Louisiana. *Pediatrics, 111* (2), 328–331.

Lee, A. (2002). *Preliminary test results on lithium batteries used in residential smoke alarms*. Washington, DC: U.S. Consumer Product Safety Commission.

Lee, A., Midgett, J., & White, S. (2004). *A review of the sound effectiveness of residential smoke alarms*. Washington, DC: U.S. Consumer Product Safety Commission.

Lyons, R., Sander, L., Weightman, A., Patterson, J., Jones, S. L., Rolfe, B., Kemp, A., & Johansen, A. (2003). Modification of the home environment for the reduction of injuries (CD003600). *Cochrane Database Systematic Reviews, 4*, 1–33.

MacKay, A. M., & Rothman, K. J. (1982). The incidence and severity of burn injuries following Project Burn Prevention. *American Journal of Public Health, 72* (3), 248–252.

Mallonee, S. (2000). Evaluating injury prevention programs: The Oklahoma City Smoke Alarm Project. *The Future of Children, 10* (1), 164–174.

Mallonee, S., Istre, G. R., Rosenberg, M., Reddish-Douglas, M., Jordan, F., Silverstein, P., Tunell, W. (1996). Surveillance and prevention of residential-fire injuries. *New England Journal of Medicine, 335* (1), 27–31.

Marshall, S. W., Runyan, C. W., Bangdiwala, S. I., Linzer, M. A., Sacks, J. J., & Butts, J. D. (1998). Fatal residential fires: Who dies and who survives? *Joural of the American Medical Association, 279* (20), 1633–1637.

McLoughlin, E., Marchone, M., Hanger, L., German, P. S., & Baker, S. P. (1985). Smoke detector legislation: Its effect on owner-occupied homes. *American Journal of Public Health, 75* (8), 858–862.

Neutra, R., & McFarland, R. A. (1972). Accident epidemiology and the design of the residential environment. *Human Factors, 14* (5), 405–420.

Parmer, J. E., Corso, P. S., Ballesteros, M. F. (2005). A cost analysis of a smoke alarm installation and fire safety education program. Unpublished data, National Center for Injury Prevention and Control, Atlanta, GA.

Rae, R., & Roll, D. (1985). Fire safety training with adults who are profoundly mentally retarded. *Mental Retardation, 23* (1), 26–30.

Reisinger, K. S. (1980). Smoke detectors: Reducing deaths and injuries due to fire. *Pediatrics, 65* (4), 718–724.

Rimsza M. E., Schackner R. A., Bowen K. A., & Marshall W. (2002). Can child deaths be prevented? The Arizona Child Fatality Review Program experience. *Pediatrics, 110* (1, Part 1), e11.

Rohr, K. D. (2003). *U.S. experience with sprinklers.* Quincy, MA: National Fire Protection Association.

Rosenberg, N. M., & Marino, D. (1989). Frequency of suspected abuse/neglect in burn patients. *Pediatric Emergency Care, 5* (4), 219–221.

Rowe, M., & Kedesdy, J. (1988). Fire evacuation skills training for institutionalized mentally retarded adults. *Behavioral Residential Treatment, 3,* 101–118.

Rowland, D., DiGuiseppi, C., Roberts, I., Curtis, K., Roberts, H., Ginnelly, L., Sculpher, M., & Wade, A. (2002). Prevalence of working smoke alarms in local authority inner city housing: Randomised controlled trial. *British Medical Journal, 325* (7371), 998–1001.

Runyan, C. W., Bangdiwala, S. I., Linzer, M. A., Sacks, J. J., & Butts, J. (1992). Risk factors for fatal residential fires. *New England Journal of Medicine, 37* (12), 859–863.

Schwarz, D. F., Grisso, J. A., Miles, C., Holmes, J. H., & Sutton, R. L. (1993). An injury prevention program in an urban African-American community. *American Journal of Public Health, 83* (5), 675–680.

Shai, D., & Lupinacci, P. (2003). Fire fatalities among children: An analysis across Philadelphia's census tracts. *Public Health Reports, 118* (2), 115–126.

Shults, R. A., Sacks, J. J., Briske, L. A., Dickey, P. H., Kinde, M. R., Mallonee, S., & Douglas, M. R. (1998). Evaluation of three smoke detector promotion programs. *American Journal of Preventive Medicine, 15* (3), 165–171.

Silverstein, P., & Lack, B. (1987). Fire prevention in the United States. Are the home fires still burning? *Surgical Clinics of North America, 67* (1), 1–14.

Smith, L. E., Greene, M. A., & Singh, H. A. (2002). Study of the effectiveness of the U.S. safety standard for child resistant cigarette lighters. *Injury Prevention, 8* (3), 192–196.

Stiles, N. J., Bratcher, D., Ramsbottom-Lucier, M., & Hunter, G. (2001). Evaluating fire safety in older persons through home visits. *Journal of the Kentucky Medical Association, 99* (3), 105–110.

Tanner, E. K. (2003). Assessing home safety in homebound older adults. *Geriatric Nursing, 24* (4), 250–254, 256.

Thompson, N. J., Waterman, M. B., & Sleet, D. A. (2004). Using behavioral science to improve fire escape behaviors in response to a smoke alarm. *Journal of Burn Care & Rehabilitation, 45* (2), 179–188.

Trifiletti, L. B., Gielen, A. C., Sleet, D. A., & Hopkins, K. (2005). Behavioral and social sciences theories and models: Are they used in unintentional injury prevention research? *Health Education Research, 20* (3), 298–307.

Turner, C., Spinks, A., McClure, R., & Nixon, J. (2004). Community-based interventions for the prevention of burns and scalds in children (CD004335). *Cochrane Database of Systematic Reviews, 3,* 1–15.

United States Department of Health and Human Services. (2000). *Healthy people 2010. With understanding and improving health and objectives for improving health* (2nd ed., 2 vols.). Washington, DC: U.S. Government Printing Office.

University of Ulster. (2001). Second international symposium on human behavior in fire: Understanding human behavior for better fire safety design. Cambridge, MA.

University of Ulster. (2004). Third international symposium on human behavior in fire: Public fire safety—professionals in partnership. Belfast, UK. London: Interscience Communications.

Viscusi, W. K., & Cavallo, G. O. (1994). The effect of product safety regulation on safety precautions. *Risk Analysis, 14* (6), 917–930.

Warda, L., Tenenbein, M., & Moffatt, M. E. K. (1999a). House fire injury prevention update. Part 1. A review of risk factors for fatal and non-fatal house fire injury. *Injury Prevention, 5* (2), 145–150.

Warda, L., Tenenbein M., & Moffatt, M. E. K. (1999b). House fire injury prevention update. Part II. A review of the effectiveness of preventive interventions. *Injury Prevention, 5* (3), 217–225.

Watson, M., Kendrick, D., Coupland, C., Woods, A., Futers, D., & Robinson, J. (2005). Providing child safety equipment to prevent injuries: Randomised controlled trial. *British Medical Journal, 330* (7484), 178.

Weese, B. (1995). Fire and burn safety: Important issues for caregivers. *Caring, 14* (9), 40–42, 44.

Ytterstad, B., Smith, G. S., & Coggan, C. A. (1998). Harstad injury prevention study: Prevention of burns in young children by community based intervention. *Injury Prevention, 4* (3), 176–180.

Ytterstad, B., & Sogaard, A. J. (1995). The Harstad injury prevention study: Prevention of burns in small children by a community-based intervention. *Burns, 21* (4), 259–266.

Chapter **7**

Interventions to Prevent Sports and Recreation-Related Injuries

Julie Gilchrist, Gitanjali Saluja, and Stephen W. Marshall

7.1. INTRODUCTION

Participation in sports, recreation, and exercise is an important part of a healthy, physically active lifestyle; however, injuries due to sports and recreational activities are a significant public health problem. Injuries can occur as a result of organized sports activities in schools, clubs, or leagues; but many injuries also occur in informal settings, such as sports played in backyards or neighborhoods. In this chapter, we address injuries related to sports, such as basketball, football, and soccer; recreational activities, such as biking, skating, skiing, and playground activities; and exercise and training activities, such as weight training, aerobics, and jogging. Although swimming and other water sports are recreational activities, drowning prevention is addressed in another chapter.

Because participants engage in sports, recreation, and exercise mainly for fun and fitness, the risks inherent in these activities may not be recognized, and injury prevention measures are often overlooked. More than 11,000 people receive treatment in U.S. emergency departments (EDs) each day for injuries sustained while participating in recreational activities (Gotsch, Annest, Holmgreen, & Gilchrist, 2002). In addition, many injuries in sports and recreation are not treated in the emergency department but rather in acute care clinics, orthopedic offices, sports medicine clinics, and primary-care providers' offices. The social and economic costs associated with these injuries are high. An estimated 7 million participants seek medical care each year in the United States for injuries they sustain while participating in sports and recreational activities (Conn, Annest & Gilchrist, 2003). More than 20% of those injured lose at least 1 day of work or school due to their injuries. Participants often cite injuries as a reason that they stop taking part in potentially beneficial physical activities (Finch, Owen & Price, 2001; Hootman et al., 2003; Koplan, Powell, Sikes, Shirley, & Campbell, 1982). Furthermore, some injuries common in these activities such as traumatic brain injuries and knee injuries can have long-term consequences such as epilepsy (Thurman, Alverson, Dunn, Guerrero, & Sniezek, 1999) or premature osteoarthritis (Feller, 2004), respectively.

Injury surveillance in the United States suggests that the sports and recreational activities most commonly associated with injuries vary by age but include basketball, bicycling, exercising (e.g., aerobics, jogging, and weight training), football, baseball/softball, soccer, skating (ice/in-line/roller), snow sports, gymnastics/cheerleading, playground activities, and horseback riding. It is not currently possible to compare risks across activities because population-based participation estimates (or exposures) are not available. Given the fact that these are popular activities and public health mandates since the 1950's include promotion of regular exercise, the potential exposure to injury risk associated with these activities is high.

Injury risk varies by many factors. Traditionally, these are classified as either intrinsic or extrinsic to the individual. Intrinsic factors are personal qualities or characteristics. Some, such as age and gender, cannot be readily altered; however, others, such as level of fitness and playing skill, can be modified to reduce injury risk. For example, pre-season conditioning programs can improve athlete fitness and reduce injury risks, even in children. Extrinsic risk factors, on the other hand, are risk factors in the environment in which an individual participates. They are common to all participants and can include things such as the risk inherent in each activity, the physical attributes of the environment where the activity takes place, and even the weather. For instance, untethered movable soccer goal posts pose a risk for all players. Many of these risk factors in fitness activities have been identified through studies during military physical training. Table 7.1 presents a summary of common intrinsic and extrinsic risk factors identified by previous authors (Jones, Reynolds, Rock, & Moore, 1993).

Unfortunately, the risk factors and injury rates for each activity have not been fully delineated. Information regarding relative risks among different age groups and in different activities is sparse. Basic information on risk and protective factors and effectiveness of prevention programs for many activities is also lacking.

Researching sports- and recreation-related injuries and prevention measures can be difficult for a number of reasons. First, the nature of participation varies greatly. For instance, basketball is a very popular activity; it can be highly organized and competitive such as NCAA Division I basketball or played alone or with friends in driveways, playgrounds, or gyms at religious centers and schools. Each level of play has some risks that are similar and some that are different. Second, exposure information to provide adequate denominators is currently lacking. Current ED data systems provide estimates of the number of injuries seen in U.S. hospital EDs; however, without valid population-based information on exposure to sports and recreational activities, meaningful injury rates can not be calculated, and risks cannot be compared across groups or activities. Third, as noted previously, many injuries are not treated in EDs. As many as 40% of medically treated injuries may be seen outside of an ED (Conn et al., 2003; Gotsch et al., 2002). Fourth, the studies that have been conducted have used a wide variety of definitions of injury and exposure to sports/recreation; and as a result, comparisons of risks and rates across studies are difficult. For example, some studies capture any injury that affected participation, even if for only a few minutes, whereas others only capture injuries that required medical care, an ED visit or hospitalization. Finally, sports- and recreation-

Table 7.1. Intrinsic and Extrinsic Risk Factors for Musculo-skeletal Injuries Associated with Weight-Bearing Exercise and Activity[a]

Intrinsic Factors

Sex
Age (extremes)
Previous injury
Behavioral factors
    Smoking
    Previous physical activity/lifestyle (sedentary)
Physical fitness
    Aerobic endurance (low)
    Muscle endurance (low)
    Strength (low or imbalanced)
    Flexibility (extremes or imbalanced)
    Body composition (extremes)
Anatomic abnormalities
    High arches
    Bowed legs
    Leg-length discrepancies
Musculoskeletal disease
    Osteoporosis
    Arthritis

Extrinsic Factors

Training parameters (excessive or rapid increase)
    Duration
    Frequency
    Intensity
Environmental conditions (extremes or irregular)
    Terrain
    Surfacing
    Weather
Equipment (e.g., worn or improperly fitting footwear)

[a]Reprinted with permission from Jones et al. (1993).

related injury prevention often has been based on anecdotal evidence. Thus many of the interventions used today have not been subjected to rigorous trials and have become entrenched as common practice often without formal scientific evaluation using study designs such as randomized controlled trials. For example, stretching before strenuous exercise has long been encouraged as a means to prevent injury; however, trials and epidemiological studies of pre-exercise stretching have produced inconsistent results regarding any injury prevention effect (MacAuley & Best, 2002; Thacker, Gilchrist, Stroup, & Kimsey, 2004). Consensus by experts in the field can be a valid way to address some injury issues; however, practices resulting from consensus, while potentially beneficial, will not be addressed in this chapter.

Despite these challenges, several effective measures have been identified to reduce injury risk. Similar to infectious diseases, the occurrence of an injury is the result of interplay between the host (the participant), the vector or vehicle (the sport or activity), and the environment (both physical and sociocultural) in which the activity takes place.

Sleet (1994) described examples of the targeted use of strategies designed to reduce sports injuries related to the host, vector, and environment and how these strategies may overlap. The three types of strategies each target different causative factors in sports injury. The education/behavior change strategies primarily target changes in host or individual risk behavior. Policy/enforcement strategies primarily target the environment through changes in laws, policies, regulations, and compliance. Engineering/technology strategies primarily target the agent or vector of injury (i.e., the activity) and modify or reduce the amount of energy transferred. An adaptation of this model is presented in Figure 7.1. Categorization of interventions is complex—for instance, a helmet may be engineered to minimize energy transfer during an activity (vector); there may be a rule or law requiring its use (environment); but ultimately, the participant (host) must decide to wear it. Effective or promising strategies have been identified to alter aspects of each of these entities to reduce injury risks in common sports and recreational activities (Table 7.2). However, for many interventions in this area, research either hasn't been conducted or findings are conflicting, limiting science-based recommendations.

The remainder of this chapter addresses example interventions in each of the areas in the model, highlighting a few that have been shown to be effective or that show promise. This is not a systematic review of all sports-injury prevention interventions but rather seeks to highlight proven or promising interventions that are of special interest from a public health perspective and to identify measures that have been proven ineffective or for which further study is necessary (Table 7.2). Several excellent systematic reviews are available on the Internet, which provide in-depth information for specific sports (Harborview Injury Prevention and Research Center, 2005; Scanlan et al., 2001).

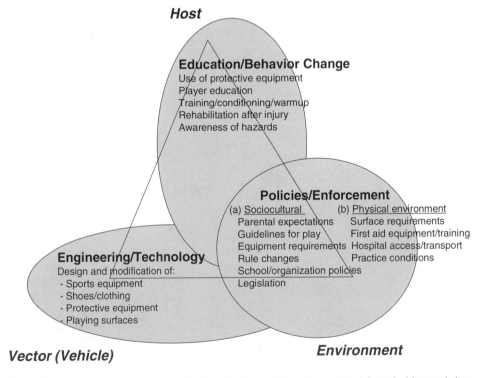

Figure 7.1. Intervention Strategies and Methods for Sports Injury Prevention. Adapted with permission from Sleet (1994).

Table 7.2. Examples of Injury Prevention Interventions in Common Activities

Activity	Proven	Promising/Potential	Not Evaluated, Insufficient or Conflicting Evidence
Baseball/softball	Breakaway bases Reduced-impact balls Faceguards/protective eyewear	Batting helmets Pitch count	Chest protectors
Basketball	Mouthguards	Ankle disk training Semirigid ankle stabilizers (especially with history of instability) Protective eyewear	Preventive knee braces
Bicycling	Helmet use (educational campaigns, laws, and subsidies all increase use)	Bike paths/lanes Retractable handlebars	Lighting on bike trails
Football	Helmets and other equipment Ankle braces rather than taping Minimizing cleat length Rule changes (no spearing, etc.) Playing field maintenance Preseason conditioning Cross-training reduces overuse Coach training/experience	Limiting practices with contact	Preventive knee braces Body pads
General	Fitness/conditioning	Return to play guidelines Attention to training parameters	Preexercise stretching Coaching factors related to injury prevention
Ice hockey	Helmet with full face shield down Rules (fair play, no checking from behind, no high sticking) Increased ice size	Enforcement of rules Discouraging fighting	Body pads
In-line skating/ skateboarding Playgrounds	Wrist guards Knee/elbow pads Shock-absorbing surfacing Height standards Maintenance standards	Helmets	
Running/jogging	Altered training regimen	Shock-absorbing insoles	Reflective clothing
Skiing/ snowboarding	Training to avoid risk situations Binding adjustment Wristguards in snowboarding	Helmets	
Soccer	Anchored, padded goal posts Shin guards Movement training (proprioceptive, neuromuscular, and plyometric training) Strength training		Head gear "Fair head" rule

7.2.   STRATEGIES TO AFFECT THE VECTOR (THE ACTIVITY)

The vector is the means by which energy is transmitted to the participant, causing injury. In the most general sense, the activity itself is the vector. More specifically, attributes of the activity serve as vectors: other athletes, the playing equipment, and even the playing surface (Fig. 7.1).

Strategies to alter the activity to increase safety generally are outside the realm of what an individual participant can undertake. This is the area in which science and technology can have a great effect in altering the energy transfer in sports and recreation by minimizing or eliminating it through the development of protective gear (e.g., helmets, pads), changes in sports equipment (e.g., bats, balls), through rules changes that alter how participants interact (e.g., spearing and checking rules, age/weight guidelines), or changes in policies to improve the quality of the playing surfaces (e.g., well-maintained surfaces with few undulations or hollows). Rules changes and other policies are addressed in the next section on altering the environment through policy, legislation, and enforcement.

Protective gear modifies the activity by preventing energy transfer above the injury threshold of a vulnerable portion of the body (e.g., the brain). Helmets, mouth guards, shoulder/knee/elbow pads, protective eyewear, and shin guards are examples of equipment that, in at least one activity, has been shown to protect the athlete by dissipating impact forces across the entire area of the pad, guard, or helmet, thereby vastly reducing the amount of force transmitted to a single vulnerable anatomical structure (such as the head or eye) (Table 7.2). However, the design and introduction of protective equipment are important so that protective gear does not interfere with the activity; no one wants to don a suit of armor to play a game of soccer or go for a run.

One alternative is to subtly modify the sports equipment used in the activity so that the energy transfer, although not completely prevented, is reduced or diverted in some way. For example, bicycle handlebars have been identified as responsible for serious abdominal injuries even from low-speed crashes (Winston et al., 1998). Using information from a surveillance system of traumatic injuries in a children's hospital ED and from on-site crash reports, engineers developed retractable handlebars to address this issue; they collapse on impact but spring back after the force is removed. This modification is not standard in the marketplace, but the design and technology exist to alter this risk, and the modification is under consideration to be included in new performance standards for handlebars (Arbogast, Cohen, Otoya, & Winston, 2001; Winston et al., 2002).

Several interventions in baseball and softball have used this concept of making sports equipment more yielding and less rigid. The observation by an orthopedic surgeon that many of his patients with broken ankles were injured during sliding in recreational baseball and softball led to the development of breakaway bases. Subsequently, research trials have documented their effectiveness in preventing these injuries not only among recreational players but also among collegiate and professional athletes (Janda et al., 1993; Janda, Wojtys, Hankin, & Benedict, 1988; Sendre, Keating, Hornak, & Newitt, 1994). Reduced-impact balls in baseball present an example of an equipment modification that moderates the force transferred to the participant during a contact with a ball. These balls are less stiff than a traditional baseball, and flatten out more when they make impact with an athlete's body, thereby moderating the force of impact; their use has been shown to decrease the risk of injury in youth baseball (Crisco, Hendee, & Greenwald, 1997; Marshall,

Mueller, Kirby, & Yang, 2003). In general, modifications of the sports equipment have been more successful when they reduce the risk of injury without reducing the participants' enjoyment of the recreational activity.

It is worth noting, however, that even subtle changes in equipment may have an effect on injury risk. In the 1960s, epidemiological research identified that increased cleat length was related to increased risk of knee injuries in football. This led to refinements in footwear for athletes that facilitate the rapid acceleration, deceleration, and side- and cross-cutting moves while minimizing the risk of injury (Robey, Blyth, & Mueller, 1971). It is quite possible there are other modifications to footwear that could reduce further the risk of lower limb injuries, however, the biomechanics of the interaction between surface and shoe are complex and poorly understood (Milburn & Barry, 1998). In a review of interventions to prevent shin splints in runners, shock-absorbent insoles were identified as showing some promise in reducing this debilitating overuse injury (Thacker, Gilchrist, Stroup, & Kimsey, 2002). In addition, knee braces have been proposed as a prophylactic intervention to prevent soft-tissue injury to these joints. Complexities regarding usage patterns and quality of fit surround the studies of prophylactic knee braces, and the evidence is equivocal at best (Albright, Saterbak, & Stokes, 1995; Thacker et al., 2003; Yang et al., 2005). There is considerably more evidence in support of ankle braces (Thacker et al., 1999).

7.3. STRATEGIES TO AFFECT THE SOCIOCULTURAL AND PHYSICAL ENVIRONMENT

The participant and the activity interact within the environment in which the activity is played. The environment refers to the actual physical space and location in which an activity takes place, including access to care in the event of an injury (i.e., proximity to medical staff or medical facilities). In addition, it refers to the sociocultural environment, which includes expectations of behavior; social norms; and policies governing the activity and their enforcement (Fig. 7.1).

7.3.1. Physical Environment

The physical environment in which an activity takes place can affect the likelihood of injury. Examples of strategies that alter the environment in which athletes participate include building bicycle paths, improving field conditions and padding, and removing obstacles near the area of play. For instance, maintenance of the playing field in football has been shown to reduce injury risk (Robey et al., 1971). The introduction of softer, impact-absorbing surfaces under playground equipment combined with ensuring that equipment meets height and maintenance standards (U.S. Consumer Product Safety Commission [CPSC], 2003) has decreased the number of serious injuries, including head injuries, due to falls (Norton, Nixon, & Sibert, 2004).

7.3.2. Sociocultural Environment

7.3.2.1. Policy

Policy changes (including rules, policies, legislation, and regulation) can be very effective in encouraging changes to reduce injury risks, not only in those participants covered by the policies but also in changing social norms (Schieber, Gilchrist,

& Sleet, 2000). Policies may be limited to a particular team or group (e.g., all bicycle club members must wear helmets on club rides) or may include legislation that encompasses all members of the population (e.g., state or local bicycle helmet laws). They may affect how the game is played (e.g., no heading in soccer under 10 years of age) or even who can participate (e.g., age and weight limits in children's football). Finally, they can govern standards for the equipment used and the environment in which activities take place (e.g., standards for playground safety).

Many activities have organizations, associations, or governing bodies that make recommendations or set requirements for the conduct of the activity. Common resources include governing bodies such as the National Collegiate Athletic Association (www.ncaa.org), and the National Federation of State High Schools Associations (www.nfhs.org); federal agencies such as the U.S. Consumer Product Safety Commission (www.cpsc.gov) and the Centers for Disease Control and Prevention (CDC) (www.cdc.gov); and professional organizations in medicine and health care, such as the National Athletic Trainers Association (www.nata.org), the American Academy of Pediatrics (www.aap.org), the American College of Sports Medicine (www.acsm.org), and the American Academy of Orthopedic Surgeons (www.aaos. org). These organizations and agencies may provide general injury prevention suggestions or recommendations regarding training; the set up and maintenance of the field of play and surrounding area; the gear that may be recommended, required, optional, or disallowed during participation; the rules of play; and the standards expected regarding any provision of medical care (Saluja, Marshall, Gilchrist, & Schroeder, 2006). In addition, specific sporting bodies provide recommendations for their sport. For example, USA Baseball recommendations to limit the number of pitches that youth pitchers throw ("pitch counts") show promise in the prevention of overuse injuries. Participants and coaches should be familiar with the various recommendations available regarding injury prevention in their chosen activity.

Rules of engagement and requirements regarding environment, gear, equipment, and participants represent fundamental policies for sports. In some situations, rule changes have been informed by injury data and research. Examples of effective policy changes include banning spearing (i.e., making initial contact with the head) in football and banning high sticking and checking from behind in ice hockey (Mueller, Cantu, & Van Camp, 1996; Watson, Singer, & Sproule, 1996). Furthermore, limiting practices in which there is full contact in NCAA football and introducing policies in support of the use of protective eyewear into women's lacrosse are both based on NCAA injury surveillance and show promise for injury prevention (R. W. Dick, personal communication, 2004). Research regarding the environment in ice hockey also has demonstrated that larger ice surfaces are associated with fewer injuries (Watson, Nystrom, & Buckolz, 1997). When the sport is played under fair play rules (where additional points are awarded when teams compete without excessive penalties) rather than standard rules, the injury rate, penalty rate, and severity of penalties significantly decline (Roberts, Brust, Leonard, & Herbert, 1996).

Schools are an ideal place to teach and advocate safe behavior for youth. The CDC (2001), in collaboration with specialists from universities and from national, federal, state, local, and voluntary agencies and organizations developed a comprehensive set of school health guidelines to prevent unintentional injuries, youth violence, and suicide. Among the guidelines, there are specific recommendations for safe physical education, sports, and recreational activities, including actions schools can take to develop, teach, implement, and enforce safety rules (Table 7.3).

Table 7.3. What Schools Can Do to Provide Safe Physical Education and Extracurricular Physical Activity Programs[a]

- Develop, teach, implement, and enforce safety rules
- Promote unintentional injury prevention and nonviolence through physical education and physical activity program participation
- Ensure that spaces and facilities for physical activity meet or exceed recommended safety standards for design, installation, and maintenance
- Hire physical education teachers, coaches, athletic trainers, and other physical activity program staff members who are trained in injury prevention, first aid, and CPR and provide them with ongoing staff development

Additional strategies to develop, teach, and enforce safety rules:

- Require physical assessment before participation
- Provide developmentally appropriate activities
- Ensure proper conditioning
- Provide student instruction regarding the biomechanics of specific motor skills
- Appropriately match participants according to size and ability
- Adapt rules to the skill level of young persons and the protective equipment available
- Avoid excesses in training
- Modify rules to eliminate unsafe practices
- Ensure that injuries, including concussions, are healed before allowing further participation
- Establish criteria, including clearance by a health care provider, for reentering play after an injury

[a]Adapted from CDC (2001) and Barrios, Sleet, and Mercy (2003).

Other CDC (2003, 2005a) materials provide coaches and school administrators with tools to create and maintain an action plan for prevention of traumatic brain injury and concussion.

7.3.2.2. Policy and Legislation

For recreational activities in which there is no governing administrative body, policy and legislation represents the major form of regulation of the social environment. Injury prevention legislation in sports and recreation has most commonly been focused on bicycle helmets and, more recently, protective gear in small-wheeled sports (i.e., in-line skating, skateboarding, scootering). These are typical activities that may involve interaction with motor vehicles, resulting in severe or fatal injuries. The first bicycle helmet law was passed in Victoria, Australia, in 1990 after a decade of targeted education campaigns. Following passage of the legislation, helmet use increased, but researchers also noted a decrease in bicycle riding (CDC, 1993). Since then in the United States, 16 states have passed helmet legislation primarily affecting children. Any policy or legislative action should be accompanied by education and enforcement to increase compliance by increasing understanding of the necessity of the rule and the consequences of inaction.

7.3.2.3. Other Factors

A large number of other factors in the social environment are not well understood—at least in terms of injury interventions—but are assumed to be powerful predictors of injury risk. These include coaching factors, expectations of behavior and social norms in the school or team environment, and parental attitudes. Coaching factors include level of training, experience, certification, and attitudes toward injury vs. achievement in sport. One study in football suggests that coaches who are over 30 years of age, have an advanced degree, and who have experience playing collegiate football have players with lower injury rates (Blyth & Mueller 1974); however, this relationship has not been examined for other activities. Thus the influence of these factors on injury risk—and how best to intervene to influence them—is currently unknown. Cultural expectations of behavior and social norms toward injury vary widely among different types of physical activity and level of competition. In some sports, such as rugby, injuries are almost regarded as a "badge of honor"; the first stop for the injured athlete is the club bar, rather than the physician's office. Experience from other fields suggests strategies to change this type of attitude, including peer or influential leaders to increase levels of professionalism in the sport. In addition, education of all those involved that injuries have potential life-long consequences, that they are preventable, and that injury prevention need not distract from the enjoyment or achievement in sports or recreation may assist in changing the social norms around injuries in sports, recreation, and exercise.

7.4. STRATEGIES TO AFFECT THE HOST (THE PARTICIPANT)

Many factors influence host susceptibility to injury. Some factors such as age, sex, and ability may not be easily alterable; however, others, such as the use of personal protective equipment, physical fitness and conditioning, warmup, rehabilitation after injury, and awareness of environmental hazards can be influenced to alter risk. Strategies to alter identified modifiable intrinsic risk factors (e.g., improving skill or fitness level) and participant behaviors that modify extrinsic risk factors likely to result in injury (e.g., choosing not to play on surfaces that are uneven or on terrain that is irregular) will help reduce injury. Probably, the most well known behavior to reduce sports-related injury is the decision to use protective gear. However, other measures, such as appropriate choice of activity and environment and appropriate training and conditioning for the chosen activity, also are important (Fig. 7.1).

7.4.1. Personal Protective Equipment

For all sports and recreational activities, use of appropriate protective gear is crucial and may be the most familiar personal injury prevention measure. In recreational and exercise activities, interventions to encourage acceptance and use of personal protective gear are especially important because, in these activities as opposed to organized sports, a participant may have little control over the environment and participation generally is not governed by rules and policies. Appropriate gear use is multifaceted and includes (1) obtaining the appropriate gear for the desired activity, (2) ensuring that it fits properly, (3) ensuring that it is well maintained and replaced when needed, and (4) using it consistently and properly.

Bicycle helmets are a familiar example of protective gear in a recreational activity. More than 700 bicyclists are killed each year, almost two thirds from head injuries (CDC, 1995, 2005b). Furthermore, an estimated 38,000 bicyclists are treated each year in emergency departments for brain injuries that occurred while cycling (unpublished data, National Electronic Injury Surveillance System—All Injury Program, CDC, 2005). Bicycle helmets have been proven effective in preventing both head and brain injury (Thompson, Rivara, & Thompson, 2000). Research and programmatic efforts over the past two decades have been focused largely on strategies to increase helmet use. Thompson, Sleet, and Sacks (2002) describe the foundational behavioral science research necessary for successful promotion programs, include a summary of research on these programs, and conclude that campaigns should be multifaceted and organized around a behavioral model to ensure a logical cohesive program. Additional CDC (1995) recommendations regarding bicycle helmet promotion include establishing a coalition, conducting awareness and education campaigns, using incentives (e.g., giveaways, coupons, and rebates), and encouraging helmet legislation mandating use. Similar promotion principles might be used to promote helmet use in other sports and settings.

Based on similar injury patterns and risk factors, helmets are also currently recommended for activities such as in-line skating, skateboarding, horseback riding, and winter sports (i.e., skiing and snowboarding) (CPSC, 1999, 2006). There has been some discussion about head protection gear in soccer; however, no controlled studies that support or refute the benefit of helmets in soccer have been identified (Institute of Medicine, 2002). The CPSC (2006) developed information to assist participants in choosing an appropriate helmet for their activity. In addition, helmets with full face shields in ice hockey have been shown to significantly reduce risk of facial and dental injuries, without an increase in the risk of neck injuries, concussions, or other injuries (Benson, Mohtadi, Rose, & Meeuwisse, 1999).

Encouraging the appropriate use of protective gear beyond helmets is important in preventing injuries to body parts other than the head. Wrist guards are effective in preventing injuries in activities during which the participant might fall on outstretched hands, such as in-line skating, skateboarding, and snowboarding (Idzikowski, Janes, & Abbott, 2000; Schieber et al., 1996). Ski poles with bowed grips were found to decrease thumb injuries in skiers who fall, and proper fitting and testing of ski bindings also reduced falls and injuries (Hauser, 1989). Finally, additional protection with knee and elbow pads have been proven effective in in-line skating and may be beneficial for other roller sports (e.g., skateboarding and roller skating) (Schieber et al., 1996). Organized team sports generally have specific gear that is recommended by the sponsoring organization, such as faceguards in youth baseball and mouth guards in basketball. These two recommendations are based on scientific studies of gear use in the sport (Labella, Smith, & Sigurdsson, 2002; Marshall et al., 2003); however, other recommendations for gear from sports organizations may be based on laboratory or other types of studies or expert consensus (Zvijac & Thompson, 1996; Vinger, Parver, Alfaro, Woods, & Abrams, 1997).

7.4.2. Physical Fitness and Conditioning

In recreation and fitness activities, as well as in team sports governed by rules and policies, participants can take an active role in minimizing the risk of injury. For instance, a review of military and civilian studies demonstrate that participants with the lowest levels of physical fitness are at increased risk of injury when compared to more fit counterparts participating at a similar level (Gilchrist, Jones, Sleet, & Kimsey, 2000). Attention to appropriate conditioning has been examined in football and demonstrated to reduce injury risk (Cahill & Griffith, 1978; Jones et al., 1993). The frequency, duration, and intensity of training are directly related to both the training effect and to injury risk. However, training in of itself presents an injury risk. Studies in runners indicate that a training threshold exists, above which increased training contributes substantially to increased injury risk but not to improved fitness levels (Pollock et al., 1977; Jones & Knapik, 1999). Thus attention to these parameters when planning training and practice regimens can limit acute and overuse injuries.

Some training programs have been designed to prevent specific injuries in certain high-risk sports. For instance, anterior cruciate ligament (ACL) injuries are common in sports such as basketball, soccer, volleyball, and handball, which require jumping, cutting, and rapid deceleration. Women are at an increased risk of ACL injury compared to their male counterparts in the same activities (Griffin et al., 2000). Training programs targeting improved balance, flexibility, strength, and/or neuromuscular control to avoid high-risk positions in basketball, volleyball, handball, and soccer have been developed and shown to be effective (Caraffa, Cerulli, Porjetti, Asia, & Rizzo, 1996; Gilchrist et al., 2004; Heidt, Sweeterman, Carlonas, Traub, & Tekulve, 2000; Hewett, Lidenfeld, Riccobene, & Noyes 1999; Myklebust et al., 2003; Olsen, Myklebust, Engebresten, Holme & Bàhr, 2005; Wedderkopp, Kaltoft, Holm, & Froberg, 2003). Most of these training programs were developed for a particular sport but could be adapted to other activities.

7.4.3. Warming Up and Stretching Before Exercise

Warmup and stretching exercises are common preparticipation practices in many recreational and sporting activities. Undertaking an appropriate warmup before a strenuous activity has been shown to decrease injury risk (Bixler & Jones, 1992). Warming up should consist of slowly increasing a participant's heart rate and body temperature, and moving through the expected range of motion of the activity (i.e., gentle golf swing, lower-speed pitch). Several recent systematic reviews of preexercise stretching as a means to prevent injuries concluded that insufficient evidence exists to recommend initiating routine preexercise stretching (Herbert & Gabriel, 2002; Shrier, 1999; Thacker et al., 2004). However, reviews of military risk factor studies demonstrate that those participants who are the least flexible and the most flexible are at an increased risk of injury during physical training, and stretching has been shown to increase flexibility (Gilchrist et al., 2000, Thacker et al., 2004). Thus one might hypothesize that maintaining flexibility in the midrange through a stretching program might reduce injury risk. On the other hand, if one is already very flexible, then perhaps stretching is not necessary or may be harmful. Further research is needed regarding the effect of stretching in populations of differing flexibility.

7.4.4. Rehabilitation After Injury

Participants also should ensure adequate rehabilitation and recovery time after an injury. For instance, in a review of the prevention of ankle sprains, the most commonly identified risk factor for a sprained ankle was a history of an ankle sprain. In particular, it appears that the greatest risk is within 6 months of the injury, suggesting that altering participation or use of a semirigid orthotic may reduce reinjury risk during this time (Thacker et al., 1999). In addition, participants sustaining a concussion and subsequently returning to physical competition before they have fully recovered are more susceptible to a second concussion (Guskiewicz et al., 2003) and possibly even have an elevated risk of sudden death from brain injury (Cantu, 1998a). Adequate recovery time after concussion is critical, and it is strongly recommended that patients seek medical evaluation by a health care provider familiar with the assessment and management of concussion to assist in the decision regarding returning to play (CDC, 1997). Because recovery occurs slowly, many recommend waiting at least 1 week following the total abatement of symptoms, not 1 week from the injury, before returning to full participation (American Academy of Neurology, 1997; Cantu, 1998b; Guskiewicz et al., 2004). Adherence to return to play guidelines shows promise in preventing consequences from concussion; however, further research is needed in this area.

7.4.5. Awareness of Environmental Hazards

In addition to choosing an appropriate activity and preparing themselves with the best available training and equipment, participants should also be attentive to the environment in which they engage in their chosen activity. For instance, a helmeted bicyclist on a bike path is likely at lower risk for injury than a helmeted bicyclist riding on the roadside with motor-vehicle traffic. In addition, an ice hockey game on an ungroomed frozen pond may result in more injuries than a game among the same participants in a well-groomed ice rink. Although some participants may not be able to change to another venue, they should be attentive to their current surroundings and make any possible changes to reduce injury risk (e.g., removing tripping hazards on and near the edges of a basketball court).

As illustrated in Figure 7.1, strategies affecting the vector, environment, and host often overlap. Education/behavior change strategies targeting the host, for example, may also have an effect on strengthening existing policies and enforcement by persuading policy makers, coaches, and school personnel to develop and enforce safe rules of play or treatment guidelines. It may also lead to the development of safer sports equipment and playing surfaces by educating manufacturers and sellers.

7.5. IMPLICATIONS FOR PUBLIC HEALTH PRACTICE

Public health policy currently encourages daily moderate to vigorous physical activity to improve the health and fitness of the population; this often involves participation in sports and recreational activities. Practitioners involved in physical activity promotion should be aware of injuries as both a barrier to and a potential outcome of physical activity. Practitioners have the opportunity to reduce the burden of these injuries by influencing the choices and behaviors of participants, by influencing the sociocultural and physical environment in which they participate, and by encouraging changes and innovations in design and engineering modifications of equipment, protective gear, and playing surfaces. The continued examination of these three elements contributing to sports injury will lead to improvements in the safety of sports and recreation participation.

Practitioners should caution participants about injury potential and include injury prevention messages in any physical-activity promotion materials. Practitioners and participants should follow current evidence-based recommendations from reputable organizations and agencies and should encourage the adoption of appropriate protective gear, sports equipment, and rules for participation. In addition, practitioners should reach out to other organizations and agencies that are working in physical activity promotion, sports, or recreation. Together, these interested parties can encourage decision makers in their schools and communities to work for safer public spaces for exercise and recreation, for safer equipment, and for policies encouraging safer behaviors to protect those at risk. For instance, many school and community playgrounds do not meet current safety standards for shock-absorbing surfacing, restrictions on equipment height, and equipment maintenance. Finally, practitioners can encourage the collection and examination of sports participation rates and injury information in their schools and communities to identify high-risk activities and help develop a plan of action for safe participation in sports and recreation.

7.6.   RESEARCH IMPLICATIONS

Injuries in sports and recreation are a diverse group of health consequences. Participants are varied in age, skill, development, level of participation, and choice of activity. Injuries can be short lived or have long-term consequences. While improvements have been made in surveillance of these injuries through the use of ED data, there continues to be a need for improved surveillance methods. Because ED information lacks details on the circumstances of the injury, the characteristics of the participant, and the exposure of the participant, comparisons across age groups and activities still are not possible. This information would allow the identification of individuals or activities of greater risk.

Specific research needs for many activities and several injuries have been identified (CDC, 2002a; Gilchrist et al., 2000; Harborview Injury Prevention and Research Center, 2005; Scanlan et al., 2001; Thacker et al., 1999; Thacker et al., 2003). Currently, information either is lacking or is conflicting regarding the effectiveness of certain protective gear (e.g., chest protectors in baseball, head gear in soccer), some environmental interventions (e.g., improved lighting on bike trails), and some proposed rule changes (e.g., the "fair head" rule in soccer). In addition to continuing efforts to examine these issues, research studies examining behavioral and social factors related to injury prevention would be useful. For instance, what influence do parents', players', coaches', and officials' attitudes toward injury prevention and competitiveness have on injury incidence? Finally, more and better information on the costs of sports injury is needed, including the cost effectiveness, cost benefit, and cost utility of preventive interventions to modify risk and protective factors associated with the host, environment, and vector (activity).

7.7.   CONCLUSIONS

Physical activity, through participation in sports and recreational activities, is an integral part of a healthy lifestyle. While these activities do not often result in fatalities, resultant injuries do represent a large burden on the health care system and often result in long-term consequences (i.e., osteoarthritis). Thus public health attention to these injuries is important. Changes in personal behavior and environmental conditions can help reduce many injuries (MacKay & Liller, 2006). For all sports and recreational activities, use of appropriate protective gear is crucial. Helmets are recommended for activities such as bicycling, in-line skating, skateboarding, horseback riding, and winter sports (e.g., skiing and snowboarding). Standard sports equipment (e.g., bicycle handlebars, baseballs) can be modified to reduce the risk of injury. Appropriate physical fitness and conditioning is also important. Sports participants should train for their chosen activity and should not undertake an activity for which they are not well prepared. Training should be well planned because some studies indicate that overtraining will increase the risk of injury without improving performance. Specific training programs also can be beneficial in improving balance, flexibility, strength, and neuromuscular control. While an effective warmup appears to reduce injury risk, the data on the effect of stretching before exercise are conflicting, and insufficient evidence exists to either recommend initiating or discontinuing routine preexercise stretching at this point.

It is important to advocate for improved safety in sports and recreation. Policy changes, including rules, policies, legislation, and regulation can be effective in encouraging implementation of effective interventions to reduce injury risks. Many activities have organizations, associations, and governing bodies that make recommendations or set requirements for the conduct of the activity. Schools are frequently amenable to changes designed to improve safety in athletic activities. Implementation of effective interventions in schools and sporting facilities has the potential for great impact because half of the injuries occur in these sites (Conn et al., 2003).

In addition to implementing widely what is already known to be effective, attention also should turn toward identifying additional safety measures. Some interventions that are common practice have not yet been evaluated (e.g., ski helmets) and others are known to be ineffective yet are still used (e.g., taping healthy ankles to prevent ankle sprain). Programs promoting physical activity should also include information on preventing activity-related injury. Improved dissemination of effective interventions should be considered where widespread uptake and use is lacking (Chapter 28). However, effective interventions have yet to be indentified for many injuries; many research priorities have been identified and just await support to be undertaken.

In summary, participation in sports and physical activity is important to maintaining the health of Americans. However, more attention to the safety aspects of all sports and recreational activities is needed so that the health benefits of participation are not offset by increases in injuries and their consequences.

REFERENCES

Albright, J. P., Saterbak, A., & Stokes, J. (1995). Use of knee braces in sports. *Sports Medicine, 20,* 281–301.

American Academy of Neurology. (1997). Practice parameter: The management of concussion in sports (summary statement). *Neurology, 48,* 581–585.

Arbogast, K. B., Cohen, J., Otoya, L., & Winston, F. K. (2001). Protecting the child's abdomen: A retractable bicycle handlebar. *Accident Analysis & Prevention, 33* (6), 753–757.

Barrios, L. C., Sleet, D. A., & Mercy, J. A. (2003). CDC school health guidelines to prevent unintentional injuries and violence. *American Journal of Health Education, 34* (5), S62–S64.

Benson, B. W., Mohtadi, N. G., Rose, M. S., & Meeuwisse, W. H. (1999). Head and neck injuries among ice hockey players wearing full face shields vs half face shields. *Journal of the American Medical Association, 282,* 2328–2332.

Bixler, B., & Jones, R. L. (1992). High-school football injuries: effects of a post-halftime warm-up and stretching routine. *Family Practice Research Journal, 12* (2), 131–139.

Blyth, C. S., & Mueller, F. O. (1974). Football injury survey 3. Injury rates vary with coaching. *Physician & Sportsmedicine, 2* (10), 71–78.

Cahill, B. R., & Griffith, E. H. (1978). Effect of pre-season conditioning on the incidence and severity of high school football knee injuries. *American Journal of Sports Medicine, 6* (4), 180–184.

Cantu, R. C. (1998a). Second-impact syndrome. *Clinics in Sports Medicine, 17* (1), 37–44.

Cantu, R. C. (1998b). Return to play guidelines after a head injury. *Clinics in Sports Medicine, 17* (1), 45–60.

Caraffa, A., Cerulli, G., Porjetti, M., Aisa, G., & Rizzo, A. (1996). Prevention of anterior cruciate ligament injuries in soccer. A prospective controlled study of proprioceptive training. *Knee Surgery, Sports Traumatology, Arthroscopy, 4* (1), 19–21.

Centers for Disease Control and Prevention. (1993). Mandatory bicycle helmet use—Victoria, Australia. *Morbidity & Mortality Weekly Report, 42* (18), 359–363.

Centers for Disease Control and Prevention. (1995). Injury-control recommendations: Bicycle helmets. *Morbidity & Mortality Weekly Report, Recommendations & Reports, 44* (RR-1), 1–18.

Centers for Disease Control and Prevention. (1997). Sports-related recurrent brain injuries—United States. *Morbidity & Mortality Weekly Report, 46* (10), 224–227.

Centers for Disease Control and Prevention. (2001). School health guidelines to prevent unintentional injuries and violence. *Morbidity & Mortality Weekly Report, Recommendations & Reports 50* (RR-22), 1–46.

Centers for Disease Control and Prevention. (2002). CDC injury research agenda. Atlanta, GA: National Center for Injury Prevention and Control.

Centers for Disease Control and Prevention. (2003). *Heads up: Brain injury in your practice.* Atlanta, GA: National Center for Injury Prevention and Control.

Centers for Disease Control and Prevention. (2005a). *Heads up: Concussion in high school sports.* Atlanta, GA: National Center for Injury Prevention and Control.

Centers for Disease Control and Prevention, National Centers for Injury Prevention and Control. (2005b). Web-based injury statistics query and reporting system (WISQARS). Retrieved August 26, 2005, from www.cdc.gov/ncipc/wisqars.

Conn, J. M., Annest, J. L., Gilchrist, J. (2003). Sports and recreation related injury episodes in the US population, 1997–99. *Injury Prevention, 9,* 117–123.

Crisco, J. J., Hendee, S. P., & Greenwald, R. M. (1997). The influence of baseball modulus and mass on head and chest impacts: A theoretical study. *Medicine & Science in Sports & Exercise, 29,* 26–36.

Feller, J. (2004). Anterior cruciate ligament rupture: Is osteoarthritis inevitable? *British Journal of Sports Medicine, 38,* 383–384.

Finch, C., Owen, N., & Price, R. (2001). Current injury or disability as a barrier to being more physically active. *Medicine & Science in Sports & Exercise, 33* (5), 778–782.

Gilchrist, J., Jones, B. H., Sleet, D. A., & Kimsey, C. D. (2000). Exercise related injuries among women: Strategies for prevention from military and civilian studies. *Morbidity & Mortality Weekly Report, Recommendations & Reports, 49* (RR-2), 13–33.

Gilchrist, J., Mandelbaum, B. R., Melancon, H., Ryan, G. W., Griffin, L. Y., Silvers, H. J., Watanabe, D. S., & Dick, R. W. (2004). A Randomized controlled trial to prevent non-contact anterior cruciate ligament injuries in female collegiate soccer players. Paper presented at the *American Orthopedic Society for Sports Medicine Annual Meeting.* San Francisco, CA.

Gotsch, K., Annest, J. L., Holmgreen, P., & Gilchrist, J. (2002). Nonfatal sports- and recreation-related injuries treated in emergency departments, United States, July 2000–June 2001. *Morbidity & Mortality Weekly Report, 51* (33), 736–740.

Griffin, L. Y., Agel, J., Albohm, M. J., Arendt, E. A., Dick, R. W., Garrett, W. E., Garrick, J. G., Hewett, T. E., Huston, L., Ireland, M. L., Johnson, R. J., Kibler, W. B., Lephart, S., Lewis, J. L., Lindenfeld, T. N., Mandelbaum, B. R., Marchak, P., Teitz, C. C., & Wojtys, E. M. (2000). Noncontact anterior cruciate ligament injuries: Risk factors and prevention strategies. *Journal of the American Academy of Orthopaedic Surgeons, 8,* 141–150.

Guskiewicz, K. M., Bruce, S. L., Cantu, R. C., Ferrara, M. S., Kelly, J. P., McCrea, M., Putukian, M., & McLeod, T. C. (2004). Recommendations on management of sport-related concussion: Summary of the National Athletic Trainers' Association position statement. *Neurosurgery, 55* (4), 891–895.

Guskiewicz, K. M., McCrea, M., Marshall, S. W., Cantu, R. C., Randolph, C., Barr, W., Onate, J. A., & Kelly, J. P. (2003). Cumulative effects associated with recurrent concussion in collegiate football players: The NCAA concussion study. *Journal of the American Medical Association, 290,* 2549–2555.

Harborview Injury Prevention and Research Center. (2005). Best practices: Recreational injuries. Retrieved August 26, 2005, from http://depts.washington.edu/hiprc/practices/topic/recreation/index.html.

Hauser, W. (1989). Experimental prospective skiing injury study. In C. D. Mote Jr., R. J. Johnson, & M. H. Binet (Eds.), *Skiing trauma and safety: Seventh international symposium, ASTM STP 1022* (pp. 18–24). Philadelphia: American Society for Testing and Materials.

Heidt, R. S. Jr., Sweeterman, L. M., Carlonas, R. L., Traub, J. A., & Tekulve, F. X. (2000). Avoidance of soccer injuries with preseason conditioning. *American Journal of Sports Medicine, 28* (5), 659–662.

Herbert, R. D., & Gabriel, M. (2002). Effects of stretching before and after exercising on muscle soreness and risk of injury: A systematic review. *British Medical Journal, 325,* 468–470.

Hewett, T. E., Lidenfeld, T. N., Riccobene, J. V., & Noyes, F. R. (1999). The effect of neuromuscular training on the incidence of knee injury in female athletes: A prospective study. *American Journal of Sports Medicine, 27* (6), 699–706.

Hootman, J. M., Macera, C. A., Ainsworth, B. E., Addy, C. L., Martin, M., & Blair, S. N. (2003). Epidemiology of musculoskeletal injuries among sedentary and physically active adults. *Medicine & Science in Sports & Exercise, 34* (5), 838–844.

Idzikowski, J. R., Janes, P. C., & Abbott, P. J. (2000). Upper extremity snowboarding injuries. Ten-year results from the Colorado snowboard injury survey. *American Journal of Sports Medicine, 28* (6), 825–832.

Institute of Medicine. (2002). *Is soccer bad for children's heads? Summary of the IOM workshop on neuropsychological consequences of head impacts in youth soccer.* Washington, DC: National Academy Press.

Janda, D. H., Mackesy, D., Maguire, R., Hawkins, R. J., Fowler, P., & Boyd, J. (1993). Sliding-associated injuries in college and professional baseball—1990–1991. *Morbidity & Mortality Weekly Report, 42* (12), 229–230.

Janda, D. H., Wojtys, E. M., Hankin, F. M., & Benedict, M. E. (1988). Softball sliding injuries. A prospective study comparing standard and modified bases. *Journal of the American Medical Association, 259,* 1848–1850.

Jones, B. H., & Knapik, J. J. (1999). Physical training and exercise-related injuries: Surveillance, research, and injury prevention in military populations. *Sports Medicine, 27,* 111–125.

Jones, B. H., Reynolds, K. L., Rock, P. B., & Moore, M. P. (1993). Exercise-related musculoskeletal injuries: Risks, prevention and care. In J. L. Durstine, A. C. King, P. L. Painter, J. L. Roitman, L. D. Zwiren, & W. L. Kenny (Eds.), *Resource manual for guidelines for exercise testing and prescription* (pp. 378–393, 2nd ed.). Philadelphia: Lea & Febiger.

Koplan, J. P., Powell, K. E., Sikes, R. K., Shirley, R. W., & Campbell, C. C. (1982). An epidemiologic study of the benefits and risks of running. *Journal of the American Medical Association, 248* (23), 3118–3121.

Labella, C. R., Smith, B. W., & Sigurdsson, A. (2002). Effect of mouthguards on dental injuries and concussions in college basketball. *Medicine & Science in Sports & Exercise, 34* (1), 41–44.

MacAuley, D., & Best, T. M. (2002). Reducing risk of injury due to exercise: Stretching before exercise does not help. *British Medical Journal, 325,* 451–452.

MacKay, M., & Liller, K. (2006). Behavioral considerations for sports and recreational injuries in children and youth. In A. C. Gielen, D. A. Sleet, & R. DiClemente (Eds.), *Injury and violence prevention: Behavior change theories, methods and applications.* San Francisco: Jossey-Bass.

Marshall, S. W., Mueller, F. O., Kirby, D. P., & Yang, J. (2003). Evaluation of safety balls and faceguards for prevention of injuries in youth baseball. *Journal of the American Medical Association, 289* (5), 568–574.

Milburn, P. D., & Barry, E. B. (1998). Shoe-surface interaction and the reduction of injury in rugby union. *Sports Medicine, 25,* 319–327.

Mueller, F. O., Cantu, R. C., & Van Camp, S. P. (1996). *Catastrophic injuries in high school and college sports.* Campaign, IL: Human Kinetics.

Myklebust, G., Engebretsen, L., Brækken, I. H., Skjølberg, A., Olsen, O. E., & Bahr, R. (2003). Prevention of anterior cruciate ligament injuries in female team handball players: A prospective intervention study over three seasons. *Clinical Journal of Sports Medicine, 13,* 71–78.

Norton, C., Nixon, J., & Sibert, J. R. (2004). Playground injuries to children. *Archives of Disease in Childhood, 89,* 103–108.

Olsen, O. E., Myklebust, G., Engebretsen, L., Holme, I., & Bahr, R. (2005). Exercises to prevent lower limb injuries in youth sports: Cluster randomized controlled trial. *British Medical Journal, 330* (7489), 449.

Pollock, M. L., Gettman, L. R., Milesis, C. A., Bah, M. D., Durstine, L., & Johnson, R. B. (1977). Effects of frequency and duration of training on attrition and incidence of injury. *Medicine & Science in Sports & Exercise, 9,* 31–36.

Roberts, W. O., Brust, J. D., Leonard, B., & Herbert, B. J. (1996). Fair-play rules and injury reduction in ice hockey. *Archives of Pediatrics & Adolescent Medicine, 150* (2), 140–145.

Robey, J. M., Blyth, C. S., & Mueller, F. O. (1971). Athletic injuries: Application of epidemiologic methods. *Journal of the American Medical Association, 217,* 184–189.

Saluja, G., Marshall, S. W., Gilchrist, J., & Schroeder, T. (2006). Sports and recreational injuries. In Liller, K. (Ed). *Injury prevention for children and adolescents* (pp 253–254). Washington, DC.: American Public Health Association.

Scanlan, A., MacKay, M., Reid, D., Olsen, L., Clark, M., McKim, K., & Raina, P. (2001). Sports and recreation injury prevention strategies: Systematic review and best practices. Retrieved August 25, 2005, from www.injuryresearch.bc.ca/Publications/Reports/SportSystematicReport.pdf.

Schieber, R. A., Branche-Dorsey, C. M., Ryan, G. W., Rutherford, G. W. Jr., Stevens, J. A., & O'Neil, J. (1996). Risk factors for injuries from in-line skating and the effectiveness of safety gear. *New England Journal of Medicine, 335* (22), 1630–1635.

Schieber, R. A., Gilchrist, J., & Sleet, D. A. (2000). Legislative and regulatory strategies to reduce childhood unintentional injuries. *Future of Children, 10* (1), 111–136.

Sendre, R. A., Keating, T. M., Hornak, J. E., & Newitt, P. A. (1994). Use of the hollywood impact base and standard stationary base to reduce sliding and base-running injuries in baseball and softball. *American Journal of Sports Medicine, 22,* 450–453.

Shrier, I. (1999). Stretching before exercise does not reduce the risk of local muscle injury: A critical review of the clinical and basic science literature. *Clinical Journal of Sports Medicine, 9,* 221–227.

Sleet, D. A. (1994). Injury prevention. In P. Cortese & K. Middleton (Eds.), *The comprehensive school health challenge: Promoting health through education.* (pp. 443–489). Santa Cruz, CA: ETR Associates.

Thacker, S. B., Gilchrist, J., Stroup, D. F., & Kimsey, C. D. (2002). The prevention of shin splints in sports: A systematic review of literature. *Medicine & Science in Sports & Exercise, 34* (1), 32–40.

Thacker, S. B., Gilchrist, J., Stroup, D. F., & Kimsey, C. D. (2004). The impact of stretching on sports injury risk: A systematic review of the literature. *Medicine & Science in Sports & Exercise, 36* (3), 371–378.

Thacker, S. B., Stroup, D. F., Branche, C. M., Gilchrist, J., Goodman, R. A., & Porter-Kelling, E. (2003). Prevention of knee injuries in sports. A systematic review of the literature. *Journal of Sports Medicine & Physical Fitness, 43* (2), 165–179.

Thacker, S. B., Stroup, D. F., Branche, C. M., Gilchrist, J., Goodman, R. A., & Weitman, E. A. (1999). The prevention of ankle sprains in sports: A systematic review of the literature. *American Journal of Sports Medicine, 27* (6), 753–760.

Thompson, D. C., Rivara, F. P., & Thompson, R. (2000). Helmets for preventing head and facial injuries in bicyclists (CD001855). *Cochrane Database of Systematic Reviews,* (2).

Thompson, N. J., Sleet, D., & Sacks, J. J. (2002). Increasing the use of bicycle helmets: Lessons from behavioral science. *Patient Education and Counseling, 46* (3), 191–197.

Thurman, D. J., Alverson C., Dunn, K. A., Guerrero, J., & Sniezek, J. E. (1999). Traumatic brain injury in the United States: A public health perspective. *Journal of Head Trauma Rehabilitation, 14* (6), 602–615.

U.S. Consumer Product Safety Commission. (1999). *Skiing helmets: An evaluation of the potential to reduce head injury.* Washington, DC: Author.

U.S. Consumer Product Safety Commission. (2003). *Handbook for public playground safety* (Publication No. 325). Washington, DC: Author.

U.S. Consumer Product Safety Commission. (2006). *Which helmet for which activity?* Washington, DC: Author.

Vinger, P. F., Parver, L., Alfaro, D. V. 3rd., Woods, T., & Abrams, B. S. (1997). Shatter resistance of spectacle lenses. *Journal of the American Medical Association, 277* (2), 142–144.

Watson, R. C., Singer, C. D., & Sproule, J. R. (1996). Checking from behind in ice hockey: A study of injury and penalty data in the Ontario University Athletic Association Hockey League. *Clinical Journal of Sport Medicine, 6* (2), 108–111.

Watson, R. C., Nystrom, M. A., & Buckolz, E. (1997). Safety in Canadian junior ice hockey: The association between ice surface size and injuries and aggressive penalties in the Ontario Hockey League. *Clinical Journal of Sport Medicine, 7* (3), 192–195.

Wedderkopp, N., Kaltoft, M., Holm, R., & Froberg, K. (2003). Comparison of two intervention programmes in young female players in European handball—With and without ankle discs. *Scandinavian Journal of Medicine & Science in Sports, 13* (6), 371–375.

Winston, F. K., Shaw, K. N., Kreshak, A. A., Schwarz, D. F., Gallagher, P. R., & Cnaan, A. (1998). Hidden spears: Handlebars as injury hazards to children. *Pediatrics, 102* (3, part 1), 596–601.

Winston, F. K., Weiss, H. B., Nance, M. L., Vivarelli-O'Neill, C., Strotmeyer, S., Lawrence, B. A., & Miller, T. R. (2002). Estimates of the incidence and costs associated with handlebar-related injuries in children. *Archives of Pediatrics & Adolescent Medicine, 156* (9), 922–928.

Yang, J., Marshall, S. W., Bowling, J. M., Runyan, C. W., Mueller, F. O., & Lewis, M. A. (2005). Use of discretionary protective equipment and rate of lower extremity injury in high school athletes. *American Journal of Epidemiology, 161* (6), 511–519.

Zvijac, J., & Thompson, W. (1996). Basketball. In D. J. Caine, C. G. Caine, & K. J. Lindner (Eds.), *Epidemiology of Sports Injuries* (pp. 86–97). Champaign, IL: Human Kinetics Publishers, Inc.

Violence Prevention

Chapter **8**

Interventions to Prevent Child Maltreatment

Deborah A. Daro and Karen P. McCurdy

8.1. INTRODUCTION

The term *child maltreatment* has been used by advocates and policy makers to describe a set of individual behaviors toward children as well as a set of social conditions (Daro, 1989; Helfer, Kempe, & Krugman, 1997). Parental behaviors considered as abusive or neglectful include, among others, the willful or intentional physical beating of a child; the failure to provide for a child's basic emotional and physical needs; overt emotional abuse of a child through continuous belittling, inappropriate control, or extreme inconsistency; and the sexual mistreatment of a child or use of a child for sexual pleasure. Social norms and public policies that condone and, sometimes, promote corporal punishment or high levels of violence and sexually explicit language in the media as well as child poverty, inadequate housing, failing educational systems, and limited access to preventive health care also represent, in the eyes of some, society's collective maltreatment of its children (Garbarino, 1997; Straus, 1994). Given this diversity in perspectives, it is understandable that the field has struggled with defining the problem's scope, consequences, and appropriate interventions.

Setting aside the issue of social conditions and inadequate welfare and support systems, the number of children directly abused or neglected is substantial. One of the earliest and most rigorous studies on the annual incidence of maltreatment estimated that in 1968 between 2 and 4 million families either failed to act or used physical force with the intent of hurting, injuring, or killing their children (Gil, 1970). Since that time, repeated household surveys and national incidence studies consistently document a problem of substantial proportion and one that affects children of all ages and socioeconomic groups (Finkelhor, Ormrod, Turner, & Hamby, 2005; Gelles & Straus, 1988; Sedlak & Broadhurst, 1996). Indeed, state and local child protective services (CPS) agencies investigated or assessed an estimated 1,800,000 referrals alleging child abuse or neglect in 2002. These referrals included more than 3 million children and, of those, approximately 869,000 (12.3 per 1,000) were determined to be victims of maltreatment (U.S. Department of Health and Human Services [HHS], 2004).

The consequences of maltreatment vary, depending on a child's age; the duration and severity of the abuse; the co-occurrence of other forms of maltreatment; and other conditions known to be harmful to a child's immediate well-being and subsequent development, such as domestic violence, substance abuse, and parental mental health (Chalk, Gibbons, & Scarupa, 2002). Maltreatment's immediate physical effects range from relatively minor trauma (e.g., bruises, cuts) to serious and permanent injuries such as broken bones; intracranial and intraocular brain hemorrhages; and changes in the part of the brain linked to memory, emotions, and basic drives (Conway, 1998; Kempe, Silverman, Steele, Droememuller, & Silver, 1962; Perry, 2001). Medical neglect can result in minor developmental delays and common childhood illnesses going undiagnosed or untreated. Over time, these conditions can result in permanent physical impairment (e.g., hearing loss) or more profound delays in a child's cognitive and social development (Gaudin, 1999).

In addition, studies have documented direct affects of maltreatment on a young victim's cognitive development, including language deficits, reduced cognitive functioning, and attention deficit disorders (Kendall-Tackett & Eckenrode, 1996). Although it is unclear if such disorders are a direct result of maltreatment or a consequence of other economic or social deprivations, maltreatment victims often do poorly in school, leading to high drop-out rates and limited long-term economic self-sufficiency (Courtney, Terao, & Bost, 2004; HHS, 2003).

And victims of all forms of maltreatment often present with adult histories of physical and mental health disorders, including depression, hopelessness, and low self-esteem (Egeland & Stroufe, 1981; Jungmeen & Cicchetti, 2003; Kendall-Tackett, 2003; Lamphear, 1985). Such victims can develop antisocial behavior and physical aggression and struggle to establish and maintain trusting and supportive relationships throughout their lives (Morrison, Frank, Holland, & Kates, 1999; Widom & Maxfield, 2001).

Over the years, child maltreatment researchers and practitioners have explicitly recognized that most maltreatment results from a complex web of factors found within a person's personality, family history, and community context (Garbarino, 1977; Bronfenbrenner, 1979; Belsky, 1980). Ecological theory, with its acknowledgment that individual, familial, community, and societal factors interact to increase or decrease the likelihood of child maltreatment, now represents the most commonly accepted theory of maltreatment (Cicchetti & Rizley, 1981). Unfortunately, most prevention programs have the capacity to address only a fraction of these causal factors, a reality that can complicate efforts to assess a program's effectiveness. No single intervention will successfully remediate the consequences of all types of maltreatment, nor will it spare all children from initial or repeated abuse or neglect. Selecting the appropriate intervention is largely in the hands of practitioners and those allocating scarce public and private resources. The purpose of this chapter is to outline the continuum of choices available to these decision makers in a way that makes the best use of what we have learned.

8.2.   BRIEF HISTORY OF PREVENTION

Over the past 30 years, efforts to prevent child maltreatment have moved through three stages: public recognition of the problem, experimentation with a wide range of prevention programs addressing one or more factors believed to increase a child's risk for maltreatment, and the evolution of systems designed to better integrate these diverse efforts (Cohn, 1987; Daro & Cohn-Donnelly, 2002a).

Programmatic efforts to prevent child abuse and neglect have followed two distinct paths: interventions targeting reductions in physical abuse and neglect (including emotional neglect and attachment disorders) and interventions targeting reductions in child sexual abuse (Daro, 1989; Daro & Cohn-Donnelly, 2002b). Programs in the first group began with an emphasis on parental knowledge or parental behavior as the "cause" of maltreatment, with services designed to address the cause (e.g., parent education workshops). Such programs have evolved in concert with the ecological paradigm to addressing the broader context in which the parent–child relationship develops. It is common for today's prevention programs to focus on parental-support networks, health care access, and parent–child interaction patterns, in addition to the more traditional emphasis on parental behavior or knowledge. Furthermore, these programs tend to focus on new parents, offering assistance when a child is born or a woman is pregnant (Daro, 2000). Subsequent prevention services are then added to this universal base in response to the specific emerging needs presented by the growing child or the evolving parent–child relationship (Guterman, 2001; Melton & Berry, 1994).

In contrast to efforts to prevent physical abuse or neglect, the target population for sexual abuse prevention has been potential victims, not potential perpetrators. Three factors contributed to this pattern: the social discomfort surrounding sexuality, the difficulty in developing voluntary treatment options for offenders, and the absence of clear risk factors identifying potential perpetrators or victims (Daro, 1994). Strategies within this framework include a number of educational-based efforts, provided on a universal basis, to children on the distinction between good, bad, and questionable touching and the concept of body ownership or the rights of children to control who touches their bodies and where they are touched (Wurtele & Miller-Perrin, 1992). As children mature, these classes cover a broader range of concepts, such as appropriate dating behavior, gender stereotypes, and nonaggressive conflict resolution strategies (Wolfe, MacPherson, Blount, & Wolfe, 1986). These educational programs also offer children and youth service options or referrals if they have been abused or are involved in an abusive peer relationship. Although most of these efforts include some type of orientation or instruction for both the parents and school personnel on how to detect and respond to suspected cases of sexual assault, their primary emphasis is making children less vulnerable.

Several policy and contextual factors have influenced the structure and focus of the current pool of child maltreatment prevention services. At the center of this shift is a general dissatisfaction with many therapeutic interventions, particularly with the ability of services to alter the trajectory of families with extensive histories of serious physical abuse and neglect. Extensive reviews of a wide range of treatment modalities find very few with strong, empirical evidence of effectiveness (Saunders, Berliner, & Hanson, 2003). Those interventions that have demonstrated the greatest promise are generally embedded in ecological theories of human development and cognitive learning theories, offer intensive services, and have a strong research base (Henggeler, Melton, Brondino, Scherer, & Hanley, 1997; Kolko, 2002; Lutzker, 2000). In addition, a child's first 3 years of life has become a major focus among those seeking better outcomes for children in numerous cognitive, emotional, and social domains (Carnegie Task Force on Meeting the Needs of Young Children [CTF], 1994; Shonkoff & Phillips, 2000). Given that the highest prevalence rates for both child maltreatment reports and placement in foster care involve children under the age of 1 year (Wulczyn, Barth, Yuan, Jones Harden, & Landsverk, 2005), the importance of early and thoughtful intervention for the birth to 3 population has become even more salient.

Today, the concept of prevention is moving away from the notion of a single-response agency or targeted intervention and more toward a communitywide system of shared responsibility and mutual support. As Melton, Thompson, and Small (2002) noted, achieving child protection becomes a shared, moral responsibility "not merely to prevent wrongdoing, but to achieve positive obligations as well" (p. 11). When this moral responsibility is jointly shared by every resident and every agency, a community can begin building the type of reciprocity and mutual support viewed by many as essential to achieving a higher standard of care for children (Melton & Berry, 1994). Although such systems are far from operational in any community, the goal of altering both the individual and the context provides a programmatic and policy response more reflective of the ecological theory often cited as the most appropriate in explaining the cause of child maltreatment.

8.3.   CHAPTER PREVIEW

The purpose of this chapter is to focus on the documented effects of a number of universal and targeted prevention services and, to the extent possible, identify those program features associated with more robust outcomes. In judging the effectiveness of the various interventions we reviewed, we primarily focused on interventions that had evidence of a reduction in child abuse and neglect reports and other child safety outcomes, such as reported injuries and accidents. In addition to these outcomes, we identified programs with documented effects on risk factors that correlate with child maltreatment, including parent characteristics, child characteristics, and the parent–child relationship. We believe that reviewing programs in light of both their distal and proximate outcomes is important as it reflects the ecological framework that guides most prevention programs and has the greatest utility for moving the field forward.

In light of the growing attention being given to early intervention services, our review pays special attention to the evidence surrounding programs that target parents of newborns and young children. Our data base involved a detailed review of meta-analyses conducted on specific program models (e.g., home visitation programs, child assault prevention efforts) as well as broad categories of programs (e.g., family-support efforts, early intervention programs). These data were augmented by an examination of specific evaluation studies conducted on both single-site as well as nationally replicated programs. We also reviewed Web-based summaries of model or exemplary programs as a secondary source for identifying evaluations beyond those typically included in academic, meta-analyses such as Blueprints for Violence Prevention (Center for the Study and Prevention of Violence) and Substance Abuse and Mental Health Services Administration (SAMHSA)'s National Registry for Effective Programs.

Following this presentation, the chapter identifies the key programmatic and policy recommendations emerging from our review. This section pays particular attention to questions of appropriate target populations, scope, critical outcomes, staff characteristics, and replication methods. In addition, the chapter addresses the key research and evaluation questions central to improving our ability to design, implement, and integrate preventive services. The chapter concludes with a set of general recommendations regarding the importance of developing more community-focused interventions.

8.4.   INTERVENTIONS AND THEIR EVIDENCE BASE

Table 8.1 summarizes the range of interventions we examined and their relative success in achieving measurable reductions on direct indictors of child maltreatment as well as proximate indicators of this construct. As noted earlier, this choice reflects the overall goals of most prevention programs and the theory that changing parental or child attitudes and behaviors will prevent child maltreatment. Maltreatment indicators include both reported and substantiated CPS cases of abuse or neglect and proxy measures of abuse and neglect such as emergency room visits and hospitalization for injuries or accidental ingestions (Hahn, Mercy, Bilukha, & Briss, 2005). Related outcomes consist of observational measures of attachment, measures of parental attitudes, knowledge and behavior, and child outcomes such as cognition and social-emotional development.

Whenever possible, we rely on meta-analyses to assess the effectiveness of prevention efforts. It should be noted that differences in meta-analytic techniques can lead to disparate findings. The meta-analyses reviewed here all share two approaches that help increase their comparability: (1) poorly designed studies (e.g., no comparison group) are excluded, and (2) nonpublished studies or government reports are included. In addition, when differences arise, we discuss the procedural differences that may have led to divergent findings.

Table 8.1. Summary of Effectiveness of Child Maltreatment Prevention Strategies[a]

Type of Prevention Strategy	Reports of Abuse or Neglect and Proxy Measures[b] (injuries, accidents, emergency room visits)	Related Outcomes[c]
Products		
Soft baby carriers	3	4
Physical environments	3	3
Behavioral interventions		
Individual/parent level		
Newsletters and print materials	3	2
Videotapes	3	4
Parent education and support	3	4
Family level		
Early home visitation	5	5
School level		
Sexual abuse prevention	4	4
Community level	3	3
Societal level		
Media campaigns	3	3

[a] The scale is as follows: 5, effective (supported by two or more well-designed studies or systematic review); 4, promising (supported by one well-designed study, similar to effective intervention, expert consensus of benefits); 3, insufficient evidence (not enough research, insufficient evidence, mixed evidence); 2, not effective (no effect found in two or more well-designed studies or systematic review); 1, harmful (negative effect found in two or more well-designed studies or systematic review).
[b] Examples include injuries, accidents, and emergency room visits.
[c] Examples include parental attitudes, knowledge and behaviors, parent–child interactions, and child outcomes.

8.4.1.   Products

Although products are not traditionally a part of child maltreatment prevention strategies, one product, soft baby carriers, represents a promising strategy for enhancing mother–child attachment and maternal sensitivity, two factors believed to protect against maternal neglect (Anisfeld, Cusper, Nozyce, & Cunningham, 1990). A randomized study of soft baby carriers versus infant seats found that the use of soft baby carriers significantly increased maternal responsiveness and secure attachment in infants as compared to the use of infant seats (Anisfeld et al., 1990). Two related randomized controlled studies support this approach. Hunziker & Barr (1986) found that increased maternal carrying of young infants, whether by arms or soft baby carriers, significantly reduced infant crying and fussiness and increased periods of infant content. Furthermore, Tessier et al. (1998) reported that skin-to-skin contact between treatment mothers and their low birth weight infants significantly increased maternal competence and sensitivity as compared to control mothers receiving traditional hospital services. As a group, the studies report positive effects on both mother and child of strategies that promote early periods of close, physical contact.

8.4.2.   Behavioral: Individual Focus

8.4.2.1.   Media

Videotapes have been successfully used to educate parents around many important child health issues (Glascoe, Oberklaid, Dworkin, & Trimm, 1998). Our search produced only one study of relevance to early child maltreatment prevention efforts. Black and Teti (1997) examined the effect of a culturally sensitive video-tape depicting both successful and unsuccessful strategies for parents to employ when feeding infants. Findings from a randomized study of the video's impact on first-time African American teen mothers demonstrated that treatment mothers reported significantly more positive parental attitudes and more parent–child inter-action during feedings than control mothers. The treatment mothers also received significantly higher ratings on an observational measure of involvement during a feeding session. As other research corroborates the use of videotapes for stimulat-ing behavioral change for parents of children with conduct disorders (Webster-Stratton, 1994), the research suggests that videotapes are a promising strategy that prevention programs should consider incorporating into their program arsenal.

In contrast to videotapes, prevention programs are more likely to include print materials as part of their effort to educate parents about normative child develop-ment, activities to promote learning, and the physical needs of infants. Insufficient evidence exists to support this strategy. Although early studies suggested some posi-tive effects, lack of comparison groups, single point in time measures, sole reliance on parental reports, and low response rates characterized much of this research (Cudabak, et al., 1985; Riley, Meinhardt, Nelson, Salisbury, & Winnett, 1991). A more rigorous study using comparison groups reported little effects on parental attitudes (Laurendeau, Gagnon, Desjardins, Perreault, & Kischuk, 1991).

8.4.2.2.   Parent Education and Support Groups

Educational and support services delivered to parents in the context of center-based programs or in group settings have been used in a variety of ways to address the risk factors associated with child abuse and neglect. At least one national survey estimates that more than 100,000 groups of parents meet every year in the United States to attend parent education classes, to provide mutual support to other parents, and to advocate for better services or public policy options (Carter, 1995).

Although the primary focus of these interventions is often on the parent, virtually all of the most frequently replicated models include opportunities for structured parent–child interactions and many incorporate parallel interventions for children. This multicomponent approach is particularly true when the program is offered to families through public education systems, early education programs such as Head Start, or day-care centers. Common features of these group-based efforts include weekly discussions for 8–14 weeks with parents around specific parenting topics (e.g., discipline, cognitive development, communications); group-based sessions with the children that provide parents with an opportunity to discuss issues or share feelings; parent–child interaction sessions to model the skills being presented to parents; and regular opportunities for all participants to share meals and important family celebrations, such as birthdays and graduations. In addition, specific instructions to children might also be incorporated into the regular classroom curriculum, further reinforcing the concepts. Because of the important role educators and day-care providers play in reinforcing and modeling positive adult–child interactions, these models also include specific teacher or staff training components on the program's goals and behavior expectations. In almost all instances, these models draw on the family-support philosophy, which emphasizes the enhancement of protective factors in addition to the reduction of negative behaviors (Dunst, 1995).

Solid empirical evidence supporting the method's efficacy in reducing maltreatment risk is limited but growing (Baker, Piotrkowski, & Brooks-Gunn, 1999; Carter & Harvey, 1996; Chalk & King, 1998; Daro & Cohn-Donnelly, 2002b; Wolfe, 1994). Repeated randomized trials of the Incredible Years, a multifaceted, developmentally based curricula for parents, teachers, and children delivered in both primary school and early education settings, found that participants demonstrated more positive affective response and a corresponding decrease in the use of harsh discipline, reduced parental depression and improved self-confidence, and better communication and problem solving within the family (Webster-Stratton, 1998; Webster-Stratton, Reid, & Hammond, 2001). Significant aspects of the model include group-based parenting skills training; classroom management training for teachers; and peer support groups for parents, children, and teachers. A meta-analysis of a broad range of family support services provided to families with children of all ages conducted by Abt Associates, found that these types of group-based parenting education and support produced larger effects than home visitation services in affecting children's cognitive outcomes and social emotional development (Layzer, Goodson, Bernstein, & Price, 2001).

In contrast to these relatively short-term interventions, other prevention efforts using a group format provide services for multiple years. For example, MELD (formerly the Minnesota Early Learning Design) is a 2-year curriculum in which groups of 10–20 mothers of newborns meet weekly to discuss various parenting and personal issues, such as health care, child development, child guidance, family management, and personal growth. Core techniques include large-group presentations, small-group discussions, modeling, and socialization before and after the meetings. Evaluations of this strategy have found the following service features central to achieving positive outcomes: group facilitation by parents who have experienced life situations similar to those of group members, long-term service availability (e.g., 2 or more years), persistent focus on parent strengths, emphasis on making decisions that produce long-term solutions to problems rather than achieving a "quick-fix," and a commitment to ongoing staff training and supervision (Hoelting, Sandell, Letourneau, Smerlinder, & Stranik, 1996).

The success of these efforts, however, is far from universal (Layzer et al., 2001). Many high-risk families find it difficult to sustain involvement in structured group programs due to logistical barriers, such as poor transportation, adjusting to a fixed schedule, and limited access to child care (Daro, 1993). Also, group-based services can be difficult to tailor to the individual needs of all participants. If the issue being addressed is general, with broad application across populations, such as how to access a given service or how to anticipate a specific parenting challenge, this inability to personalize the service is less salient. However, if parents face complex problems, the inability to provide personal guidance can reduce program effectiveness (Daro & Cohn-Donnelly, 2002b).

8.4.2.3. Child Assault Prevention Programs

In contrast to efforts designed to alter the behaviors of those who might commit maltreatment, a category of programs emerged in the early 1980s designed to alter the behavior of potential victims. Often referred to as child assault prevention or safety education programs, these efforts present children with specific information on the topic of physical abuse and sexual assault, how to avoid risk situations, and, if abused, how to respond. A key feature of these programs is their universal service-delivery systems, often being integrated into school curricula or into primary-support opportunities for children (e.g., Boy Scouts, youth groups, recreation programs). Although certain concerns have been raised regarding the appropriateness of these efforts (Gilbert, 1988; Reppucci & Haugaard, 1989), the strategy continues to be widely available in many school districts and to have increasingly adopted a more general focus on assisting children in avoiding a broad range of abusive behaviors, including peer aggression and violence prevention.

Repeated meta-analyses and other qualitative reviews of evaluations conducted on these programs have determined the method is effective in conveying safety education to children and providing children a set of skills in avoiding or minimizing the risk of assault (Berrick & Barth, 1992; Daro, 1994; MacMillan, MacMillan, Oxford, Griffith, & MacMillan, 1995; Rispens, Aleman, & Goudena, 1997). Equally important, these programs have offered children who have been victimized the language tools and procedures necessary for accessing help and reducing the risk of subsequent maltreatment (Kolko, Moser, & Hughes, 1989; Hazzard, 1990).

Although the average effect sizes (ES) noted by Berrick and Barth (1992) were modest (ES < 0.20) and limited to knowledge gains, more robust findings emerged from the meta-analysis by Rispens, Aleman, & Goudena (1997). Their review revealed significant and large effect sizes at both the postintervention (ES: 0.71) and follow-up (ES: 0.61) data collection points. Variation in these patterns most likely reflects differences in the pool of evaluations included in the two reviews. Because Rispens and co-worker's meta-analysis used studies with more rigorous designs (e.g., control groups, sufficient data for the computation of effect size, dependent variables that included knowledge of child abuse and acquisition of self-protection skills), greater confidence can be placed in those findings.

Both the descriptive reviews and meta-analyses of this strategy found that gains are unevenly distributed across concepts and participants. On balance, children have greater difficulty in accepting the idea that abuse can occur at the hands of someone they know than at the hands of strangers (Finkelhor & Strapko, 1992). Among younger participants, the more complex concepts such as secrets and dealing with ambiguous feelings often remain misunderstood (Gilbert, Duerr Berrick, LeProhn, & Nyman, 1990), although the most recent meta-analysis found that younger children (i.e., those under the age of 5.5 years) initially benefited more than older children from these programs (Rispens et al., 1997) in both knowledge and skills. However, this finding disappears at follow-up, suggesting younger children have more difficulty retaining knowledge and skills over time.

Some have attributed the 40% decline in reported cases of child sexual abuse between 1992 and 2000 to the widespread implementation of these programs, along with more consistent efforts to screen adults, providing direct intervention with children and aggressive prosecution of offenders (Finkelhor & Jones, 2004). Although it is impossible to fully understand the extent to which decreased reports reflect an absolute decrease in the total incidence, the reduction in reports offers possible evidence of the effects of universal efforts to provide most personal education or to craft a safer environment for children.

8.4.3.   Behavioral: Relationship Focus

8.4.3.1   Early Home Visitation

Home visitation, a service-delivery strategy that has been around since the late 1800s, has gained some distinction in recent decades (Gomby, Culross & Behrman, 1999). Many prevention-focused, home visiting programs target parents of newborns or young children. In such early home visitation programs, four common objectives have been identified: to prevent child abuse and neglect, to improve child health, to optimize child functioning and development, and to enhance parental care-giving abilities (McCurdy, 1995). Often, the home visitor seeks to achieve these objectives by offering education regarding infant health and development, modeling positive adult–child interactions, providing social support, and assisting the parent in achieving life outcomes such as further education.

Early home visiting services can vary on a number of program dimensions, including initiation and length of services, provider education and training, target population, and program size. Although such variation can obscure efforts to isolate the "true" effects of early home visitation as a method to prevent child maltreatment, meta-analytic techniques can assess the overall effect of home visiting on parents and children and calculate how these effects vary across certain program dimensions.

Three recent meta-analyses of early home visitation programs present similar findings regarding effectiveness—that home visiting programs significantly prevent child abuse and neglect in families with children 3 years old or younger, as measured by CPS reports or by proxy measures of maltreatment, including injuries, accidents, and emergency room visits. The two meta-analyses that investigated other indicators of child and family functioning also report positive and significant effects of home visiting; however, these analyses produce somewhat different estimates of effect size.

Hahn and co-workers' (2003) examination of 26 home visiting programs reports a 39% reduction in child abuse and neglect by visited parents as compared to the control group, with prevention measured by CPS reports and reported injuries. The results from two other meta-analyses corroborate this finding. In their examination of 60 home visiting programs, Sweet and Appelbaum (2004) document a significant reduction in potential abuse and neglect as measured by emergency room visits and treated injuries, ingestions, and accidents (ES: 0.239, p < .001). The effect of home visitation on reported or suspected maltreatment was moderate but insignificant (ES: 0.318), though failure to find significance may be due to the limited number of effect sizes available for analysis of this outcome ($k = 7$). Geeraert, Van den Noorgate, Grietens, and Onghena (2004) focused their meta-analysis on 43 programs with an explicit focus on preventing child abuse and neglect for families with children under 3 years of age. Though programs varied in service-delivery strategy, 88% ($n = 38$) used home visitation as a component of the intervention. This meta-analysis notes a significant, positive overall treatment effect on CPS reports of abuse and neglect and on injury data (ES: 0.26, $p < .001$).

While these latter two studies also report significant effects of home visitation on child and family functioning, the effect size varies. Sweet and Appelbaum (2004) note that home visitation produced significant but relatively small effects on the mother's behavior, attitudes, and educational attainment (ES: ≤0.18). In contrast, Geeraert et al. (2004) find stronger effects on indicators of child and parent functioning, ranging from 0.23 to 0.38. In assessing why these findings diverge, it seems likely that the authors' program selection processes partially contributed to these differences. Sweet and Appelbaum examine a greater number of programs (60 vs. 43), which potentially increases the accuracy of the overall effect size estimates. However, Geeraert and colleagues include 18 post-2000 evaluations not covered by Sweet and Appelbaum. These newer evaluations assess a broader array of child- and family-functioning indicators.

Two meta-analyses reported contradictory findings regarding the provider education and training on overall effectiveness. Hahn et al. (2003) discerned greater effects on child maltreatment indicators by professional visitors (nurse and mental-health workers) as compared to paraprofessional visitors, though paraprofessional visitors who provided visits for 2 or more years achieve consistent and positive effects. Sweet and Appelbaum (2004) found stronger effects on child abuse potential when paraprofessionals delivered the services as compared to professionals and nonprofessionals.

No other common program dimensions are investigated by all three meta-analyses. Overall, the studies note that the timing of service initiation, multiple- vs. single-component program structure (Hahn et al., 2003), actual service length, child age at service initiation (Sweet & Appelbaum, 2004), and year of study publication (Geeraert et al., 2004) did not significantly influence the effect of home visitation services. Sweet and Appelbaum (2004) report that the receipt of more visits corresponded to greater effect sizes in child cognition, but not in measures of potential child abuse, parental behavior, or maternal education.

In terms of targeting services to specific types of parents, Sweet and Appelbaum (2004) note differential effects; however, little consistency exists across the observed outcomes. For example, programs focusing on low-income parents yielded greater effects on potential child abuse but weaker impacts on parental behavior. A fourth meta-analysis of early home visitation programs by Guterman (1999) also addresses this issue of target population. Guterman's analyses suggest greater effects on CPS reports and other maltreatment proxies by 12 home visiting programs with population-based enrollment (i.e., services targeted to families with demographic markers such as single parenthood) as compared to 7 screening-based home visiting programs (i.e., services targeted to families based on risk-assessment scores). Tests of significance were not presented.

8.4.3.2   Characteristics of Effective Family Support Programs

In this section, we review two recent meta-analyses that assess a variety of prevention-oriented, family-support programs with the explicit goal of exploring the effect of assorted program and study elements on treatment effectiveness. The first meta-analysis, by MacLeod and Nelson (2000), examines a range of family-support programs they characterize as proactive (i.e., interventions targeted to all parents or to high-risk, nonabusive parents, with service delivery beginning either before the child's birth or in the first few years of life) or reactive (i.e., programs serving families with confirmed instances of maltreatment). Our analysis is limited to findings drawn from the analysis of 34 proactive family-support programs. The second meta-analysis, by Bakersman-Kraneburg, van Ijzendoorn, and Juffer (2003), examines 88 programs designed to increase maternal sensitivity and secure attachments.

MacLeod and Nelson (2000) report that multicomponent programs produced the largest total effect sizes in all outcome areas (ES: 0.58), followed by home visiting programs (ES: 0.41) and parent-support groups (ES: 0.38) while media interventions exerted only small effects (ES: 0.13). Follow-up effects were significantly higher than end of treatment effects for those studies that included a follow-up component.

Next, their multivariate analyses identified several moderator variables associated with differential effects of home visiting programs. For child maltreatment outcomes, service length and intensity had a curvilinear pattern with outcomes. Moderate amounts of home visiting (i.e., 25–30 months with 13–32 home visits), resulted in the greatest effects on the prevention of substantiated cases of child maltreatment and accidents and injuries. However, the reverse was true for parent behavior outcomes where moderate amounts of visits (13–50) led to significantly lower effects on parental behavior than fewer ($\leq$12) or more home visits (>50).

Some unexpected findings emerged. MacLeod and Nelson report that home visiting programs that also sought to provide social support were less successful at reducing maltreatment than home visitation programs without this component. Similarly, the parent–child environment was less likely to be changed when the home visiting program provided concrete supports (e.g., money, clothing). These results may suggest that too broad a program focus dilutes program effectiveness.

Maternal sensitivity and attachment security have been linked to neglectful and abusive behavior (Egeland & Erickson, 1993), and the meta-analysis by Bakersman-Kraneburg et al. (2003) highlights some program and participant characteristics that promote these proximate outcomes. In this analysis, 88 programs targeting families with children younger than 54 months of age are examined. The programs covered a range of intervention strategies (from viewing videos to receiving home visits), target populations (from clinical to low-risk parents), and provider credentials (ranging from no provider to professional provider). All evaluations relied on observational measures of sensitivity or attachment to assess effectiveness. Overall, the meta-analysis found moderate program effects on maternal sensitivity (ES: 0.44, $p < .001$) and positive though small effects on attachment security (ES: 0.19, $p < .05$).

For the 81 interventions assessing maternal sensitivity, several program, participant, and study attributes influenced effectiveness. First, a program focus on maternal sensitivity was more effective that other objectives, such as increasing maternal support, altering parental cognitive representations, or some combination of these three foci. Other program characteristics—such as the use of videos or video feedback, service length of less than 16 sessions, service initiation after the child reached 6 months, and the inclusion of fathers in the intervention—produced significantly stronger effects. For multiproblem families, nonprofessional providers were more effective than professional providers.

In terms of participant characteristics, these programs were more effective with clinical than with nonclinical samples. No differences emerged by low socioeconomic status, teen parenthood, premature birth, or multiproblem status. Finally, study characteristics influenced effect size because randomized studies yielded a lower, though still moderate, effect size (ES: 0.33) than nonrandomized studies (ES: 0.61), and studies with low attrition rates reported stronger effects.

Of the 29 programs assessing parent–child attachment, a focus on maternal sensitivity produced stronger effects than any other program foci. In contrast to the findings with maternal sensitivity, the use of videos was found to weaken the program's effect on attachment patterns. Service length, age of child, provider credentials, and randomization procedures did not moderate effect size.

8.4.4.   Behavioral: Community or Societal Focus

8.4.4.1.   Community Partnerships

Community partnerships often serve to encourage multiple entities (e.g., child protection agencies, social service agencies, community organizations, and community residents) to work together to protect children and support families (Annie E. Casey Foundation, 2003; CWS Stakeholders Group, 2003; Farrow, 1997; Waldfoqel, 1998). Other partnerships focus more explicitly on building resident involvement in community protection or galvanizing within local communities a greater emphasis on achieving mutual reciprocity between individual residents (Dodge et al., 2004; Melton et al., 2002).

Measuring the collective effects of a community partnership on child maltreatment requires both individual-level and community-level data. To date, insufficient evidence exists to evaluate the effect of such partnerships on CPS system performance or on community norms. However, findings from at least one community-based strategy are encouraging. In Vermont, regional partnerships, under the direction of the state's Team for Children, Families and Individuals, have greatly expanded the availability of family-support services for all pregnant women and young children. Since implementing these partnerships, the state has experienced service expansion and a significant reduction in the rates of reported child abuse and neglect as well as improvements in other indicators of child well-being (Center for the Study of Social Policy [CSSP] 2001; Hogan, 2001).

8.4.4.2.   Public Awareness Effort

Using public awareness campaigns to mobilize the public has long been regarded as a vital component of a comprehensive child maltreatment prevention strategy (Cohn Donnelly, 1997). The values and attitudes that a people hold about children and how to raise them, the behaviors they engage in as parents toward their own and other children, and the degree to which they support or fail to support certain public policies all help explain the existence of child abuse and its increase or decrease over time. To influence societal beliefs about parenting, public-awareness campaigns attempt to reach out to large numbers of individuals in a consistent manner using everyday communication media (e.g., television, radio, newspapers and magazines, billboards, the Internet).

Studies of awareness levels suggest that public service campaigns have effectively educated the public as to the existence of child maltreatment and its potential effects on victims. In the mid-1970s, only 10% of the general public reported an awareness of child abuse (Cohn Donnelly, 1997). This percent grew to over 90% by the early 1980s (Daro & Gelles, 1992). These later surveys also demonstrated that the general public had a more sophisticated understanding of the different types of child maltreatment, its individual and societal causes, and the need to take action to prevent its occurrence (Daro & Gelles, 1992).

In achieving the more ambitious goal of changing parental attitudes and behaviors, the evidence to date is mixed. In conjunction with the Advertising Council, Prevent Child Abuse America conducted a nationwide series of educational campaigns using TV, print, radio, and billboard public service announcements with editorial assistance from the media (e.g., Op-Ed pieces, columns in "Dear Abby") targeted sequentially at physical abuse/hitting, verbal abuse/yelling, and emotional neglect/ignoring. The combined campaigns garnered between $20 and $60 million a year worth of exposure in donated time and space.

The effect from the first two of these three waves suggests some success. Since 1988, parents participating in annual public opinion polls have reported a steady reduction in the use of both corporal punishment and verbal forms of aggression in disciplining their children (Daro & Gelles, 1992). However, these same studies find that the proportion of parents who report hitting their child with an object or injuring their child in the course of "normal discipline" have remained constant. Each year, roughly 10% of parents will hit their children with a belt or other implement and 1% admit to bruising or physically injuring their child (Daro & Gelles, 1992). In addition, related studies of the use of mass media to identify developmental delays found little effect on parental knowledge or attitudes (Kurtz, 1982; Kurtz, Devaney, Strain, & Sandler, 1982).

8.5. POLICY AND PRACTICE IMPLICATIONS

Program evaluations and meta-analytic studies of child abuse prevention programs present a fairly positive picture. Most important, our review found evidence that early home visitation strategies are effective at reducing the likelihood that children will be reported as victims of child abuse and neglect or that they will need treatment for physical injuries or accidents. When the pool of relevant indicators are extended to include proximal indicators of a reduction in abuse potential or an increase in core protective factors, a number of additional strategies surface as promising. Products designed to improve parental sensitivity such as soft baby carriers, interventions to enhance parental knowledge through videotapes and support groups, and strategies to protect children through child assault prevention programs show positive results. Among this second group of strategies, it is important to note that the reduction in risk behaviors or attitudes by the participants may enhance family functioning, yet have little effect on aggregate rates of physical abuse and neglect. Because some argue that program effectiveness can be proven only by reductions in child maltreatment rates (Chaffin, 2004), the field itself needs to achieve consensus on acceptable indicators of prevention.

Although our review also sought to identify the service components most likely to result in meaningful change, our efforts in this regard met with limited success. In attempting to answer whether prevention programs should begin before the child's birth, provide multiple services, rely on professional providers, last for 2 or more years, or target specific families, we were stymied by the lack of rigorous research and definitional clarity available to address these questions. The bulk of evidence suggests, however, that the definition and measurement of the target outcome is a critical factor in determining which service component leads to change. For example, strategies that seem to work in preventing maltreatment reports are not necessarily ones that work to enhance child functioning

In addition to these issues, our review suggests another source of analytic confusion. Many home visitation and parent education program assessed in our review embrace multiple strategies, yet are typically classified as single-component models. Similarly, many programs identified as "paraprofessional" consist of providers with academic degrees in addition to nonprofessional providers. Given the growing trend among prevention services to offer multiple components and hire diverse staff, such classifications may become less salient in the future.

8.6.   RESEARCH IMPLICATIONS

Our review suggests several areas in which additional research is needed if prevention efforts are to maximize their potential. First, greater clarity is needed regarding the most accurate and appropriate way to measure prevention of child maltreatment. If maltreatment reports continue to be viewed as the ultimate and most accurate indictor of prevention effectiveness, greater consistency is needed in how such reports are documented, including more careful identification and tracking of the type of maltreatment involved (e.g., physical abuse, neglect, sexual abuse, multiple forms of abuse), the actual perpetrator (e.g., parent or other adult), and the relative severity of the mistreatment.

Second, longitudinal research studies are needed that track the extent to which initial progress on various proximate outcomes is both sustained over time and sufficiently robust to reduce subsequent reports of maltreatment or involvement with child protective services. To the extent prevention programs embrace the public health model and ecological theories of maltreatment, targeted outcomes for such interventions will include a dual focus on both risk and protective factors. Understanding how changes in these factors reduce subsequent abusive or neglectful behavior is essential both in building better theory in the field of maltreatment and in enhancing program and policy effectiveness and efficacy.

While independent, rigorous program evaluations can provide evidence of a model's efficacy, developing and taking interventions to scale demand the articulation of specific quality standards and the capacity to monitor program adherence to these standards. Effective programs will be ones that operate under a framework in which information is continuously collected and fed back into the decision-making process. Strengthening our knowledge base and understanding of prevention programming requires more consistent and rigorous attention to such issues as the characteristics of the target population, the rate at which programs successfully enroll and retain their population, the content of the services provided families, and, the nature of the participant–provider relationship.

8.7. CONCLUSIONS

Despite the emphasis prevention advocates place on altering community context and building a collective sense of responsibility for child protection (Melton & Berry, 1994), most child maltreatment prevention efforts remain focused on changing individual attitudes and behaviors. Efforts to reduce child abuse and neglect rates largely target individual characteristics such as parenting skills or knowledge and the parent–child relationship. When such efforts are carefully implemented, risk can be reduced and positive outcomes achieved; however, effects on aggregate rates of maltreatment may be small.

For many of the most at-risk families, however, access to these types of services remains limited (Daro, 1993). And when at-risk families reside in high-risk communities marked by violence, poor social infrastructure, and limited economic opportunities, the odds of successfully protecting a child from harm are greatly reduced. Overcoming these obstacles will require prevention programs to become more community focused in their programming imagery. As noted earlier, calls for this type of integration between individual and contextual reforms is longstanding. Although preliminary efforts in the area of community capacity building are under way, they have not yet produced significant findings with respect to abuse reduction or the development of more robust levels of social capital (Wandersman & Florin, 2003; Dodge et al., 2004).

At present, the vast majority of public and social investment in addressing the problem of child abuse is focused on tertiary care. In the absence of any dramatic shift in mission, agency directors and line staff have no incentive to retool their operations or to alter their funding streams to accommodate the alternative service-delivery methods and values represented by prevention advocates. Prevention efforts will remain marginalized and, ultimately, ineffective until this imbalance is corrected.

REFERENCES

Anisfeld, E., Casper, V., Nozyce, M., & Cunningham, N. (1990). Does infant carrying promote attachment? An experimental study of the effects of increased physical contact on the development of attachment. *Child Development, 61,* 1617–1627.

Annie E. Casey Foundation. (2003). *Making connections: A neighborhood transformation family development initiative.* Baltimore, MD: Author.

Baker, A., Piotrkowski, C., & Brooks-Gunn, J. (1999). The home instruction program for preschool youngsters (HIPPY). *The Future of Children, 9* (1), 116–133.

Bakermans-Kranenburg, J., van Ijzendoorn, J., & Juffer, F. (2003). Less is more: Meta-analyses of sensitivity and attachment interventions in early childhood. *Psychological Bulletin, 129* (2), 195–215.

Belsky, J. (1980). Child maltreatment: An ecological integration. *American Psychologist, 35,* 320–335.

Berrick, J., & Barth, R. (1992). Child sexual abuse prevention: Research review and recommendations. *Social Work Research & Abstracts, 28,* 6–15.

Black, M., & Teti, L. (1997). Promoting meal-time communication between adolescent mothers and their infants through videotape. *Pediatrics, 99,* 432–437.

Bronfenbrenner, U. (1979). *The ecology of human development: Experiments by nature and design.* Cambridge, MA: Harvard University Press.

Carnegie Task Force on Meeting the Needs of Young Children. (1994). *Starting Points: Meeting the needs of our youngest children.* New York: Carnegie Corporation of New York.

Carter, N. (1995). *Parenting education in the United States: An investigative report.* Philadephia: Pew Charitable Trusts.

Carter, N., & Harvey, C. (1996). Gaining perspective on parenting groups. *Zero To Three*, *16* (6), 1, 3–8.

Center for the Study and Prevention of Violence, Institute of Behavioral Science. Blueprints for Violence Prevention: University of Colorado at Boulder. Retrieved December 2, 2005, from www.colorado.edu/cspv/blueprints/matrix/matrix.pdf

Center for the Study of Social Policy. (2001). *Building capacity for local decision-making: Executive summary.* Washington, DC: Author.

Chaffin, M. (2004). Is it time to rethink Healthy Start/Healthy Families? *Child Abuse & Neglect*, 28, 589–595.

Chalk, R., Gibbons, A., & Scarupa, H. (2002). *The multiple dimensions of child abuse and neglect: New insights into an old problem* (Child Trends Research Brief). Washington, DC: Child Trends.

Chalk, R., & King, P. (Eds.). (1998). *Violence in families: Assessing prevention and treatment programs.* Washington, DC: National Academy Press.

Cicchetti, D., & Rizley, R. (1981). Developmental perspectives on the etiology, intergenerational transmission, and sequelae of child maltreatment. In R. Rizley & D. Cicchetti (Eds.), *New directions for child development: Developmental perspectives in child maltreatment* (pp. 32–59). San Francisco: Jossey-Bass.

Cohn, A. (1987). Our national priorities for prevention. In R. Helfer & C. H. Kempe (Eds.), *The battered child*, 4th ed. (pp. 444–445). Chicago: University of Chicago Press.

Cohn Donnelly, A. (1997). An overview of prevention of physical abuse and neglect. In M. E. Helfer, M. Kempe, & R. Krugman (Eds.), *The battered child*, 5th ed. (pp. 579–593). Chicago: University of Chicago Press.

Conway, E. (1998). Nonaccidental head injury in infants: The shaken baby syndrome revisited. *Pediatric Annals*, 27, 677–690.

Courtney, M., Terao, S., & Bost, N. (2004). *Midwest evaluation of the adult functioning of former foster youth: Conditions of youth preparing to leave state care.* Chicago: Chapin Hall Center for Children.

Cudabak, D., Darden, C., Nelson, P., OBrien, S., Pinksy, D., & Wiggins, E. (1985). Becoming successful parents: Can age-paced newsletters help? *Journal of Family Relations*, *34*, 271–275.

CWS Stakeholders Group. (2003). *Child welfare services redesign: Draft final report.* Sacramento: California Department of Social Services.

Daro, D. (1989). *Confronting child abuse: Research for effective program design.* New York: Free Press.

Daro, D. (1993). Child maltreatment research: Implications for program design. In D. Cicchetti & S. Toth (Eds.), *Child abuse, child development, and social policy* (pp. 331–367). New York: Ablex Publishing.

Daro, D. (1994). Prevention of childhood sexual abuse. *The Future of Children*, *4* (2), 198–223.

Daro, D. (2000). Child abuse prevention: New directions and challenges. In D. Hansen (Ed.), *Motivation & child maltreatment. Vol. 46: The Nebraska symposium on motivation* (pp. 161–220). Lincoln: University of Nebraska.

Daro, D., & Cohn Donnelly, A. (2002a). Charting the waves of prevention: Two steps forward, one step back. *Child Abuse & Neglect*, 26, 731–742.

Daro, D., & Cohn Donnelly, A. (2002b). Child abuse prevention: Accomplishments and challenges. In J. Myers, L. Berliner, J. Briere, T. Hendrix, C. Jenny, & T. Reid (Eds.), *APSAN handbook on child maltreatment* (pp. 431–448, 2nd ed). Thousand Oaks, CA: Sage.

Daro, D., & Gelles, R. (1992). Public attitudes and behaviors with respect to child abuse prevention. *Journal of Interpersonal Violence*, *7* (4), 517–531.

Dodge, K., Berlin, L., Epstein, M., Spitz-Roth, A., O'Donnell, K., Kaufman, M., Amaya-Jackson, L., Rosch, J., & Christopoulos, C. (2004). The Durham Family Initiative: A preventive system of care. *Child Welfare*, *83* (2), 109–128.

Dunst, C. (1995). *Key characteristics and features of community-based family support program.* Chicago: The Family Resource Coalition.

Egeland, B., & Erickson, M. (1993). Attachment theory and findings: Implications for prevention and intervention. In S. Kramer & H. Parens (Eds.), *Prevention in mental health: Now, tomorrow, ever?* (pp. 21–50). Northvale, NJ: Aronson.

Egeland, B., & Stroufe, L. (1981). Developmental sequelae of maltreatment in infancy. In R. Rizley & D. Cicchetti (Eds.), *New directions for child development: Developmental perspectives in child maltreatment* (pp. 77–92). San Francisco: Jossey-Bass.

Farrow, F. (1997). *Child protection: Building community partnerships . . . Getting from here to there.* Cambridge, MA: John F. Kennedy School of Government, Harvard University.

Finkelhor, D., & Jones, L. (2004). Explanations for the decline in child sexual abuse cases. *Juvenile Justice Bulletin.* (pp. 11–12).

Finkelhor, D., Ormrod, R., Turner, H., & Hamby, S. (2005). The victimization of children and youth: A comprehensive, national survey. *Child Maltreatment*, *10* (1), 5–25.

Finkelhor, D., & Strapko, N. (1992). Sexual abuse prevention education: A review of evaluation studies. In D. Willis, E. Holder, & M. Rosenberg (Eds.), *Child abuse prevention.* (pp. 150–167). New York: Wiley.

Garbarino, J. (1977). The human ecology of child maltreatment: A conceptual model for research. *Journal of Marriage & the Family, 39,* 721–735.

Garbarino, J. (1997). The role of economic deprivation in the social context of child maltreatment. In M. E. Helfer, R. Kempe, & R. Krugman (Eds.), *The battered child* (5th ed). (pp. 49–60). Chicago: University of Chicago Press.

Gaudin, J. (1999). Child neglect: Short-term and long-term outcomes. In H. Dubowitz (Ed.), *Neglected children: Research, practice, and policy* (pp. 89–108). Thousand Oaks, CA: Sage.

Geeraert, L., Van den Noorgate, W., Grietens, H., & Onghena, P. (2004). The effects of early prevention programs for families with young children at risk for physical child abuse and neglect: A meta-analysis. *Child Maltreatment, 9* (3), 277–291.

Gelles, R., & Straus, M. (1988). *Intimate violence: The causes and consequences of abuse in the American family.* New York: Simon & Schuster.

Gil, D. (1970). *Violence against children: Physical child abuse in the United States.* Cambridge, MA: Harvard University Press.

Gillbert, N. (1988). Teaching children to prevent sexual abuse. *The Public Interest, 93,* 3–15.

Gilbert, N., Duerr Berrick, J., LeProhn, N., & Nyman, N. (1990). *Protecting young children from sexual abuse: Does preschool training work?* Lexington, MD: Lexington Books.

Glascoe, F., Oberklaid, F., Dworkin, P., & Trimm, F. (1998). Brief approaches to educating patients and parents in primary care. *Pediatrics, 101* (6), 10–18.

Gomby, D., Culross, P., & Behrman, R. (1999). Home visiting: Recent program evaluations—analysis and recommendations. *The Future of Children, 9* (1), 4–26.

Guterman, N. (1999). Enrollment strategies in early home visitation to prevent physical child abuse and neglect and the "universal versus targeted" debate: A meta-analysis of population-based and screening-based programs. *Child Abuse & Neglect, 23,* 863–890.

Guterman, N. (2001). *Stopping child maltreatment before it starts: Emerging horizons in early home visitation services.* Thousand Oaks, CA: Sage.

Hahn, R., Bilukha, O., Crosby, A., Fullilove, M., Liberman, A., Moscicki, E., Snyder, S., Tuma, F., Schofield, A., Corso, P., & Briss, P. (2003). First reports evaluating the effectiveness of strategies for preventing violence: Early childhood home visitation. *MMWR: Recommendations & Reports, 52,* 1–9.

Hahn, R., Mercy, J., Bilukha, O., & Briss, P. (2005). Assessing home visiting programs to prevent child abuse: Taking the silver and bronze along with the gold. *Child Abuse & Neglect, 29,* 215–218.

Hazzard, A. (1990). Prevention of child sexual abuse. In R. Ammerman & M. Hersen (Eds.), *Treatment of family violence* (pp. 354–384). New York: John Wiley.

Helfer, M. E., Kempe, R., & Krugman, R. (Eds.). (1997). *The battered child* (5th ed). Chicago: University of Chicago Press.

Henggeler, S., Melton, G., Brondino, M., Scherer, D., & Hanley, J. (1997). Multisystemic therapy with violent and chronic juvenile offenders and their families: The role of treatment fidelity in successful dissemination. *Journal of Consulting and Clinical Psychology, 65,* 821–833.

Hoelting, J., Sandell, E., Letourneau, S., Smerlinder, J., & Stranik, M. (1996). The MELD experience with parent groups. *Zero To Three, 16* (6), 9–18.

Hogan, C. (2001). *The power of outcomes: Strategic thinking to improve results for our children, families and communities.* Washington, DC: National Governors Association.

Hunziker, U., & Barr, R. (1986). Increased carrying reduces infant crying: A randomized controlled trial. *Pediatrics, 77,* 641–648.

Jungmeen, K., & Cicchetti, D. (2003). Social self-efficacy and behavior problems in maltreatment children. *Journal of Clinical Child & Adolescent Psychology, 32,* 106–117.

Kempe, C. H., Silverman, F., Steele, B., Droegemueller, W., & Silver, H. (1962). The battered child syndrome. *Journal of the American Medical Association, 181,* 17–24.

Kendall-Tackett, K. A. (2003). *Treating the lifetime health effects of childhood victimization: A guide for mental health, medical and social service professionals.* New York: Civic Research Institute.

Kendall-Tackett, K., & Echenrode, J. (1996). The effects of neglect on academic achievement and disciplinary problems: A developmental perspective. *Child Abuse & Neglect, 20,* 161–169.

Kolko, D. (2002). Child physical abuse. In: J. Myers, L. Berliner, J. Briere, T. Hendrix, C. Jenny, & T. Reid, (Eds.), *APSAN handbook on child maltreatment* (pp. 21–54, 2nd ed). Thousand Oaks, CA: Sage.

Kolko, D., Moser, J., & Hughes, J. (1989). Classroom training in sexual victimization awareness and prevention skills: An extension of red flag/green flag people program. *Journal of Family Violence, 4,* 11–35.

Kurtz, D. (1982). Using mass media and group instruction for preventive mental health in rural communities. *Social Work Research & Abstracts, 18* (3), 41–48.

Kurtz, D., Devaney, B., Strain, P., & Sandler, H. (1982). Effects of mass-media and group instruction on increasing parent awareness of early identification. *Journal of Special Education. 16* (3), 329–339.

Lamphear, V. (1985). The impact of maltreatment on children's psychosocial adjustment: A review of the research. *Child Abuse & Neglect, 9,* 252–263.

Laurendeau, M.-C., Gagnon, G., Desjardins, N., Perreault, R., & Kischuk, N. (1991). Evaluation of an early, mass media parental support intervention. *Journal of Primary Prevention, 11* (3), 207–225.

Layzer, J., Goodson, B., Bernstein, L., & Price, C. (2001). *National evaluation of family support programs. Volume A: Meta-analysis.* Unpublished manuscript. Department of Health and Human Services, ACYF. Cambridge, MA: Abt Associates.

Lutzker, J. (2000). Balancing research and treatment in child maltreatment: The quest for good data and practical service. In D. Hansen, (Ed.), *Motivation & child maltreatment. Vol. 46: The Nebraska Symposium on Motivation* (pp. 221–224). Lincoln: University of Nebraska.

MacLeod, J., & Nelson, G. (2000). Programs for the promotion of family wellness and the prevention of child maltreatment: A meta-analytic review. *Child Abuse & Neglect, 24,* 1127–1149.

MacMillan, H., MacMillan, J., Offord, D., Griffith, L., & MacMillan, A. (1994). Primary prevention of child sexual abuse: A critical review. Part II. *Journal of Child Psychology & Psychiatry, 35,* 857–876.

McCurdy, K. (1995). *Home visiting.* Washington, DC: National Resource Center on Child Abuse and Neglect.

Melton, G., & Berry, F. (Eds.). (1994). *Protecting children from abuse and neglect: Foundations for a new national strategy.* New York: Guilford Press.

Melton, G., Thompson, R., & Small, M. (Eds.). (2002). *Toward a child-centered, neighborhood-based child protection system.* Westport, CT: Praeger.

Morrison, J., Frank, S., Holland, C., & Kates, W. (1999). Emotional development and disorders in young children in the child welfare system. In J. Silver, B. Amster, & T. Haecker (Eds.), *Young children & foster care: A guide for professionals* (pp. 33–64). Baltimore, MD: Brookes.

Perry, B. (2001). The neurodevelopmnetal impact of violence in childhood. In D. Schetky & E. Benedek (Eds.), *Textbook of child and adolescent forensic psychiatry.* Washington, DC: American Psychiatric Press.

Reppucci, N., & Haugaard, J. (1989). Prevention of child sexual abuse: Myth or reality. *American Psychologist, 44*(10), 1266–1275.

Riley, D., Meinhardt, G., Nelson, C., Salisbury, M., & Winnett, T. (1991). How effective are age-paced newsletters for new parents? A replication and extension of earlier studies. *Family Relations, 40,* 247–253.

Rispens, J., Aleman, A., & Goudena, P. (1997). Prevention of child sexual abuse victimization: A meta-analysis of school programs. *Child Abuse & Neglect, 21,* 975–987.

Saunders, B., Berliner, L., & Hanson, R. (Eds.). (2003). *Child physical & sexual abuse: Guidelines for treatment.* Charleston, South Carolina: National Crime Victims Research and Treatment Center.

Sedlek, A, & Broadhurst, D. (1996). *Third national incidence study of child abuse and neglect (NIS-3): Executive summary.* Washington, DC: U.S. Department of Health and Human Services, National Center on Child Abuse and Neglect.

Shonkoff, J., & Phillips, D. (2000). *From neurons to neighborhoods: The science of early childhood development.* Washington, DC: National Academy Press.

Straus, M. (1994). *Beating the devil out of them: Corporal punishment in American families.* Lexington, MD: Lexington Books.

Substance Abuse and Mental Health Services Administration (SAMSA). National Registry of Effective Programs. www.modelprograms.samhsa.gov

Sweet, M., & Appelbaum, M. (2004). Is home visiting an effective strategy? A meta-analytic review of home visiting programs for families with young children. *Child Development, 75,* 1435–1456.

Tessier, R., Cristo, M., Velez, S., Giron, M., Ruiz-Palaez, J., Charpak, Y., & Charpak, N. (1998). Kangaroo mother care and the bonding hypothesis. *Pediatrics, 102,* 17–25.

U.S. Department of Health and Human Services. (2003). *National survey of child and adolescent well-being: Baseline report for one year foster care sample.* Washington, DC: U.S. Government Printing Office.

U.S. Department of Health and Human Services, Administration on Children, Youth and Families. (2004). *Child maltreatment 2002.* Washington, DC: U.S. Government Printing Office.

Waldfogel, J. (1998). *The future of child protection: How to break the cycle of abuse and neglect.* Cambridge, MA: Harvard University Press.

Wandersman, A., & Florin, P. (2003). Community interventions and effective prevention. *American Psychologist, 58* (6–7), 441–448.

Webster-Stratton, C., Reid M. J., & Hammond, M. (2001). Preventing conduct problems, promoting social competence: A parent and teacher training partnership in Head Start. *Journal of Clinical Child Psychology, 30* (3), 238–302.

Webster-Stratton, C. (1994). Advancing videotape parent training: A comparison study. *Journal of Consulting and Clinical Psychology, 62,* 583–593.

Webster-Stratton, C. (1998). Preventing conduct problems in head start children: Strengthening parent competencies. *Journal of Consulting and Clinical Psychology, 66,* 715–730.

Widom, C., & Maxfield, M. (2001, February). An update on the "cycle of violence." *National Institute of Justice Research Brief,* pp. 1–8.

Wolfe, D. (1994). The role of intervention and treatment services in the prevention of child abuse and neglect. In G. Melton & F. Berry, (Eds.), *Protecting children from abuse and neglect: Foundations for a new national strategy* (pp. 224–303). New York: Guilford Press.

Wolfe, D., MacPherson, T., Blount, R., & Wolfe, V. (1986). Evaluaiton of a brief intervention for educating school children in awareness of physical and sexual abuse. *Child Abuse & Neglect, 10,* 85–92.

Wulczyn, F., Barth, R., Yuan, Y., Jones Harden, B., & Landsverk. (2005). *Beyond common sense: Child welfare, child well-being, and the evidence for policy reform.* New York: Aldine-Transaction.

Wurtele, S., & Miller-Perrin, C. (1992). *Preventing child sexual abuse: Sharing the responsibility.* Lincoln: University of Nebraska Press.

Chapter **9**

Interventions to Prevent Youth Violence

Denise C. Gottfredson and Erin L. Bauer

9.1. INTRODUCTION

This chapter summarizes research on interventions to reduce or prevent the perpetration of youth violence. Youth violence is defined broadly to include acts of interpersonal aggression, ranging in seriousness from crimes against individuals (e.g., robbery, assault) to aggressive behaviors, such as hitting, bullying, and, for younger students, biting and hurling objects at others. This definition explicitly includes aggressive acts of younger children that have been shown to be precursors of later, more serious and violent delinquency (see Tolan and Gorman-Smith [1998] for a summary of such precursors). By defining youth violence to include these precursor behaviors, we are able to consider a broader array of early prevention intervention strategies targeting these earlier behaviors.

The chapter begins with a description of youth violence and a brief history of interventions to reduce it. It then provides a broad-brush snapshot of the types of interventions that have been studied for effects of youth violence and related outcomes, including brief descriptions of the most effective approaches. It concludes with implications for future prevention research and public health practice and policy.

9.2. YOUTH VIOLENCE

Juvenile arrest rates are often used to measure youth violence. Most juvenile arrests are for crimes of a relatively nonserious nature. In 2002, juveniles between the ages of 10 and 19 years, accounting for approximately 14% of the population, were responsible for 26% of all arrests, greater than their share. The disproportionality was greatest for serious property crimes (e.g., burglary, larceny/theft, motor-vehicle theft, and arson, for which youths in this age bracket accounted for 41% of the arrests) and for vandalism (49% of the arrests). Youths were also overrepresented, but less so, among arrests for serious, violent crimes—they accounted for 24% of all arrests for murder, forcible rape, robbery, and aggravated assault. Arrest records also show that males are far more likely than females to be arrested, especially for serious, violent crimes; but this gender gap has been declining for approximately three decades. Cook and Laub (2002) show that the male to female ratio for arrests for violent crimes, which was greater than 10 in 1970, had steadily declined to approximately 4 by 1999. Although violent crime is still committed far more by males than by females, females seem to be catching up. Arrest rates are also higher in urbanized areas than in rural areas (Federal Bureau of Investigation [FBI], 2002).

Arrest data, however, underestimate the amount of crime because they count only crimes that have been detected by the police. Less than 1% of chargeable offenses are actually recorded by the police (Williams & Gold, 1972). Self-reports are a useful supplemental source of data on youth crime and violence. The Youth Risk Behavior Surveillance Survey (YRBSS), a survey conducted biannually in schools in 32 states and certain localities by the Centers for Disease Control and Prevention (CDC), provides statistics regarding violent youth behavior. This survey yields prevalence rates for physical fighting and weapon use from a national sample of students in grades 9 through 12. The 2003 survey shows that fighting is common among high school students: 33% of students (40.5% of males and 25.1% of females) surveyed had been in a physical fight in the last year. Almost a fifth (17.1%) of students had carried a weapon (e.g., gun, knife, or club) in the past month, with males (26.9%) far more likely than females (6.7%) to have done so; 6.1% of students had carried a gun in the past month. This estimate is in line with that from another national survey (Sheley & Wright, 1998) showing that in 1996, approximately 3% of 10th and 11th grade males possessed a revolver or automatic or semiautomatic handgun and that 6% had carried a gun outside the home in the past year. It is interesting that half of the males in this study reported obtaining a gun would be little or no trouble.

These data sources converge in implying that although violent behavior in the form of fighting is common among young people, very serious violent crime is rare. Males are far more likely to engage in violent behavior than females, and the most serious forms of violent crime are more likely to occur in urban areas than in suburban or rural areas.

9.3. BRIEF HISTORY OF YOUTH VIOLENCE PREVENTION EFFORTS

The youth violence prevention landscape has changed drastically in the last quarter century. In 1977, Wright and Dixon published a review of juvenile delinquency prevention program reports. The results were disappointing. From approximately 6600 program abstracts, empirical data were available from only 96. Of the 96 empirical reports, only 9 used random assignment of subjects, inferential statistics, outcome measures of delinquency, and a follow-up period of at least 6 months. Of those 9, only 3 reported positive outcomes, and these three were based on the three smallest sample sizes among the 9 reports. The authors concluded that the literature was low in both scientific and policy utility. By contrast, today dozens of summaries of research on prevention practices are available, all concluding that at least some forms of preventive activities have been demonstrated effective for reducing youth violence and related youth outcomes such as delinquent behavior, conduct disorder, and substance use.

The *nature* of youth violence prevention interventions also changed in the same period. Early interventions primarily involved social work and counseling (e.g., Miller, 1962; Powers & Witmer, 1951; Reckless & Dinitz, 1972). Today, preventive interventions tend to be directed toward reducing a broad array of empirically demonstrated risk factors for subsequent problem behavior that involve not only individual characteristics (e.g., weak attachments to pro-social others, low levels of commitment to achieving educational goals, weak moral beliefs in the validity of conventional rules for behavior, poor academic achievement, low self-control) but also characteristics of families, schools, peer groups, and communities. Indeed, modern-day prevention practices tend to be multilevel and multicomponent in nature. Methods used to study the effects of these programs and policies have also become much more sophisticated in recent years.

9.4.   CHAPTER ORGANIZATION AND METHODOLOGY

We relied primarily on secondary sources and meta-analyses in writing this chapter. We summarized programs, practices, and policies that were either designed to prevent or reduce youth violence or that were evaluated for such effects. Interventions targeting violence reduction for general populations or adult populations were not the focus of this review, but they were discussed if they seemed especially relevant for youth violence prevention. The youth violence interventions were classified into one of the three main types of interventions addressed in this volume: products, environmental, or behavioral. The majority of interventions for youth violence are behavioral, focusing on changing the behaviors of individuals, organizations, or communities. Within the behavioral category, interventions were further classified into one of five groups: society level, community level, school level, family/parent, or individual. It is important to note this categorization pertains to the factor(s) directly manipulated rather than to the location of the manipulation. For example, a school-based program that seeks primarily to increase self-control was classified with the *individual* interventions; whereas a school-based intervention that seeks to reduce violence by manipulating the fairness and clarity of school rules was classified with the *school-level* interventions.

We further classified studies by the outcomes reported for each intervention. Studies were classified as having effects on (1) youth violence/aggression, (2) associated outcomes, or (3) both. The associated outcome category includes a broader set of problem behavior outcomes known to be highly correlated with violence and aggression, including delinquent behavior, conduct problem behavior, and low self-control. Studies reporting outcome measures that included items measuring violence or aggression combined with items measuring other forms of problem behavior were classified as associated outcomes. When relying on secondary sources, we sometimes had limited information about the exact nature of the outcome variable(s). If we were uncertain whether a study actually demonstrated effects on violence or aggression, we classified it as targeting associated outcomes. Conclusions for each type of intervention, based on the hierarchy of evidence described elsewhere in this volume, are summarized in Table 9.1.

Table 9.1. Summary of Effectiveness of Youth Violence Prevention Strategies

Type of Prevention Strategy	Violence/Aggression[a]	Related Outcomes[a]
Products and physical environments	3	3
Behavioral interventions		
Society-level interventions		
Media campaigns	3	3
Reducing exposure to violence	3	3
Community-level interventions		
Policing	3	3
Community mobilization	3	3
Voucher programs for public-housing residents	4	4
School-level interventions		
School and discipline management interventions	3	5
Establishing norms or expectations for behavior	5	5
Family/parent interventions		
Child education/training plus parent training	5	5
Family-skills training	3	5
Individual interventions		
Instruction focusing on social competency using cognitive-behavioral methods	5	5
Other instructional programs	3	2
Behavioral/cognitive-behavioral strategies	5	5
Counseling, social work, other therapeutic	3	3
Mentoring, tutoring, work-study	3	3
Recreational, community service, leisure activities	3	3
After-school programs with emphasis on social competency skill development	3	4

[a]The scale is as follows: *5*, Effective (supported by two or more well-designed studies or systematic review); *4*, promising (supported by one well-designed study); *3*, insufficient (not enough evidence *or* mixed evidence—strong studies show both effective and not effective); *2*, not effective (no effect found in two or more well-designed studies or systematic review); *1*, harmful (negative effect supported by two or more well-designed studies or systematic review).

9.5.   REVIEW OF INTERVENTIONS BY LEVEL OF EVIDENCE

9.5.1.   Products and Physical Environments

There is little research on the effects of products on youth violence or associated outcomes, with the exception of one study on the use of metal detectors in schools. Ginsberg and Loffredo (1993) conducted a survey on a representative sample of high school students in New York City to compare the frequency of weapon carrying in schools with and without metal detectors. They found that, although students in schools with metal detectors were half as likely to carry a weapon to school as students in schools without metal detectors, metal detectors in schools may not affect weapon carrying in other locations. Eck (2002) reviewed the effects of a variety of products on the prevention of crime in high-crime locations, such as apartment buildings, subway stations and airports. For example, closed-circuit television may reduce the incidence of violent crime in open public spaces because it enables "designated guardians" to observe people and contact the police when necessary (Armitage, Smyth, & Pease, 1999). Other research shows passenger screening and the use of metal detectors lead to a reduction in aircraft hijacking (Easteal & Wilson, 1991; Landes, 1978). Although Eck (2002) did not specifically address youth violence, these products found to be effective in reducing crime in general could be studied to determine their effects on youth violence. Although research on the effects of structural changes to the physical environmental interventions on youth violence is rare, Eck identified several promising strategies that must be further investigated to determine effects on youth violence.

9.5.2. Behavioral

Behavioral interventions to reduce or prevent youth violence fall into five broad categories: society (laws, policies, broad cultural norms), communities, schools, parent/family, and individuals. In fact, the majority of effective and promising interventions for youth violence focus on changing features of schools, families, or individuals. All five behavioral categories are reviewed here, but more emphasis is placed on interventions that target schools, families, and individual behaviors and attitudes related to violence.

9.5.2.1. Society-Level Interventions

The society-level interventions we describe are media campaigns and the effects of reducing exposure to violence in the media.[1]

9.5.2.1.1. Media Campaigns.   The majority of media campaigns directed at youth have been directed toward reducing cigarette use or alcohol consumption, such as Partnership for a Drug Free America (Catalano, Arthur, Hawkins, Berglund, & Olson, 1998). Several studies have been conducted to determine the effect of media campaigns on youth substance use. Derzon and Lipsey (2002) examined evaluations of 72 media campaigns and found small changes in youths' knowledge, attitudes, and behavior regarding substance use. They found small reductions in alcohol, tobacco, and marijuana use among adolescents. Although studies show media campaigns have limited effectiveness alone, they are more effective in conjunction with classroom curricula (Catalano et al., 1998). Biglan, Brennan, Foster, and Holder (2004) and Catalano et al. (1998) indicated there were no evaluations of media campaigns developed to affect antisocial or violent behavior. Because media campaigns are a promising strategy for reducing substance use, they should be explored and studied for their effects on youth violence.

9.5.2.1.2. Reducing Exposure to Violence in the Media.   The effects of youth exposure to violence—through exposure to television as well as to other forms of media such as computers, movies, video games, and music videos—has been a concern for several decades (U.S. Public Health Service [USPHS], 2001). The majority of research conducted on children's exposure to violence in the media examined its effects on verbal and physical violence (USPHS, 2001). Paik and Comstock (1994) conducted a meta-analysis of 217 empirical studies on the effect of media violence and aggressive behavior on youths. They found exposure to media violence led to a temporary increase in aggressive, and in some cases violent, behavior among youths. Several longitudinal studies have shown a long-term relationship between exposure to media violence during childhood and future aggressive behavior during adolescence and adulthood (Eron, Huesmann,

---

[1]Laws and policies addressing violence were considered but are not discussed here because they are covered in another chapter in this volume.

Lefkowitz, & Walder, 1972; Huesmann & Eron, 1986; Huesmann, Lagerspetz, & Eron, 1984; Lefkowitz, Eron, Walder, & Huesmann, 1977; Milavsky et al., 1982). Research has yet to be published on the effects of exposure to violence on the Internet and in music videos on youth behavior (USPHS, 2001). Anderson and Bushman (2001) conducted a meta-analysis of the studies on the effect of violent video games on youth aggression. They found the effect of violent video games was small for physical aggression and moderate for aggressive thinking, although more research needs to be conducted in this area.

Although this research on the association of exposure to violence and subsequent violence suggests that reducing exposure to violence will reduce violence, we know of no studies that have actually tested interventions designed to reduce such exposure. Such interventions might, for example, train parents to limit their childrens' television watching or change the type of movies they watch. Until such research demonstrates that such intervention is possible and effective, we conclude that the evidence is insufficient to support claims of effectiveness for efforts to reduce exposure to violence.

In summary, because studies on the effects of media campaigns primarily focus on substance use, insufficient evidence is available to support the effectiveness of society-level interventions on youth violence. Research shows, however, that media campaigns against substance use are effective. These types of interventions should be further studied to determine effects on youth violence. Further research, especially employing experimental manipulations, is also needed to more completely determine the effects of reducing exposure to violence in the media on youth violence/aggression and associated outcomes.

9.5.2.2.   Community-Level Interventions

Several community-level interventions are effective for reducing crime in general, but few target youth violence. The community-level interventions we discuss are policing strategies, community mobilization, and voucher programs. Some additional interventions that ordinarily take place in the community—such as after-school programs and mentoring—primarily focus on altering individual-level risk factors for engaging in subsequent violent acts. They are discussed later.

9.5.2.2.1. Policing Strategies.   Community interventions are classified as policing strategies if the police actually carry out the intervention and if they focus on altering one or more community-level variables. The majority of these interventions do not specifically target youth violence. Sherman and Eck (2002) described several of these interventions including increased directed patrols, proactive arrests, problem-oriented policing, and community-oriented policing. Directed patrols, a concentration of patrols in high-crime areas, or hot spots, and during predetermined times of heightened criminal activity, are an effective crime prevention intervention. Proactive arrests, or police-initiated arrests, are also an effective crime prevention intervention. A third effective crime prevention intervention is problem-oriented policing, which focuses on identifying and solving the causes of crime patterns to ensure public safety and the prevention of crime. In contrast to problem-oriented policing, community-oriented policing focuses on improving the relationship between police and the community to reduce crime. Sherman and Eck (2002) classified community-oriented policing as a promising intervention due to mixed results on its effectiveness.

While directed patrols, proactive arrests, problem-oriented policing, and community-oriented policing are policing interventions designed to reduce crime, they do not specifically target youth violence. One example of targeted policing at juveniles is the Boston Gun Project implemented in 1996 (Kennedy, Piehl, & Brage, 1996). This project focused on gang-related violence and violence prevention. It used a gang-suppression strategy with an emphasis on firearms and included two components: direct law-enforcement attack on those illegally providing youths with firearms and a strong deterrent to gang violence (Braga, Kennedy, & Piehl, 1999). Deterrence was achieved through multiple agencies, such as detached workers, social services, and drug-treatment providers (Kennedy et al., 1996; Braga et al., 1999). The response to violence included a variety of actions such as shutting down drug markets and serving warrants (Kennedy, 1997). The Boston Gun Project coincided with a reduction in youth homicide victims across Boston, a decrease in the mean number of gun assault incidents throughout the city (Braga et al., 1999), and a reduction in overall gang violence in Boston (Kennedy et al., 1996). However, a recent National Academy of Sciences report on firearms and violence (Wellford, Pepper, & Petrie, 2004) argued that it is difficult to specify the role the intervention played in the reduction of youth homicide in Boston. Therefore, we suggest the findings regarding the Boston Gun Project be interpreted with caution.

In summary, several policing strategies are effective interventions for crime prevention in general, but more research needs to be conducted on the effects of this type of intervention on youth violence and associated outcomes.

9.5.2.2.2. Community Mobilization. Similar to the policing strategies, community mobilization interventions tend to be more general. They target entire neighborhood populations rather than specifically targeting youth violence. They are, therefore, rarely evaluated specifically for effects on youth violence. However, to the extent they are effective at all, they can be expected to affect youth violence. Community mobilization strategies focus on the actions of citizens to prevent crime and include neighborhood block watch and citizen patrol (Catalano et al., 1998). Catalano et al. (1998) reviewed block watch and citizen-patrol programs and concluded these interventions did not have a significant effect on crime. Similarly, Welsh and Hoshi (2002) argued community mobilization interventions had an unknown effect on crime and the available evaluations were of low scientific rigor. Community mobilization interventions targeting substance use have been much better developed than those targeting violence. Such interventions are promising for reducing substance use (Hingson et al., 1996). We conclude there is insufficient evidence on the effectiveness of community mobilization interventions on youth violence and associated outcomes.

9.5.2.2.3. Voucher Programs. Another promising community-level intervention is voucher programs for public-housing residents, in which tenants are given vouchers they can use to rent housing in the private market in any location. The primary goals of voucher programs are to deconcentrate poverty and improve employment, education, and other opportunities for the poor by dispersing people of low socioeconomic status within more economically and socially heterogeneous communities. A recent CDC report (2002) noted results from a systematic review of family housing interventions and concluded rental voucher programs are an effective intervention for improving household safety and reducing families' exposure to violence. Evidence for effects on youth problem behaviors, delinquent acts, and arrests were less conclusive, though. Ludwig, Duncan, and Hirschfield (2001) conducted a randomized housing-mobility experiment to determine the effects of voucher programs on youth violence. They found voucher programs providing families with the opportunity to relocate to low-poverty areas led to a reduction in violent arrests among juveniles. We conclude public-housing voucher programs are a promising community-level intervention for youth violence.

9.5.2.3.   School-Level Interventions

Gottfredson, Wilson, & Najaka, (2002) identified several types of interventions seeking to reduce youth problem behavior by altering characteristics of school environments, including school and discipline management and establishing norms or expectations for behavior.[2]

9.5.2.3.1. School and Discipline Management Interventions.   School discipline management interventions include those focused on changing the decision-making processes or authority structures to enhance the organizational capacity of the school. These interventions often involve collaboration among staff and sometimes parents, students, and community members to identify problems within the school, develop potential solutions, and design activities to improve the school. One example program that shows the effectiveness of these interventions is Project PATHE (Gottfredson, 1986, 1990).

Project PATHE altered the organization and management structures in seven secondary schools between 1981 and 1983 as part of the Office of Juvenile Justice and Delinquency Prevention's (OJJDP's) alternative education initiative (Gottfredson, 1986). This intervention used a school-team approach known as program development evaluation (PDE), which is a structured organizational development method designed to help organizations plan, initiate, and sustain needed changes (Gottfredson, 1984). In Project PATHE, the intervention schools used this structured method to implement activities to increase the clarity of school rules and consistency of rule enforcement and increase students' success experiences and their feelings of belonging in the school. The students in the intervention schools reported less delinquent behavior and drug use and fewer punishments in school relative to the students in the comparison schools (Gottfredson, 1986, 1990).

Evaluations of PATHE and several other programs that alter school management or discipline management (summarized in Gottfredson et al. [2002]) lead us to conclude that this type of intervention is effective for reducing problem behaviors associated with youth violence, although there is insufficient evidence to determine the effects on youth violence/aggression per se.

School resource officer (SRO) programs have increased in popularity, especially since several well-publicized school shooting events in the middle to late 1990s highlighted the problem of school violence. These programs, we believe, fall into the category of programs just discussed. The SRO concept first emerged during the 1950s in Flint, Michigan, as part of the implementation of community policing (Girouard, 2001). The concept grew during the 1960s and 1970s, primarily in Florida, although it did not spread nationally until the mid-1990s (Girouard, 2001). Johnson (1999, p. 174) defined SROs as "uniformed police officers placed in city high schools and middle schools for the purpose of creating and maintaining

---

[2]This section taken with minor revision from Gottfredson et al. (2002).

a safe and secure school environment." The placement of SROs in schools was an attempt to prevent school fights, theft, drug and alcohol abuse, the use of weapons, and other school problems (Johnson, 1999). Johnson conducted a preliminary evaluation on the SRO program using self-report data from SROs, program administrators, and school principals. The evaluation also included a comparison of suspension rates over time. This study is not sufficiently rigorous to draw conclusions regarding the effectiveness of SRO programs on youth violence. Although there is insufficient evidence to support the effectiveness of SROs, their similarity to the larger class of effective school and discipline management programs should be noted. More rigorous research is clearly needed on SRO programs, however.

9.5.2.3.2. Establishing Norms or Expectations for Behavior.   The second type of environmentally focused school-level intervention focuses on establishing clear norms or expectations for behavior. These interventions consist of schoolwide efforts to redefine norms for behavior and to signal appropriate behavior (Gottfredson et al., 2002). These efforts include activities such as newsletters, posters, ceremonies during which students declare their intention to remain drug-free, and displaying symbols of appropriate behavior. Two examples of this type that focus on violent behavior are Bullying Prevention (Olweus, 1991, 1992; Olweus & Alsaker, 1991; Olweus, Limber, & Mihalic, 1999), and the Safe Dates Program (Foshee et al., 1996, 1998).

The Bullying Prevention Program targets students in elementary, middle, and high schools (Olweus et al., 1999). The program consists of schoolwide, classroom, and individual components to target bullying. Examples of schoolwide components are increased supervision of students at bullying "hot spots" and schoolwide conferences to discuss bullying. Classroom components are the development and enforcement of rules against bullying. The program also includes individual-level components such as counseling children identified as bullies and victims. Olweus and colleagues (1999) found the implementation of this program led to large reductions in bullying and victimization among students as well as a decline in incidents of antisocial behavior such as vandalism, fighting, and theft. An earlier evaluation of the program indicated bullying decreased by 50% among the 2500 students (aged 11–14 years) included in the study (Olweus, 1991, 1992; Olweus & Alsaker, 1991).

A second example of this type of intervention is the Safe Dates Program aimed at changing norms for dating violence among adolescents (Foshee et al., 1996, 1998). The school activities in the Safe Dates Program include a theater production performed by peers, a 10-session curriculum addressing dating violence norms, gender stereotyping and conflict management skills, and a poster contest. The community activities include special services for adolescents in abusive relationships and community service provider training. Foshee et al. (1998) evaluated the Safe Dates Program for eighth and ninth grade students and found that the students in the treatment schools reported significantly less psychological abuse and violence perpetrated against the current dating partner than the students in the control schools. Most of these effects were explained by changes in dating violence norms, gender stereotyping, and awareness of services (Gottfredson et al., 2002). These two example programs, the Bullying Prevention Program and the Safe Dates Program, were evaluated using rigorous methodology and showed significant positive effects on youth violence. Therefore, we conclude interventions that establish norms or expectations for behavior are an effective intervention for violence/aggression as well as associated outcomes.

9.5.2.4. Family/Parent Interventions

The family/parent interventions are classified into two groups: child–parent training and family focused. These groups are based on the classification of interventions provided by Webster-Stratton and Taylor (2001). Child–parent training interventions include parent-focused and child-focused interventions with a parent component. Parent-focused interventions focus primarily on parent training, such as prenatal and infancy parent education and family-management training. They sometimes also include a child component, which is often delivered in a child-care or preschool program. Child-focused interventions in this family/parent category include programs that specifically focus on child training but also include a parent component. Most child-focused interventions are covered elsewhere in this chapter. Finally, family-focused interventions target the interaction of family members and family processes, such as functional family therapy and family-strengthening programs.

9.5.2.4.1. Child–Parent Training. Child–parent training interventions include parent-focused and child-focused with parent component interventions. Parent-focused interventions consist primarily of home visitation programs, including parent training and education in a variety of areas such as proper nutrition during pregnancy; infant care and development; and managing temper tantrums, defiance, and aggressive behavior (Webster-Stratton & Taylor, 2001). One example of a parent-focused intervention is the Prenatal/Early Infancy Project (Olds, 1998; Olds, Eckenrode, & Henderson, 1997; Olds, Henderson, Phelps, Kitzman, & Hanks, 1993).

The Prenatal/Early Infancy Project was developed in Elmira by Olds et al. (1997) to improve prenatal health and outcomes of pregnancy; the care parents provide to their children and thus children's development and overall health; and women's own personal life-course development, such as education and career planning. The program included free transportation to prenatal and child doctor appointments, nurse home visits during pregnancy and early childhood, and parent education and training (Olds et al., 1993). Evaluations of this program included random assignment of mothers to treatment and control conditions (Olds et al., 1997; Olds, 1998). The program (when mothers received all components) had immediate positive effects on high-risk mothers' child abuse and neglect (Olds et al., 1997, 1998). A 13-year follow-up evaluation showed the program's positive effects on high-risk mothers' arrests and convictions as well as on children's arrests (Olds, 1998; Olds et al., 1997).

Based on the meta-analyses conducted by Farrington and Welsh (2002) and Webster-Stratton and Taylor (2001), we conclude that parent-focused programs are an effective intervention for reducing child behavior problems, delinquency, and other related outcomes. However, evidence is insufficient with respect to effects on measures of youth violence/aggression.

Child-focused interventions with a parent component focus on child training, for example in school or day care, with a minor parenting component. One example program is Linking the Interests of Families and Teachers (LIFT), an intervention to prevent conduct problems among adolescents, including antisocial behavior and involvement with delinquent peers (Reid, Eddy, Fetrow, & Stoolmiller, 1999). The program is designed for first and fifth graders living in areas with high rates of juvenile delinquency. LIFT consisted of three components: classroom component, playground component, and parenting component. The classroom component consists of lectures and role playing on a variety of social or problem-solving skills, structured group skills practice, free play, and daily rewards. The playground component calls for the separation of children into small groups and provides children with rewards for positive behavior while on the playground. The parenting component involves group and community meetings to educate parents about creating positive home environments. Reid et al. (1999) used a comparison group design and found children in the LIFT program showed a significant reduction in physical aggression on the playground compared to the control group. The program also had a positive effect on child behavior problems after 1 year. We conclude, based on the work of Farrington and Welsh (2002) and Webster-Stratton and Taylor (2001) that child-focused programs with a minor parenting component are an effective intervention for both youth violence/aggression and associated outcomes.

9.5.2.4.2. Family-Focused Interventions. Family-focused interventions target the family unit, rather than the individual members, and target the interaction of family members and family processes. One example of this intervention is Multidimensional Treatment Foster Care (MTFC) (Chamberlain & Reid, 1998). In the MTFC program, young males with a history of serious and chronic offending are placed in an alternative family setting for approximately 6 months (Chamberlain & Reid, 1998). Families recruited for the program are trained and implement an individualized program for each youth in their home to emphasize the youth's strengths and establish clear rules and boundaries. Other components of this program include weekly supervision, support meetings, family therapy for biological parents, and individual therapy. Chamberlain (1990) used a matched control group to evaluate the program and found the outcomes were better for MTFC children and families as compared to other residential treatment models. For example, adolescents were incarcerated for a shorted amount of time when they received MTFC. Youths that received MTFC were compared with adolescents in the control group that received Group Care (GC) (variations on group, individual, and family therapy). They found boys in the treatment group had fewer arrests than the control group, reported committing fewer criminal acts, and ran away or were expelled from the program less often.

We conclude there is insufficient evidence to evaluate the effectiveness of family-focused interventions on violence and aggression per se, although these interventions are effective for reducing outcomes closely associated with youth violence (Farrington & Welsh, 2002; Lipsey & Wilson, 1998; Webster-Stratton & Taylor, 2001).

9.5.2.5.   Individual Interventions

The majority of youth violence interventions aim to alter some individual characteristic or set of individual characteristics that place the individual at elevated risk for perpetrating youth violence.[3] These interventions range from interventions with preschool youths,[4] aimed at teaching them social competency skills and preparing

---

[3]This section is taken, with minor revision, from Gottfredson et al. (2002).

[4]Note that several individual-level interventions that target preschool children include a parent component and are, therefore, classified as child education/training plus parent training interventions, discussed in the previous section.

them for a successful school experience, to interventions for adjudicated adolescents that take place either in the community or in a juvenile institution. In between these extremes is a wide range of interventions for school-aged youths, some of which target the general population and others of which target specific youths who have displayed risk factors for violent behavior or some related problem behavior. Summarizing these interventions in a few pages is a challenge.

The several meta-analyses and reviews of delinquency prevention available for summary tend to focus on different segments of the youth violence landscape. For example, Gottfredson et al. (2002) focus on interventions delivered in schools; Welsh and Hoshi (2002), on interventions delivered in community settings; and Lipsey and Wilson (1998), on interventions for adjudicated youths. In summarizing these sources, we tried to retain the classification of interventions provided in Gottfredson et al. (2002), mapping results from other reviews where possible into these categories. Three additional categories were added from other sources. The five main categories of school-based prevention are instructing students; behavioral and cognitive-behavioral strategies; counseling and social work; mentoring, tutoring, and work-study experiences; and providing recreational, community service, and leisure activities. We added after-school programs as separate categories and a "comprehensive" category, which includes programs emphasizing a variety of strategies such as instruction, work-study, family-skills training, and mentoring. In the following pages, we describe each of these categories and provide one example of each type of intervention (when possible) for preschool, elementary, and adolescent children.

9.5.2.5.1. Instructing Students. Gottfredson et al. (2002) identified the broad category of "instructing students" as the most common prevention strategy used in schools. These interventions provide instruction to students to teach them factual information, increase their awareness of social influences to engage in misbehavior, expand their repertoires for recognizing and appropriately responding to risky or potentially harmful situations, increase their appreciation for diversity in society, improve their moral character, etc. Gottfredson et al. (2002) differentiated this broad group of instructional interventions according to their content and the instructional methods used. They discovered that instructional programs that had both a specific focus on social competency skill development and that used what they called "cognitive-behavioral methods" were more effective than other instructional programs. Instructional programs that use cognitive-behavioral methods depend on strategies such as the use of cues, feedback, rehearsal, and role-playing. They are more engaging for students. Those without cognitive-behavioral methods depend more on traditional methods of instruction such as workbooks, lecture, and some class discussion.

An example program of instruction with cognitive-behavioral methods for preschool students is Interpersonal Problem-Solving Skills (ICPS) (Shure & Spivak, 1979, 1980, 1982). The ICPS program uses cognitive training to help children as young as 4 years learn a variety of skills, such as how to find alternative solutions to problems, become aware of steps required to reach a goal, and consider consequences of their behavior (Gottfredson et al., 2002). ICPS is a school-based program in which teachers work with small groups of children to improve these skills. Shure and Spivak used a comparison group design to evaluate ICPS. The study consisted of over 200 African American inner-city nursery school children who received the intervention for different lengths of time. Some children received the training only in nursery school, while others continued to receive training in kindergarten, and some children had the training only in kindergarten. A fourth group did not receive the ICPS training. Shure and Spivak found students that received ICPS training in only nursery school or kindergarten improved significantly more than controls on ICPS skills and behavioral adjustment. In addition, children who received training both years had significantly higher scores on measures of ICPS, although the additional year did not result in greater differences in behavior ratings.

FAST Track (Coie, 1997; Conduct Problems Prevention Research Group [CPPRG], 1997) is one example of instruction with cognitive-behavioral methods for elementary-aged children and is the most ambitious school-based prevention effort aimed at young school children to date (Gottfredson et al., 2002). This program integrates five intervention components designed to promote competence in the family, child, and school and thus prevent conduct problems, poor social relations, and school failure, all precursors of subsequent criminal behavior, during the elementary school years. The program involves training for parents in family-management practices; frequent home visits by program staff to reinforce skills learned in the training, to promote parental feelings of efficacy, and to enhance family organization; social skills coaching for children delivered by program staff; academic tutoring for children; and a classroom instructional program, focusing on social competency skills coupled with classroom-management strategies for the teacher. An experimental evaluation showed this program had positive effects on child social cognitive skills, problem behavior recorded by trained observers, and other antisocial/aggressive behaviors. This program combines several of the most effective school-based strategies. Its positive results for such a difficult population are encouraging and attest to the need for more comprehensive, theory-based, preventive interventions implemented with careful attention to strength and fidelity.

One example of an instructional program using cognitive-behavioral methods for adolescents is Anger Control Training (Feindler, Marriott, & Iwata, 1984). This program was delivered to junior high school boys who were participating in an existing program for disruptive youths (Gottfredson et al., 2002). The 36 most disruptive of these youths were selected and randomly assigned to receive anger management training or not. The program consisted of 10 sessions delivered by a trained therapist in which students were taught to analyze the components of the provocation cycle—the antecedent anger cues, aggressive responses, and consequent events—using self-monitoring and written logs. Students also learned to replace aggressive responses with more appropriate responses, problem-solving techniques, and specific cognitive behaviors (e.g., self-instruction). Feindler et al. (1984) found experimental students improved more than controls on an interview measure of problem-solving skills and on teacher ratings of self-control. The program also had significant positive effects on mild verbal and physical misbehaviors (cursing, arguing, and shoving). For more serious infractions, the trend favored treatment students but the differences were not statistically significant.

These programs are effective interventions for both violence/aggression and associated outcomes among children of all age groups. In contrast, the evidence is mixed (at best) regarding the instructional programs that do not use cognitive-behavioral methods. Two meta-analyses have concluded that these programs are ineffective interventions for reducing youth violence/aggression and associated outcomes (Gottfredson et al., 2002; Lipsey & Wilson, 1998), but because some of the specific studies in these reviews find positive effects, we classify the evidence as mixed. The most well known program of instruction that does not rely on cognitive-behavioral methods is DARE (Drug Abuse Resistance Education). Numerous evaluations have been conducted on DARE; Gottfredson et al. (2002) concluded DARE has a trivial effect on measures of substance abuse and does not work for reducing conduct problems. The broader category of instructional programs that do not use cognitive-behavioral strategies (of which DARE is an example) has mixed evidence of effectiveness for reducing problem behaviors associated with youth violence.

9.5.2.5.2. Behavioral and Cognitive-Behavioral Strategies. Behavioral and cognitive-behavioral strategies focus on modifying behavior and on teaching "thinking skills" (Gottfredson et al., 2002). Behavior modification interventions focus directly on changing behaviors by rewarding desired behavior and punishing undesired behavior. Many programs for delinquent and at-risk populations also attempt to alter thinking skills. These "cognitive-behavioral training" interventions are based on a substantial body of research indicating that delinquents are deficient in a number of thinking skills necessary for social adaptation. Delinquents often do not think before they act, believe that what happens to them is due to fate or chance rather than to their own actions, misinterpret social cues, fail to consider alternative solutions to problems, and lack interpersonal skills necessary for effective communications.

An example of a group-based behavior management program for elementary-aged children is the Good Behavior Game (GBG) (Dolan et al., 1993). In GBG, small student teams are formed within each classroom, and the teams are rewarded for achieving behavioral standards. Because the team reward depends on the behavior of each member of the team, peer pressure is used constructively in this program to achieve positive behavior. Dolan et al. (1993) used a randomized control group design and found (when comparing with a control classroom in the same school) that GBG males were rated by their peers (but not by their teachers) as significantly less aggressive at the end of first grade. The opposite pattern was found for females: teacher ratings (but not peer ratings) of aggression were significantly lower for GBG students. Compared to control classrooms in different schools, GBG males were rated by their teachers but not by their peers as less aggressive at the end of the first grade, and none of the comparisons of GBG females, with the external controls, showed significant differences. Gottfredson et al. (2002) pooled data for males and females, teacher and peer raters, and found an overall significant effect of GBG on aggressive behavior.

Thompson and Hudson (1982) evaluated Behavioral Group Counseling for adolescents, and found the program had a significant positive effect on maladaptive behavior among adolescents in grade nine. They contrasted the effects of behavioral group counseling with a values clarification intervention delivered to orphaned ninth-grade boys in a residential home. Behavioral counseling consisted of 15 weeks of weekly meetings during which a counselor trained in behavioral counseling procedures led activities aimed at understanding problems in behavioral terms and helping students modify their behaviors. Behavioral techniques included role-playing, rational behavior therapy, environmental manipulation, and contracting. During the 15-week posttreatment phase, the behavioral counseling group had significantly fewer acts of maladaptive behavior than did the control group or placebo groups. This type of intervention is also among the most effective for adjudicated youth (Lipsey & Wilson, 1998).

We conclude based on the available research summaries that behavioral and cognitive-behavioral strategies are effective interventions for reducing youth violence/aggression and associated outcomes among all age groups.

9.5.2.5.3. Counseling, Social Work, and Other Therapeutic Interventions.

Gottfredson et al. (2002) concluded that school-based counseling approaches to crime reduction do not work for reducing antisocial behavior and that the results for these types of programs are mixed for crime outcomes. Lipsey and Wilson (1998) concluded that individual counseling is an effective intervention for recidivism among noninstitutionalized youth but that the results are mixed for institutionalized youths. This category of intervention is fairly heterogeneous, and research summaries have not yet succeeded in identifying the characteristics of more effective counseling-type programs. It is likely that different definitions of *counseling* have been used in determining which programs to even include in the category. For example, several of the interventions included in Gottfredson and co-workers' (2002) effective behavioral or cognitive-behavioral category were in fact *counseling* programs based on these effective models. These same or similar programs most likely contribute to the effectiveness of Lipsey and Wilson's (1998) individual counseling category, as they indicated that many of the most effective programs also relied on behavioral and cognitive-behavioral strategies. We conclude that the evidence at this point in time is mixed in regard to these interventions. We encourage future research to investigate this area more carefully in an attempt to understand the heterogeneous effects.

It is important to understand this category of intervention more fully because some evidence suggests that counseling interventions might actually increase youth problem behaviors. For example, Gottfredson (1987) used random assignment to evaluate the Peer Culture Development (PCD) program, a peer-group counseling program in elementary and high schools to promote the adoption of pro-social attitudes. As many negative as positive effects were found in the evaluation of the elementary version of the program. In the high school program, treatment youths reported significantly more delinquent behavior than control youths. Gottfredson concluded that the unconstrained group sessions in which youths were free to discuss their unconventional beliefs and receive validation for them may have contributed to the negative effects.

9.5.2.5.4. Mentoring, Tutoring, and Work-Study.

Mentoring, tutoring, and work-study interventions usually involve one-on-one interaction with an older, more experienced person to provide advice or assistance (Gottfredson et al., 2002). They are differentiated from counseling in that the older adult is generally not a professional counselor, and the interaction is generally not focused on the individuals' problem behavior. Welsh and Hoshi (2002) concluded that there is insufficient evidence on the effectiveness of community-based mentoring programs on youth violence/aggression and associated outcomes. Gottfredson et al. (2002) reported that only one of four evaluations of school-based mentoring programs for elementary students found a significant positive effect on violence/aggression or associated outcomes. For adolescents, Hahn, Leavitt, and Aaron (1994) using a randomized design, found the Quantum Opportunities Program (QOP) had significant positive effects after 2 years on academic and functional skills, educational expectations, graduation rates, and self-reported trouble with the police. This program provides both in- and out-of-school services to disadvantaged high school students and includes academic assistance, service activities, and a curriculum focusing on life/family skills and planning for college and jobs (Gottfredson et al., 2002). Taggart (1995) found a 70% reduction in arrests for the QOP treatment subjects relative to the control subjects in this initial study. However, a more recent replication evaluation of QOP, also using a randomized design (Maxfield, Schirm, & Rodriguez-Planas, 2002), found that, although QOP increased the likelihood of graduation and of engaging in postsecondary education or training, the program did not reduce risky behaviors or improve grades or achievement test scores.

We conclude that, with the failure of QOP to replicate positive results on problem behaviors, the evidence is mixed as to the effectiveness of mentoring, tutoring, and work-study intervention on violence/aggression and associated outcomes.

9.5.2.5.5. Recreation, Community Service, Enrichment, and Leisure Activities. Another popular type of youth violence prevention for children and adolescents is a category including recreation, community service, enrichment, and leisure activities. Wilderness challenge programs and "ropes" courses, often provided to higher-risk youths, also fit into this category. Drop-in recreation centers, after-school and weekend programs, dances, community service activities, and other events are offered as alternatives to more dangerous activities. Gottfredson et al. (2002) and Lipsey and Wilson (1998) concluded that, at best, there is insufficient evidence to determine the effectiveness of these interventions on violence/aggression and associated outcomes.

However, after-school programs can be differentiated from the larger group of recreational and leisure programs as potentially effective. These programs almost always involve a recreational component but many also provide a social skill-development component that can be expected to produce positive effects, and they have the potential to reduce association with negative peers, which is likely to occur when adolescents are left unsupervised in the afternoon hours. On the basis of three quasi-experimental evaluations of after-school programs, Welsh and Hoshi (2002) concluded that such programs are promising for reducing crime. The most rigorous of the studies they reviewed was an evaluation of a Boys and Girls Club (BGC) (Schinke, Orlandi, & Cole, 1992) in which youths in public housing units with access to the clubs were compared with youths in public housing units without access. Half of their BGCs implemented a "self-management and resistance training" program involving social competency skill instruction. The housing units with access to BGCs experienced less vandalism, and substance abuse and drug trafficking were also lower in these units.

More recently, Gottfredson, Gerstenblith, Soulé, Womer, Lu (2004) and Gottfredson, Soulé, and Cross (2004) examined the effect of after-school programs implemented in Maryland. They found one set of programs reduced delinquent behavior among middle school students, but not among elementary-aged children, and that the most successful programs focused on social skills and character development (Gottfredson, Gerstenblith, et al., 2004). In an evaluation of the subsequent Maryland After School Opportunity Fund Program, Gottfredson, Soulé, and Cross (2004) found youths increased their decision-making skills and reduced their delinquent behavior relative to the comparison group. Once again, programs with an emphasis on social problem-solving instruction were most effective for reducing delinquency and drug use.

Unfortunately, no randomized experimental study has yet assessed the effects of after-school programs on violence or related problem behaviors. However, based on the Welsh and Hoshi (2002) summary and on the more recent evaluations of after-school programs, we conclude that after-school programs that incorporate social competency skill instruction are promising for reducing problem behaviors associated with youth violence among adolescents (but not elementary school youths). There is insufficient evidence to judge their effects on violent and aggressive behavior.

9.5.2.5.6. Comprehensive Interventions. Some programs combine several of the intervention categories described above. Several broad programs (e.g., Fast Track, LIFT) were included in the categories summarized above when it seemed that one of the interventions in the set was emphasized more than others. But some programs encompass many components, all of which are emphasized. No one part seems to capture the essence of the program.

Children At Risk (CAR) is a comprehensive program that targets high-risk youths in poor neighborhoods in urban areas of the United States (Harrell, Cavanagh, & Sridharan, 1999). CAR included family counseling, family-skills training, tutoring, mentoring, after-school activities, and community policing (Farrington & Welsh, 2002). Harrell et al. (1999) evaluated the program using random assignment of youths to experimental and control conditions. After 1 year, Harrell et al. (1999) found youths participating in CAR committed fewer violent crimes than youths in control conditions. In addition, treatment youths were less likely to associate with delinquent peers, felt less peer pressure to engage in delinquency, and had more positive support from peers (Farrington & Welsh, 2002). CASASTART (Striving Together to Achieve Rewarding Tomorrows) represents the second iteration of CAR research at The National Center on Addiction and Substance Abuse at Columbia University (Harrell, Cavanagh, & Sridharan, 1998). Harrell et al. (1998) evaluated the program and found youths in the quasi-experimental group reported less drug abuse and participation in violent crimes than control youths. There are too few truly comprehensive programs to render a judgment as to their effectiveness as a group. Furthermore, the effectiveness of these comprehensive programs depends highly on the combination of components in the program. But we present this category to illustrate the potential for combining elements known to be effective alone into a much broader and possibly more potent comprehensive package.

9.6. IMPLICATIONS AND LIMITATIONS FOR PUBLIC HEALTH PRACTICE AND FUTURE PREVENTION PLANNING

Some programs are effective for reducing youth violence and aggression. Others are of unknown effectiveness for reducing these problems but have been demonstrated to reduce related forms of problem behavior and, therefore, can be considered promising for reducing youth violence as well. Other prevention activities are unlikely to make a difference in levels of crime or substance use. Clearly, legislation and funding guidelines that have the effect of shifting monies away from approaches with less research support and toward approaches with more research support should be encouraged to improve outcomes in the short run. For the long run, much more research is needed to provide a more complete picture of the broader spectrum of potential interventions to reduce youth violence. These research needs are elaborated next.

As communities move toward more effective youth violence prevention, it is important that they recognize that programs and practices are usually not implemented in a vacuum. It is far more likely that within a given organization such as a school, multiple efforts aimed at achieving the same or related outcomes will be ongoing. We encourage organizations to develop comprehensive, long-term prevention strategies to coordinate these various efforts. Models for such comprehensive strategies exist, and training and technical assistance in implementing them is available. Howell (2003), for example, discussed several models for developing a comprehensive community-based strategy that would involve delivering relevant prevention and intervention strategies throughout the life course through a variety of community organizations and institutions. His comprehensive strategy includes prevention and early intervention, a system of graduated sanctions, and a parallel continuum of treatment alternatives (Howell, 2003). He identifies several models that can be used to guide the development of such comprehensive strategies: Communities That Care (CTC) is an example of a communitywide approach for preventing assorted problem behaviors that includes research-based tools to promote positive development among youth and prevent delinquency (Hawkins, 1999). The PDE method is another technique for encouraging researchers and practitioners to work together to develop, implement, and evaluate efforts to reduce problem behaviors (Gottfredson, 1984). This method has been employed to help School Improvement Teams of teachers, parents, and school officials to reduce school disorder (Gottfredson, 1986; Gottfredson, Gottfredson, & Hybl, 1993).

As communities move away from the idea of installing stand-alone model programs and toward a more comprehensive planning of coordinated strategies for reducing youth violence, and as they begin to select strategies that have been demonstrated effective to fill out the details of their comprehensive strategy, their programs will begin to resemble the more comprehensive programs summarized above (e.g., CASASTART) that have been shown to be effective for reducing youth violence.

Another implication for prevention practice concerns the quality of implementation. Effectiveness trials of model programs are beginning to reveal that the positive effects demonstrated in efficacy trials of model programs under amenable conditions are not always evident when the same programs are implemented under more natural conditions (Alper, 2002; Cho, Hallfors, Kim, Khatapoush, & Sanchez, 2004; Gottfredson et al., in press; Gutman, Foltz, Mitlal, & Kaltenbach, 2004; Henggeler, Melton, Brondino, & Schere, 1997). One major reason for the diminished benefits is that the quality of implementation tends to be lower when programs are implemented away from the watchful eye of the program developer or his or her staff. Policy makers should require that mechanisms to monitor the quality of implementation of funded activities be established and should encourage systems to provide necessary technical assistance and organization development assistance to improve implementation. For example, effort should be invested in identifying the key features of model programs and ensuring that program implementers understand the standards for implementation. Implementation measurement keyed to these standards can be developed and recipients of public funds can be required to collect data on the extent to which these standards are met. Mechanisms for providing helpful technical assistance and organization development could then be established to help organizations reach these implementation standards.

9.7   RESEARCH GAPS

The existing research on effectiveness of interventions to reduce youth violence suggests that, although certain types of interventions are clearly effective, what we don't know about preventing youth violence still far exceeds what we do know.[5] The research base can be strengthened in the following five ways: (1) including direct measures of aggression and violence in evaluations of programs targeting related problem behaviors, (2) encouraging studies of a greater variety of program types, (3) encouraging more rigorous research designs, (4) including long-term follow-ups, and (5) more carefully measuring and reporting on the strength and fidelity of implementation.

Studies of the effects of prevention on actual measures of violent behavior are rare. Far more common are studies assessing program effects on alcohol, tobacco, or other drug use and other less serious forms of defiant behavior. For example, of the 178 studies of school-based crime prevention examined in Gottfredson et al. (2002), only 39 (22%) measured any type of criminal behavior. In comparison, 102 (57%) studies measured noncriminal forms of antisocial behavior or conduct problems, and 77 (43%) studies measured alcohol, tobacco, or other drug use. Of the minority that did measure criminal behavior, only 13 (7%) measured serious crimes committed against people as opposed to property. Often, studies will include measures of aggression or violence against individuals, but these items will be combined with associated problem behavior measures, making it impossible to determine a specific program effect on aggression and violence. This practice, although reasonable given the more general focus of many programs being studied, limits the generalizeability of program effects to violent and aggressive behavior. It may be possible to develop agreements among federal agencies funding prevention work to encourage researchers to include a short battery of items measuring aggression and violence in their studies.

Table 9.1 makes clear that at present, although a handful of prevention strategies have sufficient evidence to support claims of effectiveness, there is still insufficient evidence to draw conclusions about most prevention strategies. Most of the untested strategies are plausible, and many have already been demonstrated effective for reducing problem behaviors closely related to violence and aggression. The types of programs and practices that have been well evaluated tend to be individually oriented programs in which relatively small studies can be conducted contrasting individuals receiving and not receiving specific services. Those that are clearly understudied tend to be interventions directed toward altering larger units—community norms and school management, for example. Although rigorous studies of such interventions may be more difficult and expensive to carry out, several examples of rigorous evaluations of these types of interventions exist in fields related to youth violence (e.g., Sherman and Berk's [1984] random assignment of policing strategies for domestic violence and Wagenaar, Murray, & Toomey's [2000] random assignment of communities to a community mobilization strategy). Clearly, more effort must be directed toward obtaining rigorous evaluations of a wider variety of youth violence prevention strategies.

A third limitation is weak evaluation design. Few studies use randomized experimental research designs, one of the most effective designs for eliminating competing explanations for observed effects. Gottfredson et al. (2002) rated the

---

[5]This section is based on a similar section in Gottfredson, Wilson, and Najaka (2001).

overall methodological rigor of the 178 studies included in their review. Each treatment–comparison contrast was rated on a 5-point scale with the following anchors: (1) no confidence should be placed in the results of the evaluation because of serious shortcomings in the methodology employed; (3) methodology rigorous in some respects, weak in others; and (5) methodology rigorous in almost all respects. Generally, only randomized controlled trials were rated at level 5. Only 26 (10%) of the treatment–comparison contrasts received the highest rating of 5. The increased reliance on meta-analysis makes it possible to obtain estimates of effect sizes across a large number of studies of a given type, regardless of the methodological rigor of the studies so summarized. But confidence in the conclusions of these meta-analyses is bolstered when the set of summarized studies includes some true experiments, and when the meta-analysis is able to show that the conclusions based on all studies are in accordance with those based on the most rigorous studies. We, therefore, encourage an emphasis on funding randomized trials of a greater variety of program types.

Another limitation of existing studies of youth violence prevention is their failure to measure long-term program effectiveness. Evaluations often assess program effect immediately after the conclusion of the intervention but lack a follow-up assessment; thus they are unable either to detect effects that may be less immediate or to determine whether immediate effects deteriorate over time. Limiting outcome measurement to an immediate posttest provides a high-end estimate of program effects.

A final drawback of existing evaluations of school-based prevention practices is their failure to report on the strength of program implementation. Quality and quantity of implementation are important predictors of program effectiveness (Gottfredson, 2001; Lipsey, 1992; Wright & Dixon, 1977). Yet many researchers fail to measure these factors. Before dismissing an intervention program and its underlying program theory, it is necessary to determine whether the proposed intervention actually took place as intended. Doing so requires a careful assessment of the strength and fidelity of program implementation.

9.8. CONCLUSIONS

At the present time, the most effective strategies for reducing youth violence and associated problem behavior outcomes are as follows:

- Programs aimed at clarifying and communicating norms about behaviors— for example, by communicating norms through schoolwide campaigns (e.g., antibullying campaigns) or ceremonies.
- Comprehensive instructional programs that focus on a range of social competency skills (e.g., developing self-control, stress management, responsible decision making, social problem solving, and communication skills) and that are delivered using cognitive-behavioral methods (e.g., cues, feedback, rehearsal, and role-playing).
- Behavior modification interventions and programs that teach thinking skills to high-risk youths. These programs focus directly on changing behaviors by rewarding desired behavior and punishing undesired behavior or teaching specific cognitive skills (such as thinking before acting, correct attributions, correct cue interpretations, etc.).

- Comprehensive family interventions that deliver interventions similar to those described above but augment them with parent training in family management. This category also includes parent training interventions, including prenatal and infancy parent education and family-management training.

The following strategies are known to be effective strategies for reducing problem behavior outcomes associated with youth violence, but additional research is required to demonstrate effects on youth violence:

- School and discipline management interventions that aim to improve the general management of the school and clarify and communicate norms about behaviors by establishing school rules and improving the consistency of their enforcement (particularly when they emphasize positive reinforcement of appropriate behavior).
- Family-focused interventions that seek to improve the interaction of family members and family processes, such as functional family therapy and family-strengthening programs.

A huge investment in youth violence prevention research is needed to expand the research base on effective strategies. In the meantime, funding agencies and communities should focus their efforts on the types of interventions that are known to be effective. Until additional research is conducted that supports the efficacy of other youth violence prevention strategies, they should not be supported with public dollars.

Communities should focus efforts on developing comprehensive, coordinated strategies for youth violence prevention that incorporate elements that resemble the programs and practices that have been shown to be effective. They should also pay close attention to the quality of implementation of these practices, because the probability is high that the positive outcomes achieved when these interventions were delivered as part of highly controlled research studies will not be replicated when the same interventions are delivered under more natural conditions.

REFERENCES

Alper, J. (2002). The nurse home visitation program. In S. L. Isaacs & J. R. Knickman (Eds.), *To improve health and health care. Vol. 5: The Robert Wood Johnson anthology* (pp. 3–22). San Francisco: Jossey-Bass.

Anderson, C. A., & Bushman, B. J. (2001). Effects of violent video games on aggressive behavior, aggressive cognition, aggressive affect, physiological arousal, and prosocial behavior: A meta-analytic review of the scientific literature. *Psychological Science, 12* (5), 353–360.

Armitage, R., Smyth, G., & Pease, K. (1999). Burnley CCTV evaluation. In K. Painter & N. Tilley (Eds.), *Surveillance of public space: CCTV, street lighting and crime prevention* (pp. 225–250, vol. 10). Monsey, NY: Criminal Justice Press.

Biglan, A., Brennan, P. A., Foster, S. L., & Holder, H. D. (2004). *Helping adolescents at risk: Prevention of multiple problem behaviors.* New York: Guilford Press.

Braga, A. A., Kennedy, D. M., & Piehl, A. M. (1999). *Problem-oriented policing and youth violence: An evaluation of the Boston Gun Project.* Final report submitted to the National Institute of Justice. Cambridge, MA: John F. Kennedy School of Government, Harvard University.

Catalano, R. F., Arthur, M. W., Hawkins, J. D., Berglund, L., & Olson, J. J. (1998). Comprehensive community- and school-based interventions to prevent antisocial behavior. In R. Loeber & D. P. Farrington (Eds.), *Serious and violent juvenile offenders: Risk factors & successful interventions* (pp. 248–283). Thousand Oaks, CA: Sage.

Centers for Disease Control and Prevention. (2002). Community interventions to promote healthy social environments: Early childhood development and family housing. *Morbidity & Mortality Weekly Report, 51*(RR-1), 1–8.

Chamberlain, P. (1990). Comparative evaluation of specialized foster care for seriously delinquent youths: A first step. *Community Alternative: International Journal of Family Care, 2* (2), 21–36.

Chamberlain, P., & Reid, J. (1998). Comparison of two community alternatives to incarceration for chronic juvenile offenders. *Journal of Consulting and Clinical Psychology, 66*, 624–633.

Cho, H., Hallfors, D., Kim, H. M., Khatapoush, S., & Sanchez, V. (2004). *Findings from a randomized controlled trial of the effectiveness of an indicated prevention program.* Paper presented at the annual meeting of the Society for Prevention Research, Quebec City.

Coie, J. D. (1997). *Testing developmental theory of antisocial behavior with outcomes from the Fast Track Prevention Project.* Paper presented at the meeting of the American Psychological Association, Chicago.

Conduct Problems Prevention Research Group. (1997). *Prevention of antisocial behavior: Initial findings from the Fast Track Project.* Paper presented at the meeting of the Society for Research in Child Development, Washington, D.C.

Cook, P. J., & Laub, J. H. (2002). After the epidemic: Recent trends in youth violence in the United States. In M. Tonry (Ed.), *Crime & justice* (pp. 1–17, vol. 29). Chicago: University of Chicago Press.

Derzon, J. H., & Lipsey, M. W. (2002). A meta-analysis of the effectiveness of mass-communication for changing substance-use knowledge, attitudes, and behavior. In W. D Crano, & M. Burgoon (Eds.), *Mass media and drug prevention: Classic and contemporary theories and research,* (pp. 231–258). Mahwah, NJ: Lawrence Erlbaum Associates.

Dolan, L. J., Kellam, S. G., Brown, C. H., Werthamer-Larsson, L., Rebok, G. W., Mayer, L. S., Laudolff, J., Turkkan, J. S., Ford, C., & Wheeler, L. (1993). The short-term impact of two classroom-based preventive interventions on aggressive and shy behaviors and poor achievement. *Journal of Applied Developmental Psychology, 14*, 317–345.

Easteal, P. W., & Wilson, P. R. (1991). *Preventing crime on transport.* Canberra: Australian Institute of Criminology.

Eck, J. E. (2002). Preventing crime at places. In L. W. Sherman, D. P. Farrington, B. C. Welsh, & D. L. MacKenzie (Eds.), *Evidence-based crime prevention* (pp. 241–294). New York: Routledge.

Eron, L. D., Huesmann, L. R., Lefkowitz, M. M., & Walder, L. O. (1972). Does television violence cause aggression? *American Psychologist, 27*, 253–263.

Farrington, D. P., & Welsh, B. C. (2002). Family-based crime prevention. In L. W. Sherman, D. P. Farrington, B. C. Welsh, & D. L. MacKenzie (Eds.), *Evidence-based crime prevention* (pp. 22–55). New York: Routledge.

Federal Bureau of Investigation. (2002). *Crime in the United States, 2002.* Retrieved February 9, 2005, from www.fbi.gov/ucr/cius_02/pdf/02crime4.pdf.

Feindler, E. L., Marriott, S. A., & Iwata, M. (1984). Group anger control training for junior high school delinquents. *Cognitive Therapy & Research, 8* (3), 299–311.

Foshee, V. A., Bauman, K. E., Arriaga, X. B., Helms, R. W., Koch, G. G., & Linder, G. F. (1998). An evaluation of Safe Dates, an adolescent dating violence prevention program. *American Journal of Public Health, 88* (1), 45–50.

Foshee, V. A., Linder, G. F., Bauman, K. E., Langwick, S. A., Arriaga, X. B., Heath, J. L., McMahon, P. M., & Bangdiwala, S. (1996). The Safe Dates Project: Theoretical basis, evaluation design, and selected baseline findings. *American Journal of Preventive Medicine, 12* (5), 39–47.

Ginsberg, C., & Loffredo, L. (1993). Violence-related attitudes and behaviors of high school students—New York City 1992. *Journal of School Health, 63*, 438–439.

Girouard, C. (2001). OJJDP fact sheet: School resource officer training program. Washington, DC: U.S. Department of Justice.

Gottfredson, D. C. (1986). An empirical test of school-based environmental and individual interventions to reduce the risk of delinquent behavior. *Criminology, 24* (4), 705–731.

Gottfredson, D. C. (1990). Changing school structures to benefit high-risk youths. In P. E. Leone (Ed.), *Understanding troubled and troubling youth,* (pp. 246–271). Newbury Park, CA: Sage.

Gottfredson, D. C. (2001) *Schools and delinquency.* New York: Cambridge University Press.

Gottfredson, D. C., Gerstenblith, S. A., Soulé, D. A., Womer, S. C., & Lu, S. (2004). Do after school programs reduce delinquency? *Prevention Science, 5* (4), 253–266.

Gottfredson, D. C., Gottfredson, G. D., & Hybl, L. G. (1993). Managing adolescent behavior: A multiyear, multischool study. *American Educational Research Journal, 30*, 179–215.

Gottfredson, D. C., Kumpfer, K., Polizzi, D., Banks, D., Puryear, V., Wilson, D., Middleton, J., & Beatty, P. (in press). The Strengthening Washington D.C. Families Project: A randomized effectiveness trial. *Prevention Science.*

Gottfredson, D. C., Soulé, D. A., & Cross, A. (2004). *A statewide evaluation of the Maryland After School Opportunity Fund Program.* Final report submitted to the Maryland Department of Human Resources. College Park, MD: Department of Criminology and Criminal Justice.

Gottfredson, D. C., Wilson, D. B., & Najaka, S. S. (2001). The schools. In J. Q. Wilson, & J. Petersilia (Eds.), *Crime: Public policies for crime control* (pp. 149–190, 2nd ed). San Francisco: ICS Press.

Gottfredson, D. C., Wilson, D. B., & Najaka, S. S. (2002). School-based crime prevention. In L. W. Sherman, D. P. Farrington, B. C. Welsh, & D. L. MacKenzie (Eds.), *Evidence-based crime prevention* (pp. 56–164). New York: Routledge.

Gottfredson, G. D. (1984). A theory ridden approach to program evaluation: A method for stimulating researcher implementer collaboration. *American Psychologist, 39,* 1101–1112.

Gottfredson, G. D. (1987). Peer group interventions to reduce the risk of delinquent behavior: A selective review and a new evaluation. *Criminology, 25* (3), 671–714.

Gutman, M. A., Foltz, C., Mittal, R., & Kaltenbach, K. (2004). *Outcomes of a family-based prevention model with women in substance abuse treatment and their children: The Philadelphia Strengthening Families Project.* Unpublished manuscript. Philadelphia: Treatment Research Institute.

Hahn, A., Leavitt, T., & Aaron, P. (1994). *Evaluation of the Quantum Opportunities Program (QOP): Did the program work?: A report on the post secondary outcomes and cost-effectiveness of the QOP Program.* Unpublished manuscript. Brandeis University, Waltham, MA.

Harrell, A. V., Cavanagh, S., & Sridharan, S. (1998). *Impact of the children at risk program: Comprehensive final report II.* Washington, DC: The Urban Institute.

Harrell, A. V., Cavanagh, S. E., & Sridharan, S. (1999). Evaluation of the children at risk program: Results 1 year after the end of the program (*Research in Brief,* November). Washington, DC: National Institute of Justice, U.S. Department of Justice.

Hawkins, J. D. (1999). Preventing crime and violence through communities that care. *European Journal on Crime Policy & Research, 7,* 443–458.

Henggeler, S. W., Melton, G. B., Brondino, M. J., & Schere, D. G. (1997). Multisystematic therapy with violent and chronic juvenile offenders and their families: The role of treatment fidelity in successful dissemination. *Journal of Consulting and Clinical Psychology, 65,* 821–833.

Hingson, R., McGovern, T., Howland, J., Heeren, T., Winter, M., & Zakocs, R. (1996). Reducing alcohol-impaired driving in Massachusetts: The Saving Lives Program. *American Journal of Public Health, 86,* 791–797.

Howell, J. C. (2003). *Preventing & reducing juvenile delinquency.* Thousand Oaks, CA: Sage.

Huesmann, L. R., & Eron, L. D. (1986). *Television and the aggressive child: A cross-national comparison.* Hillsdale, NJ: Lawrence Erlbaum Associates.

Huesmann, L. R., Lagerspetz, K., & Eron, L. D. (1984). Intervening variables in the TV violence-aggression relation: Evidence from two countries. *Developmental Psychology, 20,* 746–775.

Johnson, I. M. (1999). School violence: The effectiveness of a school resource officer program in a southern city. *Journal of Criminal Justice, 27* (2), 173–192.

Kennedy, D. M. (1997). Pulling levers: Chronic offenders, high-crime settings, and a theory of prevention. *Valparaiso University Law Review, 31,* 449–484.

Kennedy, D. M., Piehl, A. M., & Braga, A. A. (1996). Youth violence in Boston: Gun markets, serious youth offenders, and a use-reduction strategy. *Law & Contemporary Problems, 59,* 147–196.

Landes, W. M. (1978). An economic study of US aircraft hijacking, 1961–1976. *Journal of Law & Economics, 21,* 1–32.

Lefkowitz, M. M., Eron, L. D., Walder, L. O., & Huesmann, L. R. (1977). *Growing up to be violent: A longitudinal study of the development of aggression.* New York: Pergamon Press.

Lipsey, M. W. (1992). Juvenile delinquency treatment: A meta-analysis inquiry into the variability of effects. In T. D. Cook, H. Cooper, D. S. Cordray, H. Hartmann, L. V. Hedges, R. J. Light, T. A. Lewis, & F. Mosteller (Eds.), *Serious and violent juvenile offenders: Risk factors and successful interventions* (pp. 86–105). Thousand Oaks, CA: Sage.

Lipsey, M. W., & Wilson, D. B. (1998). Effective intervention for serious juvenile offenders. In R. Loeber & D. P. Farrington (Eds.), *Serious and violent juvenile offenders: Risk factors and successful intervention* (pp. 248–283). Thousand Oaks, CA: Sage.

Ludwig, J., Duncan, G. J., & Hirschfield. (2001). Urban poverty and juvenile crime: Evidence from a randomized housing-mobility experiment. *Quarterly Journal of Economics, 116,* 655–679.

Maxfield, M., Schirm, A., & Rodriguez-Planas, N. (2002). The Quantum opportunity program demonstration: Implementation and short-term impacts. Washington, DC: U.S. Department of Labor.

Milavsky, J. R., Kessler, R., Stipp, H., Rubens, W. S., Pearl, D., Bouthilet, L., & Lazar, J. (Eds.). (1982). *Television and behavior: Ten years of scientific progress and implications for the eighties. Vol. 2: Technical reviews* (DHHS Publication No. ADM 82-1196). Washington, DC: U.S. Government Printing Office.

Miller, W. B. (1962). The impact of a total community delinquency control project. *Social Problems, 10* (2), 168–191.

Olds, D. L. (1998). Long-term effects of nurse home visitation on children's criminal and antisocial behavior: 15-year follow-up of a randomized trial. *Journal of the American Medical Association, 280,* 1238–1244.

Olds, D. L., Eckenrode, J., & Henderson, C. R. (1997). Long-term effects of home visitation on maternal life course and child abuse and neglect: 15-year follow-up of a randomized trial. *Journal of the American Medical Association, 278,* 637–643.

Olds, D. L., Henderson, C. R., Phelps, C., Kitzman, H., & Hanks, C. (1993). Effects of prenatal and infancy nurse home visitation on government spending. *Medical Care, 31,* 155–174.

Olweus, D. (1991). Bully/victim problems among schoolchildren: Basic facts and effects of a school based intervention program. In D. J. Pepler, & K. H. Rubin (Eds.)., *The development and treatment of childhood aggression* (pp. 411–418). Hillsdale, NJ: Lawrence Erlbaum Associates.

Olweus, D. (1992). Bullying among schoolchildren: Intervention and prevention. In R. DeV. Peters, R. J. McMahon, & V. L. Quinsey (Eds.), *Aggression and violence throughout the life span* (pp. 100–125). Newbury Park, CA: Sage.

Olweus, D., & Alsaker, F. D. (1991). Assessing change in a cohort-longitudinal study with hierarchical data. In D. Magnusson, L. R. Bergman, G. Rudinger, & B. Torestad (Eds.), *Problems and methods in longitudinal research: Stability and change* (pp. 107–132). Cambridge, UK: Cambridge University Press.

Olweus, D., Limber, S., & Mihalic, S. F. (1999). Blueprints for violence prevention, book nine: Bullying prevention program. Boulder, CO: Center for the Study and Prevention of Violence.

Paik, H., & Comstock, G. (1994). The effects of television violence on antisocial behavior: A meta analysis. *Communication Research, 26,* 124–143.

Powers, E., & Witmer, H. (1951). *An experiment in the prevention of delinquency: The Cambridge-Somerville Youth Study.* New York: Columbia University Press.

Reckless, W. C., & Dinitz, S. (1972). *The prevention of juvenile delinquency: An experiment.* Columbus: Ohio State University Press.

Reid, J. B., Eddy, J. M., Fetrow, R. A., & Stoolmiller, M. (1999). Description and immediate impacts of a preventive intervention for conduct problems. *American Journal of Community Psychology, 27* (4), 483–517.

Schinke, S. P., Orlandi, M. A., & Cole, K. C. (1992). Boys and Girls Clubs in public housing developments: Prevention services for youth at risk. *Journal of Community Psychology,* (OSAP Special Issue), 118–128.

Sheley, J. F., & Wright, J. D. (1998). *High school youths, weapons, and violence: A national survey* (National Institute of Justice *Research in Brief, NCJ-172857*). Washington, DC: National Institute of Justice, U.S. Department of Justice.

Sherman, L. W., & Berk, R. A. (1984). The specific deterrent effects of arrest for domestic assault. *American Sociological Review, 49,* 261–272.

Sherman, L. W., & Eck, J. E. (2002). Policing for crime prevention. In L. W. Sherman, D. P. Farrington, B. C. Welsh, & D. L. MacKenzie (Eds.), *Evidence-based crime prevention,* (pp. 295–329). New York: Routledge.

Shure, M. B., & Spivak, G. (1979). Interpersonal cognitive problem solving and primary prevention: Programming for preschool and kindergarten children. *Journal of Clinical Child Psychology, 8,* 89–94.

Shure, M. B., & Spivak, G. (1980). Interpersonal problem solving as a mediator of behavioral adjustment in preschool and kindergarten children. *Journal of Applied Developmental Psychology, 1,* 29–44.

Shure, M. B., & Spivak, G. (1982). Interpersonal problem-solving in young children: A cognitive approach to prevention. *American Journal of Community Psychology, 10* (3), 341–356.

Taggart, R. (1995). *Quantum opportunity program.* Philadelphia: Opportunities Industrialization Centers of America.

Thompson, D. G., & Hudson, G. R. (1982). Values clarification and behavioral group counseling with ninth-grade boys in a residential school. *Journal of Counseling Psychology, 29* (4), 394–399.

Tolan, P. H., & Gorman-Smith, D. (1998). Development of serious and violent offending careers. In R. Loeber & D. P. Farrington (Eds.), *Serious and violent juvenile offenders: Risk factors and successful interventions* (pp. 68–85). Thousand Oaks, CA: Sage.

U.S. Public Health Service. Youth violence: A Report of the Surgeon General, 2001, Retrieved January 7, 2005, from www.surgeongeneral.gov/library/youthviolence/chapter4/appendix4b.htm.

Wagenaar, A. C., Murray, D. M., Toomey, T. L. (2000). Communities mobilizing for change on alcohol (CMCA): Effects of a randomized trial on arrests and traffic crashes. *Addiction, 95* (2), 209–217.

Webster-Stratton, C., & Taylor, T. (2001). Nipping early risk factors in the bud: Preventing substance abuse, delinquency, and violence in adolescence through interventions targeted at young children (0–8 years). *Prevention Science, 2* (3), 165–192.

Wellford, C. F., Pepper, J. V., & Petrie, C. V. (2004). *Firearms and violence: A critical review.* Washington, DC: National Academic Press.

Welsh, B. C., & Hoshi, A. (2002). Communities and crime prevention. In L. W. Sherman, D. P. Farrington, B. C. Welsh, & D. L. MacKenzie, D. L. (Eds.), *Evidence-based crime prevention* (pp. 165–197). New York: Routledge.

Williams, J. R., & Gold, M. (1972). From delinquent behavior to official delinquency. *Social Problems, 20,* 209–229.

Wright, W. E., & Dixon, M. C. (1977). Community prevention and treatment of juvenile delinquency: A review of evaluation studies. *Journal of Research in Crime & Delinquency, 1,* 35–67.

Chapter **10**

Interventions to Prevent Suicidal Behavior

Kerry L. Knox

10.1. THE EPIDEMIOLOGY AND PUBLIC HEALTH BURDEN OF SUICIDE

There is now a substantial literature on risk factors for suicide in the United States (U.S. Dept of Health and Human Services, PHS, 2001; Committee on Pathophysiology & Prevention of Adolescent & Adult Suicide Board, 2002) that can be used to guide the development of prevention programs to reduce the rates of suicide in this country. There is a wealth of evidence that having a mental disorder increases the risk for both attempted suicide and suicide. However, in and of itself a mental disorder should not be equated with elevated suicide risk because the majority of individuals with a mental illness never kill themselves (Bostwick & Pankratz, 2000). Suicide is the outcome of extremely complex circumstances, and it is likely we will never be able to predict its occurrence given the putative interaction between psychiatric, psychological, physiological, social, and cultural factors. For example, there is considerable evidence that aggression and impulsivity, acute and chronic stress, trauma, and substance or alcohol use are associated with suicidality, but their effects are moderated by gender and age.

Because of the inability to predict who will kill themselves, suicide is a public health problem of considerable magnitude. In the United States in 2002 there were 31,655 deaths from suicide, making suicide the overall 11th leading cause of death (Kochanek & Smith, 2004). Suicide is now the 3rd leading cause of death for individuals aged 10–24 years (Kochanek & Smith, 2004). Since the 1950s, the rate of youth suicide has tripled, and there was an alarming gradual upswing in suicide among young African American males in the United States between 1980 and 1995 (Shaffer, Gould, & Hicks, 1994). Substantially higher rates of suicide in elders in the United States have been observed consistently for some time (Pearson & Brown, 2000).

The estimated years of potential life lost and associated economic cost due to suicide are enormous (Knox & Caine, 2005). Moreover, these estimates do not take into account the considerable cost of attempted suicide to society, the health care system, and families, although one study estimated that the total direct costs were $581 million for attempted suicides and $68 million for suicide deaths (Palmer, Revicki, Halpern, & Hatziandreu, 1995); these figures depend on reliable reports of the number of suicides and attempted suicides. Recently, the Centers for Disease Control and Prevention (CDC) reported that there were 411,128 self-harm injuries in 2003 (National Center for Injury Prevention and Control, 2005); however, there was no distinction made between events that had lethal intent and those without lethal intent. It also is essential to consider the separate effect of highly prevalent risk factors and antecedent conditions for suicide, such as mood disorders (Charney et al., 2003), hopelessness (Beck, Kovacs, & Weissman, 1975), alcohol and substance abuse or dependence (Conner, Li, Meldrum, Duberstein, & Conwell, 2003), family turmoil and domestic violence (Conner, Duberstein, & Conwell, 2000b), and unemployment (Gunnel et al., 1999). And no currently available statistical measure captures the reverberating effect of suicide and attempted suicide on family members, friends, co-workers, and employers.

This chapter begins by reviewing a typology of strategies for suicide prevention; within this typology, four theoretical domains are used as a framework for describing existing interventions. Extant interventions for suicide are then examined for published evidence of efficacy or effectiveness; interventions with demonstrable or promising evidence of efficacy or effectiveness are discussed in detail. Finally, implications and limitations for public health practice and future prevention planning and the overall gaps in the research on suicide prevention are presented.

10.2.   A TYPOLOGY OF SUICIDE PREVENTION STRATEGIES

Reducing events of suicide, like many public health problems of complex causes, will likely be unresponsive to one-dimensional strategies. Recognizing the limitations of the traditional nomenclature use of primary, secondary, and tertiary prevention for describing many current public health challenges, including suicide, this chapter makes use of the Institute of Medicine's (Mrazek & Haggerty, 1994) recommendations for prevention terminology. These are (1) universal prevention strategies designed to reduce risk and enhance protective or mitigating factors, (2) selective prevention strategies to address population-specific characteristics that place individuals at higher than average risk, and (3) indicated prevention strategies to treat individuals with precursor signs and symptoms to prevent development of full-blown disorders.

These strategies are not mutually exclusive. New evidence suggests that effective suicide prevention will likely follow the examples of efforts to reduce substance use or to prevent HIV/AIDS; Negative outcomes that are the result of a complex origin of risk factors are most likely to respond to multilayered approaches (Des Jarlais & Friedman, 1998; Latkin & Forman, 2001) For suicide prevention, it is likely that programs integrating all three prevention strategies will have the most durable effect on reducing the public health burden of suicide.

10.2.1.   The Current Theoretical Basis of Suicide Prevention

A separate but related issue to types of prevention strategies is the current thinking regarding four theoretical domains for suicide prevention. Although a comprehensive review of these orientations is not possible, the Institute of Medicine's report on suicide provides an excellent overview of psychiatric/psychological theories of suicide, biological theories, childhood trauma and developmental theories, and social/cultural theories (Committee on Pathophysiology, 2002). Our understanding of how these theoretical orientations should or could be integrated as part of prevention programs is less well developed than our understanding of the ways in which types of prevention strategies can be used to develop and evaluate interventions for suicide prevention. Prevention research in the mental health arena often has struggled to ensure that interventions are theoretically and empirically tied to known risks. However, because current knowledge holds that theory-driven interventions are more likely to be rigorously evaluated and to result in the desired outcomes, many investigators now advocate for clearer guidelines on how to accomplish this (Kellam & Langevin, 2003).

10.2.2. Universal Strategies

10.2.2.1. Laws and Policies: Means Control

The herbicide paraquat was introduced in Samoa in 1972 (Hutchinson et al., 1999), with a sudden time-tagged rise in suicide deaths. After the herbicide's removal, rates declined. Similarly, in the United Kingdom, the reduction of high levels of carbon monoxide in the coal-generated form of cooking gas led to a definable decline in deaths from suicide during the mid-1970s. The decline was notable; after several years, there was a gradual return to the preremoval baseline level as new means of committing suicide were employed. Such observations clearly raise concerns about the effect of environmental factors on the success of universal interventions for preventing suicide. However, suicidal acts are sometimes impulsive or fleeting ideas. In those cases, interventions that target individuals who are particularly vulnerable to self-injurious behavior may be especially powerful, as suggested by several investigators (Brent et al., 1994; Conner et al., 2000a). For example, alcohol intoxication is known to be associated with impulsive, angry suicides, quite often brought on by the loss of a relationship (Conner et al., 2000a). It has been observed for many years that hopelessness (Beck et al., 1975; Orbach & Bar-Joseph, 1993) is associated with heighten risk for suicide in both adults and adolescents. These psychological "state" variables (in contrast to trait variables) may be more likely to be associated with impulsive or poorly planned suicidal acts.

The recognition that poorly planned suicides may require distinct prevention strategies has also underpinned the recent UK effort to limit access to lethal doses of paracetamol (acetaminophen in the United States) and salicylates by restricting the sizes of retail packages (24 doses in blister packs, providing a smaller number of hard-to-open pills). Initial reports after the change in legislation in the UK in 1998 suggest a marked drop in deaths and in the need for liver transplants, given the extreme hepatotoxicity of paracetamol (Hawton et al., 1996). At 6 years after the legislation, there were statistically significant decreases in the rates of self-poisonings from paracetamol and fewer, hospital admissions, listings for liver transplants, and actual liver transplants after such poisoning (Table 10.1) (Hawton, 2002). The ingestion of available pills in the medicine cabinet is a common occurrence for individuals with less-than-lethal intent or ambivalent motivation; self-poisoning is the leading method of suicide attempts in the United States (approximately 216,000 cases in 2001) (Arias, Anderson, & Kung, 2003). The continued availability in the United States of this highly potent liver toxin in bottles

Table 10.1. Numbers of Suicides, Undetermined Deaths, and Deaths Resulting from Accidental Poisoning Attributable to Paracetamol and Salicylates among People Aged 12 Years and over in England and Wales before and after the Change in Law on Packaging[a,b]

Drug	Number (%) of Deaths			% Change in Incidence[d] (95% CI)	p Value	% Change in Proportional Incidence[d] (95% CI)	p Value
	Penultimate 12 Months before Change (n = 2255)	12 Months before Change (n = 2234)	12 Months after Change (n = 2086)[c]				
Paracetamol							
Alone	203 (9.0)	185 (8.3)	147 (7.0)	−21 (−34 to −5)	0.01	−18 (−33 to −1)	0.04
With other drugs	59 (2.6)	56 (2.5)	56 (2.7)	2 (−26 to 39)	0.9	5 (−24 to 44)	0.8
Salicylates							
Alone	35 (1.6)	29 (1.3)	16 (0.8)	−48 (−70 to −11)	0.02	−46 (−69 to −7)	0.03
With other drugs	4 (0.2)	8 (0.4)	3 (0.1)	−48 (−85 to 81)	0.3	−46 (−85 to 91)	0.3
Paracetamol and salicylates	11 (0.5)	5 (0.2)	9 (0.4)	18 (−47 to 163)	0.7	21 (−47 to 174)	0.6

[a]Modified with permission from Hawton (2002).
[b]September 16, 1998.
[c]These numbers were increased by 4.5% in the analyses.
[d]Comparison of 12 months after the change with the average of the 2 years before.

of 100 or more suggests one approach to reducing mortality and morbidity due to suicidal behavior.

Because the debate over firearms in the United States will likely continue for many years in political and social arenas, there is little reason to assume that universal interventions to restrict firearms will be feasible in the foreseeable future. However, there is a growing consensus that for indicated populations, such as adolescents with a previous history of self-harm, restriction of firearms may prevent deaths from suicide. Evidence for this observation is discussed later in this chapter.

10.2.2.2.   Public Health Messages

There is a paucity of evidence for the effectiveness of public health messages for preventing suicide (Chambers et al., 2004). On the one hand, public health messages may have a powerful effect on reversing social and cultural norms that serve to stigmatize suicide and related behaviors. However, concern over potential harmful effects due to media campaigns has been paramount in the United States; there is a great need for further research in this area to determine the potential of public awareness campaigns to prevent suicide. In a related vein, although media campaigns to prevent suicide have not been actively pursued as a prevention strategy, the media can play an important role in shaping the public's perception and awareness of suicide simply by reporting on death by suicide, particularly for youth and young adults. For example, there is considerable evidence that sensational reporting of a death by suicide of a celebrity may result in a flurry of suicide deaths in young people (Gould, Fisher, Parides, Flory, & Shaffer, 1996; Gould, Jamieson, & Romer, 2003). In contrast, the media is well positioned to encourage a positive public attitude in preventing suicide (Gould, 2001). A powerful intervention for decreasing suicide deaths from imitation and for increasing the mental health literacy of the public regarding suicide may be the implementation of media guidelines for reporting suicides. In Austria, media guidelines for reporting deaths from suicide and the subsequent effect on suicide rates has been evaluated by Etzersdorfer and colleagues (Etzersdorfer, Sonneck, Nagel-Kuess, 1992). These investigators found that suicide rates declined significantly after implementation of media guidelines by the Austrian Association for Suicide Prevention in 1987. Similar guidelines have been developed in United States based on the recommendations from a national workshop sponsored by the CDC (1994). The efficacy of these guidelines for preventing deaths from suicide has not yet been established and warrants further study.

10.2.2.3.   School-Based Interventions

An intuitively appealing theoretical basis for suicide prevention can be found in developmental theories, in particular those that are psychological or epidemiological based. For example, youth are more likely to exhibit irritability, acting-out behaviors, and anger than sad and depressed behaviors (Gould et al., 1996) Targeting individuals between the ages of 13 and 24 years to reduce negative behaviors, such as conduct disorders, may ultimately serve to decrease the risk for suicide. School-based suicide-prevention programs began with a number of educational curricula during the 1980s, resulting in several controlled studies to evaluate their efficacy (Eggert, Thompson, Randell, & Pike, 2002; Kalafat & Elias, 1994). Evidence of effectiveness from these early investigations is equivocal. Although some studies have reported moderate effect sizes in changed knowledge (Kalafat and Elias, 1994), others reported no change or possible negative effects. Based on these data and other observations of the limitations of purely knowledge-based curriculum, most school-based suicide-prevention programs now focus on some aspect of skills training, be it in increasing awareness of a peer's suicidal behavior or in increasing the coping skills of high-risk individuals in particular, which may have reverberating effects for reducing suicide in later years (Dolan, Kellam, Brown, & Werthamer-Larsson, 1993; Orbach & Bar-Joseph, 1993).

There are a number of school-based programs that use screening methods to identify individuals at high risk for suicide (Thompson, Eggert, Randell, & Pike, 2001). These latter programs are beginning to provide new data to suggest that a layered approach to school-based suicide prevention may be effective, especially in subpopulations of high-risk youth. However, in terms of the employment of universal strategies for effective suicide prevention, school-based programs have lacked consistent design and outcome measures. As a result, these programs have yet to form any evidence-based consensus concerning their effectiveness. A critical area of continued development for suicide prevention programs must be to develop and evaluate school-based programs with increasingly rigorous and standardized study designs.

10.2.2.4.   Gatekeeper Interventions

Gatekeeper interventions are based on identifying members of a community that are most likely to come in frequent contact with the target population (including teachers, counselors, coaches, primary-care physicians, clergy, police, or workplace co-workers). The CDC has referred to the training of "natural community helpers" (Gould & Kramer, 2001) as gatekeeper training (CDC, 1994). These natural community helpers are individuals who come in contact with the target population and therefore are potentially well positioned to identify individuals in distress and those who may be considering harming themselves. There is considerable evidence from preventive efforts in other fields that gatekeeper interventions are effective (Kelly, Lawrence, & Diaz, 1991). Although there are several promising examples of the potential effectiveness of gatekeeper interventions to reduce events of suicide and suicidal behavior (Kalafat & Elias, 1994), there are as yet no reports from controlled studies. In a cross-sectional design of high school counselors, results from Project SOAR (suicide, opinions, awareness, and relief) found that intensive suicide prevention training increased school counselors' confidence in identifying students at risk for suicide compared to counselors nationwide (King, 2000) The U.S. Air Force uses a multilayered gatekeeper program as part of a comprehensive suicide-prevention program (Knox, Litts, Talcott, Feig, & Caine, 2003). By 2002, approximately 97% of active duty air force personnel had been trained in increased awareness of detecting signs of individuals in distress and in developing the competency to appropriately refer such individuals for help. It is unknown whether this component of the program was most strongly associated with the significant drop in suicide rates seen after implementation of the full program.

It is worth noting that there are a number of grassroots efforts that have generated gatekeeper interventions. Although potentially promising, none of these gatekeeper interventions has been the subject of rigorous scientific study, limiting their usefulness for widespread dissemination in any population. One example is the ASIST program, originally developed in Alberta, Canada, which was disseminated throughout Norway as part of the Norwegian Plan for Suicide Prevention (Mehlum & Reinholdt, 2000). There is a great need for further research in this area because many organizations and institutions will likely continue to adopt gatekeeper strategies for suicide prevention, despite the lack of sufficient scientific rationale.

10.2.2.5. Screening

Screening for suicide has focused largely on adolescents in schools and health settings to identify suicidal behaviors and depression (Joiner, Pfaff, & Acres, 2002; Shaffer et al., 2004) Screening programs have used screening instruments to identify high-risk youth and/or relied on a clinician to determine whether an individual required a clinical referral for further assessment or treatment. Pena and Caine (2005) report that two such programs noted reduction in youth suicide attempts after the use of a screening instrument. In a study of the effectiveness of the Signs of Suicide (SOS) screening program, Aseltine and De Martino (2004) compared 2100 students randomly assigned to intervention control groups. They found that there was a significant reduction in self-reported suicide attempts in ninth grade youth 3 months after the program. Of note was the observation that the adolescents who were screened via SOS did not report increased help-seeking behaviors, although this had been reported in an earlier study of the same program (Aseltine, 2003). Teen Screen, which has been implemented in many schools across the nation, has been shown to have promise for identifying suicidal behaviors, although there is no demonstrable evidence that this screening program reduces suicide events (Pena & Caine, 2005).

Of critical relevance to any discussion of screening is a recent study reported by Gould et al. (2005), who report that youth who are assessed for suicidal behaviors are not at increased risk for self-harm. Although it should not be concluded from this study that screening reduces the risk of suicide, it does address the question, using a randomized controlled trial design, of whether possible iatrogenic effects reduce any potential benefit of screening programs. This is in sharp contrast to a previous study in which adverse effects were identified in several suicide-awareness programs (Shaffer et al., 1990).

10.2.3. Selective Approaches

Depression is a major risk factor for suicide and suicidal ideation in late life (Pearson, Conwell, & Lyness, 1997). This population-specific depression may place some elderly individuals at higher risk for suicide. Because the majority of older adults who die by suicide have been seen by their physician within months of their death (Conwell et al., 2000), a site- and population-specific design was incorporated in a multisite, randomized trial titled Prevention of Suicide in Primary Care Elderly: Collaborative Trial (PROSPECT). A total of 20 primary-care practices in New York City, Philadelphia, and Baltimore were randomized to either an intervention group or treatment as usual. The intervention consisted of two major components of geriatric care: improving physician knowledge for treating geriatric depression in a primary-care setting through provision of a clinical algorithm and use of depression care managers (trained social workers, nurses, and psychologists) to collaboratively work with physicians to improve treatment management. Initial outcomes on the effectiveness of the intervention for reducing suicidal ideation and depression severity were reported. Suicide itself is an infrequent event in individual primary-care practices, and the study was not designed to use reduction in completed suicide as an outcome. However, reduction in suicidal ideation, improved response to treatment for depression, lessening severity of depression, and depression remission were found in patients who received the intervention compared to patients receiving usual care (Table 10.2) (Bruce et al., 2004). The authors note certain limitations to the study (e.g., a higher baseline prevalence of suicidal ideation was reported in the intervention group compared to treatment as usual, and depression treatment was offered at no cost to participants). However, after adjusting for the difference in suicidal ideation at baseline, the effect of the intervention persisted. A major strength of the study was the relative heterogeneity of the study sample, which was greater than that generally achieved in randomized controlled trials. The study suggests that selective approaches offer powerful prevention strategies for changing the distribution of population-specific risk factors for suicide and suicidal behaviors.

Another selective intervention that has been evaluated using a quasi-experimental design with intervention and nonintervention conditions is the Zuni Life Skills Development (ZLSD) curriculum (LaFromboise, 1995) For the past 15 years, suicide has been a leading cause of death for 15- to 24-year-old American Indians and Alaska Natives. In particular, the Zuni Pueblo reservation in Arizona has experienced a significantly high rate of suicide. Failure to treat problems such as depression, alcoholism, drug abuse, and unemployment suggested that a suicide-prevention program specific to changing normative behavior in Zuni culture could potentially be effective in this community. The ZLSD curriculum was a culturally tailored intervention targeting high school students, focusing on increasing protective factors (e.g., building self-esteem, increasing communication and problem-solving skills), and reducing known risk factors (e.g., recognizing and eliminating self-destructive behavior). After implementation of the program, the suicide rate dropped significantly. There is a critical need to evaluate the effectiveness of similar programs designed for specific cultural and ethnic groups.

For example, because suicide risk in American Indians and Alaska Natives is associated with alcohol problems, suicide awareness and prevention interventions that have been incorporated into alcohol-treatment programs in these communities have been shown to effectively reduce the suicide rate 10-fold (Middlebrook, LeMaster, Beals, Novins, & Manson, 2001). As a promising approach, suicide-prevention efforts may find their place in culturally appropriate venues, such as churches, Veteran Administration centers, or agencies that serve elderly populations.

10.2.4. Indicated Approaches

The persistently mentally ill represent an underserved group of individuals, and both detectable and asymptomatic individuals bear risk markers. Although there has been promising work on identifying biological and genetic markers for suicidality, largely focusing on markers involving the serotonergic system (Mann et al., 2000), there are no data from these studies that can be used to create suicide-prevention programs that integrate such markers. Nevertheless, incorporating an understanding of the biological correlates of suicide would be an important component of any comprehensive theoretically based program.

Lamberti et al. (2001) and Lamberti and Weisman (2002) developed a community coalition with three nongovernment organizations that were ethnically oriented and two other care providers to work with the local county office of

Table 10.2. Depression Severity over Time[a,b]

	Mean (SD) HDRS Score		Group Difference in Change From Baseline (95% CI)	p Value	Omnibus Test[c]
	Intervention	Usual Care			
All depressed patients (n = 598)					Model $\chi_3^2 = 32.4$; $p < .001$
Baseline	18.61 (6.12)	17.55 (5.79)		.88	
4 months	11.24 (7.51)	13.61 (8.42)	−3.5 (−4.7 to −2.3)	<.001	
8 months	10.45 (7.39)	11.38 (7.49)	−2.1 (−3.4 to −0.9)	<.001	
12 months	9.77 (7.28)	10.35 (6.78)	−1.8 (−3.1 to −0.5)	.006	
Major depression (n = 396)					Model $\chi_3^2 = 33.1$; $p < .001$
Baseline	21.05 (5.74)	19.72 (5.53)		.89	
4 months	12.58 (7.74)	15.87 (8.44)	−4.6 (−6.2 to −3.1)	<.001	
8 months	11.69 (7.93)	12.85 (7.27)	−2.5 (−4.1 to −0.9)	.003	
12 months	10.42 (7.62)	11.21 (7.11)	−2.0 (−3.7 to −0.4)	.02	
Clinically significant minor depression only (n = 202)					Model $\chi_3^2 = 3.0$; $p = .39$
Baseline	13.69 (3.23)	13.44 (3.65)		.82	
4 months	8.34 (6.07)	9.50 (6.77)	−1.3 (−3.1 to 0.5)	.15	
8 months	7.81 (5.23)	8.72 (7.20)	−1.4 (−3.2 to 0.5)	.15	
12 months	8.39 (6.33)	8.86 (5.91)	−1.0 (−2.9 to 0.8)	.28	

[a]Modified with permission from Bruce et al. (2004).
[b]CI, confidence interval; HDRS, Hamilton Depression Rating Scale.
[c]p values calculated using Wald statistic adjusting for baseline ideation and HDRS scores.

mental health, the local criminal justice systems, and the courts to proactively treat chemically dependent seriously mentally ill persons as they were being released from jail or discharged from the local state psychiatric facility and individuals identified (by providers or the courts) at heightened risk for repeated incarceration. The program, called Project Link, involved intensively focused community case management (Lamberti et al., 2001; Weisman & Lamberti, 2002), careful evaluation of medical and psychiatric problems, and alternative supervised housing. It is distinguished by being run by a team of culturally attuned, "street-wise" clinicians and case workers who actively partner with probation and court-based personnel. During the study period, there were no assaults, suicide attempts, or other reportable incidents. Preliminary cost estimates showed that for the initial 46 participants, the monthly jail costs dropped from nearly $31,000 to $7,235 ($672 to $157 per consumer), and monthly hospitalization costs decreased from nearly $198,000 to just over $42,000 ($4,302 to $918 each). Moreover, there was a high level of consumer satisfaction. The overall annual operating budget for Project Link during its first year was $681,063, which is far less than the nearly $2.2 million in savings gleaned from reducing jail and hospital services.

Without flexible adaptation of current funding streams, programs such as Project Link can be neither developed nor sustained. Moreover, its proactive nature and high level of community integration are atypical of programs around the country. Thus its portability remains to be established. Nonetheless, it serves as a model of preventative morbidity reduction in a group of very difficult to treat individuals who have some of the highest rates of suicide. As well, this program proved to be a broadly based violence-reduction intervention in addition to demonstrably improving the lives of this patient population. The target population does not readily seek care through traditional service providers, such as community mental health centers.

Another indicated intervention with evidence of effectiveness targets youth identified through emergency departments to be at risk for suicide. Emergency department personnel were trained to provide education on restricting access to lethal means to parents of children who are assessed to be at risk for suicide. Lethal means that were tagged for restriction included firearms, medications (over-the-counter and prescribed), and alcohol. Collaboration with local law-enforcement or other appropriate organizations was recommended for eliminating or restricting access to firearms. In a prospective study of 103 children, parents who received the intervention from trained emergency department staff were significantly more likely to self-report restricting access to lethal means (Kruesi et al., 1999).

In an indicated intervention for adults who deliberately poisoned themselves, Guthrie and colleagues (2001) used a randomized two-group design to determine the effectiveness of a brief psychological intervention. They found that at the 6-month follow-up, only 9% of patients who deliberately poisoned themselves and were assigned to the intervention had harmed themselves again, compared to 28% who had harmed themselves and were assigned to treatment as usual. Cognitive-behavior therapy (CBT) has also been shown to be effective in reducing chronic suicidality in patients with borderline disorder (Linehan, Armstrong, Suarez, Allmon, & Heard, 1991). In a randomized controlled trial of adults, Brown et al. (2005) found that a 10-session cognitive therapy intervention designed to prevent suicide attempts in adults who recently attempted suicide reduced the incidence of repeat suicide attempts and the number of days until a suicide attempt (Fig. 10.1). Other outcomes (hopelessness and depression severity) were also significantly reduced in

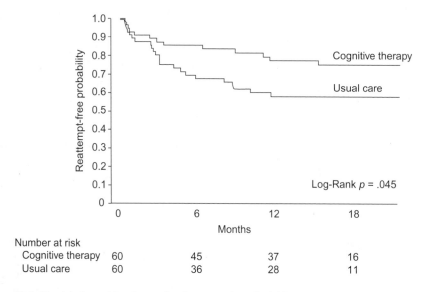

Figure 10.1. Results of cognitive therapy for the prevention of suicide attempts. (Reprinted with permission from Brown et al., 2005.)

the treatment group. In a study by Motto and Bostrom (2001), 843 people who were hospitalized because of a depressive or suicidal state were randomly assigned to two groups. The intervention group was contacted by letter at least four times a year for 5 years. The control group received no further contact. Patients were followed during the 5-year contact period and then for 10 years more. For all 5 years of the study, the contact group had a lower rate of suicide. Discontinuation of contact resulted in reversal of this prevention effect (Motto & Bostrom, 2001). In studies among elders in Italy, DeLeo and colleagues demonstrated that twice-weekly telephone support resulted in lower than expected suicide rates among elderly users. The effect persisted over time in elderly females but not in elderly males (DeLeo, Carollo, & Buono, 1995; DeLeo, Buono, & Dwyer, 2002).

Taken together, these results suggest that targeting high-risk individuals with brief behavioral interventions and supportive interventions may be an essential component of multifactorial approaches to suicide prevention. It also appears that incorporating interventions into nontraditional sites outside of the clinical setting may be a critical factor in these interventions.

10.2.5.   Multifactorial Approaches

Employment of single-strategy approaches will likely be insufficient for effectively reducing suicide and suicidal behavior in heterogeneous populations. Although the U.S. Air Force (USAF) is homogenous in terms of displaying remarkable demographic stability over time, its active-duty population is still considerably heterogeneous in regard to variability among different installations. After an alarming increase in suicide rates during the early to middle 1990s, top leadership mandated that suicide prevention had to become a USAF communitywide responsibility, instead of being viewed as a medical problem (Thomas Moorman, personal communication, June 2001). Under the urgent impetus of its then vice-chief of staff and its surgeon general, the USAF promulgated servicewide a suicide-prevention program during 1996–97, which was built through a broadly based collaborative process that drew together (and has since coordinated) a comprehensive array of community- and personnel-oriented agencies (e.g., health, mental health, public health, police, criminal investigation, legal services, family advocacy, child and youth services, air force personnel) (Litts, Moe, Roadman, Miller, & Janke, 1999). The substance of this multifactorial, integrated strategy came from the agencies that included the major stakeholders from the beginning of the program. The strategy benefited from the sustained commitment of top leadership, which has been given by four incumbents who have held the chief of staff position.

A significant and sustained drop in suicide rates was observed after communitywide dissemination of the program. Key components of the program were the ongoing commitment from leadership, as mentioned; consistent, regular, and repeated education and communication regarding suicide prevention, including confronting and addressing a possible stigma for seeking assistance for emotional and family problems (including mental health treatment); improved and sustained collaboration among community prevention agencies; and the identification and training of "everyday" gatekeepers. In addition to reducing suicides, there were significant changes in a variety of outcomes that share common risk factors with suicide, including decreased rates of accidental death and homicide, violent offenses, and severe and moderate cases of family violence, suggesting that the USAF suicide-prevention program had an overall effect on reducing the mean risk of violence in the population (Fig. 10.2).

An overall take-home message that one can infer from the USAF suicide-prevention program is as follows: Destigmatizing the idea of seeking help for mental disorders saves lives and reduces violence in the community. How this message affected the overall culture of the USAF and the day-to-day lives of its active-duty personnel remains to be defined. Demonstrating the feasibility of translating the program to civilian settings will be essential. A second implicit

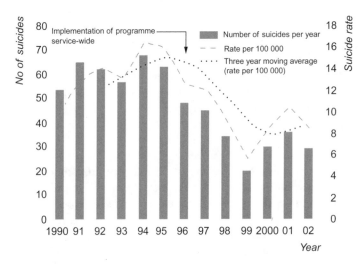

Figure 10.2. Trends in rates of suicide 1990–2002. Implementation of the U.S. Air Force suicide prevention program began in late 1995 and was fully implemented by 1997. (Date from Knox et al., 2003.)

message is also important when considering the degree to which this type of program can be effective in other settings: Successful prevention efforts may depend on the community providing accessible and effective care for those who seek help.

10.3. DISCUSSION

10.3.1. Implications of Extant Data for Public Health Practice

There finally are sufficient data regarding key risk and protective factors to shift collective attention from building awareness to undertaking direct action to reduce the loss of life and the burden of antecedent conditions and the unwanted behaviors associated with suicide. Preventing suicide will require the integration of population-oriented public health prevention measures with currently available clinical and medical interventions designed specifically to deal with the needs of high-risk individuals through prevention of early co-morbid patterns. These strategies, if developed on the foundation of promising theoretical tenets, may provide the greatest promise for suicide prevention to become institutionalized at a local level.

This type of integration has been essentially nonexistent for suicide prevention, although such approaches have been extended successfully to combat other conditions such as heart disease, stroke, cancer, and HIV/AIDS. Population-based interventions stress the need for a multilevel approach in which multiple messages are delivered through multiple channels to multiple target groups. This is a public health approach to prevention; the goal is to shift the mean population risk for suicide and related behaviors. This approach assumes that all segments of the population are generally homogenous in their response to the layers of the intervention and respond in a positive manner. However, there is a paucity of data from community-level interventions (for preventing suicide or other adverse outcomes) on the specific characteristics of a community that predict a favorable response. The role of culture in preventing suicide has only begun to be studied (Joe & Kaplan, 2001; LeMaster & Connell, 1994; Middlebrook et al., 2001), but it appears to be emerging as a critical component of developing effective suicide-prevention programs.

Prospective studies on populations thought to bear key risk and protective factors could potentially provide a more expansive epidemiological perspective across the life span. Such studies have been difficult to conduct, due in large part to concerns over human safety and ethical considerations. While appropriate precautions must be taken to protect individuals who may be at greater risk, the National Institute of Mental Health has released a report to address the ways in which standard practices of clinical trials can apply to suicidal patients as well (Pearson, Stanley et al., 2001). Such data would permit us to test which risk or protective factors give rise to differential expression of morbidity, and perhaps mortality, captured in hypothesized families of related behaviors, events, and disorders. It is well recognized that there are substantial statistical limitations in achieving sufficient statistical power in studies with a relatively low base rate outcome, such as suicide. Research currently under way by Brown and Liao (1999) on interventions designed to prevent violence and conduct disorders in children may result in useful strategies for reducing suicidal behaviors in later years. If conducted at multiple sites, longitudinal studies in children may eventually render sufficient power to detect demonstrable changes in the numbers of expected suicides.

10.3.2. Gaps in Research

The current gaps in research on suicide prevention continue to include the lack of controlled trials with demonstrable efficacy on which a critical evidence base could be built for dissemination of guidelines. However, given the limitations of achieving sufficient power, rigorous alternative designs should be incorporated into research on suicide prevention. Some of these designs have been proposed by Brown (2003). Other potential means of increasing the evidence base for suicide prevention include focusing on introducing greater rigor into the design and evaluation of effectiveness trials, which may better inform us of the feasibility of implementing prevention programs or interventions in community settings.

Much of the published literature on the epidemiology and prevention of suicide has focused on adolescents especially those in schools (Beautrais, Joyce, & Mulder, 1997; Cantor & Neulinger, 1998; Gould et al., 2003; Gould et al., 1996; Gunnell et al., 1999; Ho, Hung, Lee, Chung, & Chung, 1995; Metha, Weber, & Webb, 1998; Shaffer et al., 2004), and elders (Bruce & Pearson, 1999; Conwell & Duberstein, 2001; Luoma & Pearson, 2002; Pearson et al., 1997; Pearson & Brown, 2000). There are limited epidemiological data and evidence-based research on prevention available for other at risk subpopulations in the United States, such as men and women in the middle years of life (Knox & Caine, 2005); college students (Barrios, Everett, Simon, & Brenner, 2000; Douglas & Collins, 1997; Jobes, Jacoby, Cimbolic, & Hustead, 1997; Langhinrichsen-Rohling, Arata, Bowers, O'Brien, & Morgan, 2004); and potentially high-risk populations, such as those with severe mental illness (Lamberti & Weissman, 2002), the homeless, and the incarcerated (Goss, Peterson, Smith, Kalb, & Brodey, 2002; Lamberti et al., 2001; Tuskan & Thase, 1983). There is an immediate need for more research to address the paucity of effective efforts to prevent suicide for some groups.

10.4. CONCLUSIONS

Table 10.3 summarizes the evidence for effectiveness and efficacy of suicide-prevention efforts, organized by strategy. Recommendations for future research are as follows.

Universal strategies
- Design prospective, longitudinal studies to evaluate school-based programs (including screening), adopting increasingly rigorous and standardized study designs, such as split plot designs (classroom-based intervention and individual service-based intervention).
- Longitudinally implement and evaluate gatekeeper programs, especially through randomized control trials or dynamic wait-list designs.
- Evaluate public health messages for suicide prevention for possible iatrogenic effects (surveys and focus groups).

Selective strategies
- Implement and evaluate culturally appropriate suicide-prevention programs for groups that bear a greater than expected risk (e.g., men in the middle years of life, America Indians and Alaska Natives, homeless individuals, and juveniles).

Table 10.3. Evidence of Effective Suicide-Prevention Interventions[a]

Type of Prevention Strategy	Suicide	Related Outcomes
Products		
Universal interventions: screening instruments	3	3
Physical environments	4	4
Universal interventions: means control		
Indicated interventions: means control		
Behavioral interventions		
Universal interventions		
Laws/policies	4	4
Media campaigns/media guidelines	3	3
School-based interventions (education only)	3	3
School-based interventions (skill building)	4	4
Screening	3	3
Gatekeeper training	3	3
Selected interventions		
Life skills competency	4	4
Small groups skills training	4	4
Managing geriatric depression in primary care	4	4
Indicated interventions		
Behavioral/cognitive-behavioral strategies	5	5
Brief psychological intervention	4	4
Contact through letter or telephone	4	4

[a]The scale is as follows: 5, effective (supported by two or more well-designed studies or systematic review); 4, promising (supported by one well-designed study); 3, insufficient (not enough evidence or mixed evidence—strong studies show both effective and not effective); 2, not effective (no effect found in two or more well-designed studies or systematic review); 1, harmful (negative effect supported by two or more well-designed studies or systematic review).

- Evaluate the effectiveness of placing suicide prevention within community settings such as churches, Veteran Administration centers, substance use counseling centers, and agencies that serve elder populations.

Indicated strategies

- Identify novel sites for implementing suicide-prevention programs for high-risk individuals, such as family violence court.
- Enlarge treatment studies to include individuals with a diverse history of treatment and risk and protective factors, including as appropriate suicidal individuals.

REFERENCES

Arias, E., Anderson, R. N., & Kung, H. C. (2003). Deaths: Final data for 2001. *National Vital Statistics Reports (CDC)*, *52*, 1–116.

Aseltine, R. H. (2003). An evaluation of a school-based suicide prevention program. *Adolescent & Family Health*, *3*, 81–88.

Aseltine, R. H., & DeMartino, R. (2004). An outcome evaluation of the SOS Suicide Prevention Program. *American Journal of Public Health 94* (3), 446–451.

Barrios, L. C., Everett, S. A., Simon, T. R., & Brenner, N. D. (2000). Suicide prevention among US college students. Association with other injury risk behaviors. *Journal of American College Health*, *48*, 229–233.

Beautrais, A. L., Joyce, P. R., & Mulder, R. T. (1997). Precipitating factors and life events in serious suicide attempts among youths aged 13 through 24 years. *Journal of the American Academy of Child & Adolescent Psychiatry, 36,* 1543–1551.

Beck, A. T., Kovacs, M., & Weissman, A. (1975). Hopelessness and suicidal behavior. An overview. *Journal of the American Medical Association, 234,* 1146–1149.

Bostwick, J. M., & Pankratz, V. S. (2000). Affective disorders and suicide risk: A reexamination. *The American Journal of Psychiatry, 157,* 1925–1932.

Brent, D. A., Johnson, B. A., Perper, J., Connolly, J., Bridge, J., Bartle, S., & Rather, C. (1994). Personality disorder, personality traits, impulsive violence, and completed suicide in adolescents. *Journal of the American Academy of Child & Adolescent Psychiatry, 33,* 1080–1086.

Brown, C. H. (2003). Design principles and their application in preventive field trials. In W. J. Bukoski & Z. Sloboda (Eds.), *Handbook of drug abuse theory, science, and practice* (pp. 523–540). New York: Plenum Press.

Brown, C. H., & Liao, J. (1999). Principles for designing randomized preventive trials in mental health: An emerging developmental epidemiology paradigm. *American Journal of Community Psychology, 27,* 673–710.

Brown, G. K., Ten Have, T., Henriques, G. R., Xie, S. X., Hollander, J. E., & Beck, A. T. (2005). Cognitive therapy for the prevention of suicide attempts. *Journal of the American Medical Association, 294,* 563–570.

Bruce, M., & Pearson, J. (1999). Designing an intervention to prevent suicide: PROSPECT (Prevention of Suicide in Primary Care Elderly: Collaborative Trial). *Dialogues in Clinical Neuroscience, 1,* 100–112.

Bruce, M. L., Ten Have, T. R., Reynolds, C. F. Ill, Katz, I. I., Schulberg, H. C., Mulsant, B. H., Brown, G. K., McAray, G. J., Pearson, J. L., & Alexopoulos, G. S. (2004). Reducing suicidal ideation and depressive symptoms in depressed older primary care patients: A randomized controlled trial. *Journal of the American Medical Association, 291,* 1081–1091.

Cantor, C., & Neulinger, K. (1998). The epidemiology of suicide and attempted suicide among young Australians. *Australian & New Zealand Journal of Psychiatry, 34,* 8–14.

Centers for Disease Control and Prevention. (1994). Programs for the prevention of suicide among adolescents and young adults; and suicide contagion and the reporting of suicide: Recommendations from a national workshop. *Morbidity & Mortality Weekly Report, 40,* 633–635.

Chambers, D., Pearson, J., Lubell, K., Brandon, S., O'Brien, K., & Zinn, J. (2004). The science of public messages for suicide prevention: A workshop summary. *Suicide & Life-Threatening Behavior, 35* (2), 134–145.

Charney, D. S., Reynolds, C. F. III, Lewis, L., Lebowitz, B. D., Sunderland, T., Alexopoulos, G. S., Blazer, D. G., Katz, I. R., Meyers, B. S., Arean, P. A., Borson, S., Brown, C., Bruce, M. L., Callahan, C. M., Charlson, M. E., Conwell, Y., Cuthbert, B. N., Devanand, D. P., Gibson, M. J., Gottlieb, G. L., Krishnan, K. R., Laden, S. K., Lyketsos, C. G., Mulsant, B. H., Niederehe, G., Olin, J. T., Oslin, D. W., Pearson, J., Persky, T., Pollock, B. G., Raetzman, S., Reynolds, M., Salzman, C., Schulz, R., Schwenk, T. L., Scolnick, E., Unutzer, J., Weissman, M. M., & Young, R. C. (2003). Depression and bipolar support alliance consensus statement on the unmet needs in diagnosis and treatment of mood disorders in late life. *Archives of General Psychiatry, 60,* 664–672.

Committee on Pathophysiology & Prevention of Adolescent & Adult Suicide Board on Neuroscience and Behavioral, Institute of Medicine (2002). *Reducing suicide: A national imperative.* Washington, D.C.: National Academy Press.

Conner, K. R., Cox, C., Duberstein, P. R., Tian, L., Nisbet, P. A., & Conwell, Y. (2000a). Violence, alcohol, and completed suicide: A case-control study. *American Journal of Psychiatry, 158,* 1701–1705.

Conner, K. R., Duberstein, P. R., & Conwell, Y. (2000b). Domestic violence, separation, and suicide in young men with early onset alcoholism: Reanalyses of Murphy's data. *Suicide & Life-Threatening Behavior., 30,* 354–359.

Conner, K. R., Li, Y., Meldrum, S., Duberstein, P. R., & Conwell, Y. (2003). The role of drinking in suicidal ideation: Analyses of Project MATCH data. *Journal of Studies on Alcohol, 64,* 402–408.

Conwell, Y., & Duberstein, P. R. (2001). Suicide in elders. *Annals of the New York Academy of Sciences, 932,* 132–150.

Conwell, Y., & Lyness, J. M., Duberstein, P., Cox, C., Seidlitz, L., DiGiorgio, A., & Caine, E. D. (2000). Completed suicide among older patients in primary care practices: A controlled study. *Journal of the American Geriatrics Society, 48,* 23–29.

DeLeo, D., Buono, M. D., & Dwyer, J. (2002). Suicide among the elderly: The long-term impact of a telephone support and assessment intervention in northern Italy. *British Journal of Psychiatry, 181,* 226–229.

DeLeo, D., Carollo, G., & Buono, M. D. (1995). Lower suicide rates associated with a tele-help/tele-check service for the elderly at home. *American Journal of Psychiatry, 152,* 632–634.

Des Jarlais, D. J., & Friedman, S. R. (1998). Fifteen years of research on preventing HIV infection among injecting drug users: What we have learned, what we have not learned, what we have done, what we have not done. *Public Health Reports, 113* (suppl. 1), 182–188.

Dolan, L. J., Kellam, S. G., Brown, C. H., & Werthamer-Larsson, L. (1993). The short-term impact of two classroom-based preventive interventions on aggressive and shy behaviors and poor achievement. *Journal of Applied Developmental Psychology, 14,* 182–188.

Douglas, K. A., & Collins, J. L. (1997). Results from the 1995 National College Health Risk Behavior Survey. *Journal of American College Health, 46* (2), 55–66.

Eggert, L. L., Thompson, E. A., Randell, B. P., & Pike, K. C. (2002). Preliminary effects of brief school-based prevention approaches for reducing youth suicide—Risk behaviors, depression, and drug involvement. *Journal of Child & Adolescent Psychiatric Nursing, 15,* 48–64.

Etzersdorfer, E., Sonneck, G., & Nagel-Kuess, S. (1992). Newspaper reports and suicide. *New England Journal of Medicine, 327,* 502–503.

Goss, R. J., Peterson, K., Smith, L. W., Kalb, K., & Brodey, B. B. (2002). Characteristics of suicide attempts in a large urban jail system with an established suicide prevention program. *Psychiatric Services, 53,* 574–579.

Gould, M. S. (2001). Suicide and the media. *Annals of the New York Academy of Sciences, 932,* 200–224.

Gould, M. S., Greenberg, T., Velting, D. M., & Shaffer, D. (2003). Youth suicide risk and preventive interventions: A review of the past 10 years. *Journal of the American Academy of Child & Adolescent Psychiatry, 42,* 386–405.

Gould, M. S., Fisher, P., Parides, M., Flory, M., & Shaffer, D. (1996). Psychosocial risk factors of child and adolescent completed suicide. *Archives of General Psychiatry, 53,* 1155–1162.

Gould, M., Jamieson, P., & Romer, D. (2003). Media contagion and suicide among the young. *American Behavioral Scientist, 46,* 1269–1284.

Gould, M. S., & Kramer, R. A. (2001). Youth prevention suicide. *Suicide & Life-Threatening Behavior, 31,* 6–31.

Gould, M. S., Marrocco, F. A., Kleinman M., Thomas, J. G., Mostkoff, K., Cote, J., & Davies, M. (2005). Evaluating iatrogenic risk of youth suicide screening programs. A randomized trial. *Journal of the American Medical Association, 293* (13), 1635–1643.

Gunnell, D., Lopatatzidis, A., Dorling, D., Wehner, H., Southall, H., & Frankel, S. (1999). Suicide and unemployment in young people. Analysis of trends in England and Wales, 1921–1995. *British Journal of Psychiatry, 175,* 263–270.

Guthrie, E., Kapur, N., Mackway-Jones, K., Chew-Graham, C., Moorey, J., Mendel, E., Marino-Francis, F., Sanderson, S., Turpin, C., Boddy, G., & Tomenson, B. (2001). Randomised controlled trial of brief psychological intervention after deliberate self poisoning. *British Medical Journal, 323,* 135–138.

Hawton, K. (2002). United Kingdom legislation on pack sizes of analgesics: Background, rationale, and effects on suicide and deliberate self-harm. *Suicide & Life-Threatening Behavior, 32,* 223–229.

Hawton, K., Ware, C., Mistry, H., Hewitt, J., Kingsbury, S., Roberts, D., & Weitzel, S. (1996). Paracetamol self-poisoning: Characteristics, prevention and harm reduction. *British Journal of Psychiatry, 168,* 43–48.

Ho, T. P., Hung, S. F., Lee, C. C., Chung, K. F., & Chung, S. Y. (1995). Characteristics of youth suicide in Hong Kong. *Social Psychiatry & Psychiatric Epidemiology, 30* (3), 107–112.

Hutchinson, G., Daisley, H., Simeon, D., Simmonds, V., Shetty, M., & Lynn, D. I. (1999). High rates of paraquat-induced suicide in southern Trinidad. *Suicide & Life-Threatening Behavior, 29,* 186–191.

Jobes, D. A., Jacoby, A. M., Cimbolic, P., & Hustead, L. A. (1997). Assessment and treatment of suicidal clients in a university counseling center. *Journal of Counseling Psychology, 44* (4), 368–377.

Joe, S., & Kaplan, M. (2001). Suicide among African American men. *Suicide & Life-Threatening Behavior, 31,* 106–121.

Joiner, T. E. Jr., Pfaff, J. J., & Acres, J. G. (2002). A brief screening tool for suicidal symptoms in adolescents and young adults in general health settings: Reliability and validity data from the Australian National General Practice Youth Suicide Prevention Project. *Behaviour Research & Therapy, 40,* 471–481.

Kalafat, J., & Elias, M. (1994). An evaluation of a school-based suicide awareness intervention. *Suicide & Life-Threatening Behavior, 24,* 224–233.

Kellam, S. G., & Langevin, D. (2003). A framework for understanding "evidence" in prevention research and programs. *Prevention Science, 4,* 137–153.

Kelly, J. A., Lawrence, S., & Diaz, Y. E. (1991). HIV risk behavior reduction following intervention with key opinion leaders of population: An experimental analysis. *American Journal of Public Health, 81,* 168–171.

King, K. S. J. (2000). Project SOAR: A training program to increase school counselors' knowledge and confidence regarding suicide prevention and intervention. *Journal of School Health*, *70*, 402–407.

Knox, K. L., Litts, D. A., Talcott, G. W., Feig, J. C., & Caine, E. D. (2003). Risk of suicide and related adverse outcomes after exposure to a suicide prevention programme in the United States Air Force: Cohort study. *British Medical Journal*, *327*, 1376–1380.

Knox, K. L., & Caine, E. D. (2005). Establishing priorities for reducing suicide and its antecedents in the United States. *American Journal of Public Health*, *95* (11), 1898–1903.

Kochanek, K. D., & Smith, B. L. (2004). Deaths: Preliminary data for 2002 (Report No. 52[13]). *National Vital Statistics Reports*, pp. 1–48.

Kruesi, M. J. P., Grossman, J., Pennington, J. M., Woodward, P., Duda, D., & Hirsch, J. G. (1999). Suicide and violence prevention: Parent education in the emergency department. *Journal of the American Academy of Child & Adolescent Psychiatry*, *38*, 250–255.

LaFromboise, T. D. (1995). The Zuni Life Skills Development Curriculum: Description and evaluation of a suicide prevention program. *Journal of Counseling Psychology*, *42*, 479–486.

Lamberti, S. J., & Weisman, R. L. (2002). Preventing incarceration of adults with severe mental illness: Project Link. In G. Landsberg, M. Rock, & L. Berg (Eds.), *Seriously mentally ill offenders*. (pp. 133–143). New York: Springer.

Lamberti, J. S., Weisman, R. L., Schwarzkopf, S. B., Price, N., Ashton, R. M., & Trompeter, J. (2001). The mentally ill in jails and prisons: Towards an integrated model of prevention. *Psychiatric Quarterly*, *72*, 63–77.

Langhinrichsen-Rohling, J., Arata, C., Bowers, D., O'Brien, N., & Morgan, A. (2004). Suicidal behavior, negative affect, gender, and self-reported delinquency in college students. *Suicide & Life-Threatening Behavior*, *34*, 255–266.

Latkin, C. A., & Forman, V. L. (2001). Patterns of needle acquisition and sociobehavioral correlates of needle exchange program attendance in Baltimore, Maryland, U.S.A. *Journal of Acquired Immune Deficiency Syndromes*, *27*, 398–404.

LeMaster, P. L., & Connell, C. M. (1994). Health education interventions among Native Americans: A review and analysis. *Health Education Quarterly*, *21*, 521–538.

Linehan, M. M., Armstrong, H. E., Suarez, A., Allmon, D., & Heard, H. L. (1991). Cognitive-behavioral treatment of chronically parasuicidal borderline patients. *Archives of General Psychiatry*, *48*, 1060–1064.

Litts, D. A., Moe, K., Roadman, C. H., Miller, J., & Janke, R. (1999). Suicide prevention among active duty air force personnel—United States 1990–1999. *Morbidity & Mortality Weekly Report*, *48*, 1053–1057.

Luoma, J. B., & Pearson, J. L. (2002). Suicide and marital status in the United States, 1991–1996: Is widowhood a risk factor? *American Journal of Public Health*, *92*, 1518–1522.

Mann, J. J., Huang, Y. Y., Underwood, M. D., Kassir, S. A., Oppenheim, S., Kelly, T., Dwork, A. J., & Arango, V. (2000). A serotonin transporter gene promoter polhymorphism (5-HTTLPR) and prefrontal cortical binding in major depression and suicide. *Archives of General Psychiatry*, *57*, 729–738.

Mehlum, L., & Reinholdt, N. (2000). The Norwegian plan for suicide prevention: Follow-up project 2000–2002; Building on positive experiences. *Notwegian Journal of Suicidologi*, *5*, Supplement.

Metha, A., Weber, B., & Webb, L. D. (1998). Youth suicide prevention: A survey and analysis of policies and efforts in the 50 states. *Suicide & Life-Threatening Behavior*, *28*, 150–164.

Middlebrook, D. L., LeMaster, P. L., Beals, J., Novins, D. K., & Manson, S. M. (2001). Suicide prevention in American Indian and Alaska Native communities: A critical review of programs. *Suicide & Life-Threatening Behavior*, *31*, 132–149.

Motto, J. A., & Bostrom, A. G. (2001). A randomized controlled trial of postcrisis suicide prevention. *Psychiatric Services*, *52*, 828–833.

Mrazek, P. J., & Haggerty, R. J. (1994). Risk and protective factors for the onset of mental disorders. In *Reducing risks for mental disorders: Frontiers for preventive intervention research* (pp. 127–214). Washington, DC: National Academy Press.

National Center for Injury Prevention and Control, Centers for Disease Control and Prevention. (2005). Non-fatal self injury data for 2003. Retrieved July 10, 2005, from www.cdc.gov/ncipc/wisqars/default.htm; accessed.

Orbach, I., & Bar-Joseph, H. (1993). The impact of a suicide prevention program for adolescents on suicidal tendencies, hopelessness, ego identity, and coping. *Suicide & Life-Threatening Behavior*, *23*, 120–129.

Palmer, C. S., Revicki, D. A., Halpern, M. T., & Hatziandreu, E. J. (1995). The cost of suicide and suicide attempts in the United States. *Clinical Neuropharmacology, 18*, S25–S53.

Pearson, J. L., Stanley, B., King, C., & Fisher, C. (2001). *Issues to consider in intervention research with persons at high risk for suicidality.* Washington, D.C.: National Institute of Mental Health.

Pearson, J. L., & Brown, G. K. (2000). Suicide prevention in late life: Directions for science and practice. *Clinical Psychology Review, 20*, 685–705.

Pearson, J. L., Conwell, Y., & Lyness, J. M. (1997). Late-life suicide and depression in the primary care setting. In L. S. Schneider (Ed.), *Developments in geriatric psychiatry: New directions for mental health services,* (pp. 13–38, vol. 76). San Francisco: Jossey-Bass.

Pena, J. B., & Caine, E. D. (2005). *Screening as an approach for adolescent suicide prevention.* Paper presented at the Suicide Prevention Resource Center Regional Conference, Pittsburgh, PA.

Shaffer, D., Vieland, V., Garland, A., Rojas, M., Underwood, M. M., & Busner, C. (1990). Adolescent suicide attempters: Response to suicide-prevention programs. *Journal of the American Medical Association, 264*, 3151–3155.

Shaffer, D., Gould, M., & Hicks, R. C. (1994). Worsening suicide rate in black teenagers. *American Journal of Psychiatry, 151*, 1810–1812.

Shaffer, D., Scott, M., Wilcox, H., Maslow, C., Lucas, C., Garfinkel, R., & Greenwald, S. (2004). The Columbia Suicide Screen: Validity and reliability of a screen for youth suicide and depression. *The Journal of the American Academy of Child & Adolescent Psychiatry, 43*, 71–79.

Thompson, E. A., Eggert, L. L., Randell, B. P., & Pike, K. C. (2001). Evaluation of indicated suicide risk prevention approaches for potential high school dropouts. *American Journal of Public Health, 91*, 742–752.

Tuskan, J. J., & Thase, M. E. (1983). Suicides in jails and prisons. *Journal of Psychosocial Nursing & Mental Health Services, 21*, 29–33.

U.S. Department of Health and Human Services, Public Health Service (2001). National Strategy for Suicide Prevention: Goals and Objectives for Action. Rockville, MD: Author.

Weisman, R. L., & Lamberti, J. S. (2002). Violence prevention and safety training for case management services. *Community Mental Health Journal, 38*, 339–348.

Chapter 11

Interventions to Prevent Intimate Partner Violence

Daniel J. Whitaker, Charlene K. Baker, and Ileana Arias

11.1. INTRODUCTION

Intimate partner violence (IPV) became widely recognized as a health and social problem in the 1970s. The accumulated body of research indicates that IPV is very common. The lifetime prevalence among women for experiencing partner violence has been estimated between 22% and 28% (Straus, Gelles, & Steinmetz, 1980; Tjaden & Thoennes, 1998). IPV can result in fatal and nonfatal injuries and a wide range of adverse health consequences (Basile, Arias, Desai, & Thompson, 2004; Coker, Smith, Bethea, King, & McKeown, 2000) and substantial economic burden (National Center for Injury Prevention and Control [NCIPC], 2003). Research on causes and risk factors has implicated a range of individual psychological factors, relationship and family factors, and contextual or sociocultural factors in the development of IPV (Stith, Smith, Penn, Ward, & Tritt, 2004).

The goal of this chapter is to discuss and review the various prevention efforts that have been undertaken to reduce IPV perpetration. Our review includes strategies designed to reduce the incidence of IPV (either by preventing new cases or by preventing reperpetration) but not strategies that target *only* the negative consequences of IPV. We follow the definition of Saltzman, Fanslow, McMahon, & Shelley (1999) of *partner violence*, which includes physical violence, sexual violence and threats of physical or sexual violence and psychological/emotional abuse when it occurs within the context of prior physical or sexual violence. It should be noted that emotional and psychological abuse can result in many of the same negative consequences as physical abuse (Coker et al., 2000).

Table 11.1 describes the intervention approaches that were reviewed, along with the populations, settings, and targets of the intervention and our conclusions regarding the effectiveness of the intervention strategy. Interventions are organized by whether their focus is primary or secondary prevention. Primary prevention

Table 11.1. Intervention Descriptions, Populations, Settings, and Recommendations Regarding Effectiveness

Strategy and Summary	Populations and Settings, Social-Ecological Level	Evidence, Recommendations, and Caveats
Dating violence prevention curriculum: Most evaluated programs have used a structured curriculum based on feminist and social learning theory to target knowledge and attitudes that support intimate partner violence (IVP), and perpetration of partner violence; length varies from single-session presentations to longer programs (36 hours)	• Implemented mostly with middle and high school students, in a school-based setting • Targets both victims and perpetrators • Both primary/secondary prevention • Individual level	*Recommended*: Recommended rating applies to programs with a skills-based curriculum and community-based elements
Media campaigns: Media campaigns target attitudes, beliefs, and behaviors of broad populations; can include television, radio, posters	• Can be broad (e.g., national) or local • Target victims and perpetrators (or nonvictims, nonperpetrators) • Either primary or secondary prevention • Community level	Insufficient evidence
Couples counseling: Behavioral and cognitive-behavioral approaches have been used; typically therapy involves multiple sessions involving both partners, either as a couple therapy or group couple therapy; length has ranged from relatively brief (10 sessions) to extensive (56 sessions)	• Targets couples who wish to remain intact, and who are using low to moderate levels of violence • Involves both victims and perpetrators • Evaluated as a secondary prevention strategy • Relational level	*Promising*: Recommendation applies only to certain couples (e.g., low levels of violence); assessments of appropriateness for couples counseling is a must
Substance abuse counseling: Behavioral couples counseling or individual counseling with the goal of reducing substance use; therapy lasts anywhere from 22 to 56 sessions	• Targets substance abuse • Targets perpetrators but may involve the couple • Evaluated as a secondary prevention strategy • Individual or relational level	*Promising*: For behavioral couples counseling targeting substance use Insufficient evidence: For individual counseling
Screening for IPV: Screening is typically conducted in health care settings (e.g., primary care, OB/GYN, emergency departments) and can be conducted via interview, survey, or computer; several validated screening measures exist	• Targets victims with any level of IPV, depending on the questions • Used in a variety of health care settings • Secondary prevention • Individual level	*Insufficient evidence*: Unclear if screening alone has any effect; not clear if interventions available for referral are effective

Table 11.1. *Continued*

Strategy and Summary	Populations and Settings, Social-Ecological Level	Evidence, Recommendations, and Caveats
Community services for victims: Shelters provide victims of partner violence housing and other services (advocacy, support groups) for a period of 30–60 days; transitional housing programs provide longer-term housing (1–2 years) along with additional services, such as employment assistance, assistance with permanent housing; advocacy provides support, help accessing services such as housing, child care, and legal assistance; legal advocacy focuses specifically on navigating the legal system	• Target victims, usually with more severe IPV • Secondary prevention • Shelters and advocacy are both individual-level interventions	*Promising (advocacy only)*: Not clear which elements of advocacy are important; individual needs of victims must be considered when implementing
Police responses: Mandatory arrest policies require police to arrest the primary aggressor when responding to a domestic violence call; can sometimes result in dual arrest when primary aggressor cannot be determined	• Arrest policies target moderate to severe levels of domestic violence (which are more likely to involve police) • Focused on perpetrators • Secondary prevention • Community level	*Insufficient evidence*: Arrest may have more of an effect on individuals with greater social capital (e.g. jobs)
Court interventions: No-drop policies require prosecution of arrested domestic violence (DV) offenders regardless of victims' wishes; domestic violence courts are specialized courts dealing only with DV cases (goal is to provide better coordination); protective orders are either temporary or permanent (issued in civil courts)	• Target moderate to severe violence • All target perpetrators • Secondary prevention • No-drop policies and DV courts are community-level interventions; protective orders are individual-level interventions	Insufficient evidence
Sentencing: Batterer intervention programs (BIPs): BIPs are typically group counseling sessions for perpetrators of partner violence (usually male); most are based on feminist theory, cognitive-behavioral theory, or both; groups can range from 12 to 52 sessions	• Target moderate to severe violence • Target perpetrators • Individual level	*Promising*: More data are needed to understand who benefits
Coordinated community response: Typically focused on creating better coordination between law enforcement, courts, and social services; several strategies for creating coordination have been discussed, such as community partnering, community intervention, task forces	• Targets moderate to severe violence • Targets both perpetrators and victims • Community level	Insufficient evidence

strategies target individuals or groups where partner violence has not occurred (i.e., preventing IPV before it occurs), whereas secondary prevention interventions target known perpetrators or victims of partner violence to prevent reperpetration.

Two points are important to bear in mind when reviewing prevention strategies. First, there is variability in level, forms, severity, and motivation of IPV perpetration (Gottman & Jacobson, 1998; Holtzworth-Munroe & Stuart, 1994; Johnson, 1995). For example, IPV may consist of repeated and severe, physical, sexual, and emotional abuse, used by one partner to demean and control the other. Or it may consist of infrequent, low-severity acts (i.e., no physical injuries), used by both partners with few elements of control or coercion. Given the variability, different prevention strategies are likely needed for different forms of IPV. However, strategies and prevention programs have not typically been designed to address a specific form or type of IPV. There are almost no studies examining the efficacy of strategies as a function of the type of IPV or type of perpetrator (Saunders, 1996, is an exception). Thus we caution that interventions deemed effective or promising may be so only for certain types of partner violence. The second point is that although men and women report equal IPV perpetration (Archer, 2000), IPV prevention work has focused almost exclusively on IPV perpetrated by men against women. Thus any conclusions based on the literature reviewed may not be pertinent for female-to-male IPV or IPV among same-sex couples.

11.2. PRIMARY PREVENTION PROGRAMS

11.2.1. Dating Violence Prevention Programs

Dating violence prevention programs focus on increasing IPV knowledge, and changing IPV attitudes, beliefs, and behaviors. Most dating violence prevention programs have been based on feminist theory and/or social learning theory (Whitaker et al., 2006) and have targeted beliefs, attitudes, and behaviors that are thought to lead to IPV: awareness of IPV, acceptance of aggression, beliefs about sex roles and gender inequality, verbal and psychological aggression, communication skills, anger control and conflict in relationships, and understanding healthy relationships. Dating violence prevention programs often consist of didactic instruction, interactive activities, and skill-building exercises such as role-playing. Most evaluated dating violence prevention programs have been conducted in school settings (Whitaker et al., 2006).

Two recent reviews of dating violence prevention programs concluded that dating violence programs tend to be effective at changing attitudes, such as acceptance of aggression, but changes in behavior have not been consistently measured or demonstrated (Avery-Leaf & Cascardi, 2002; Hickman, Jaycox, and Aronoff, 2004). A systematic review (Whitaker et al., 2006) of empirical studies published since 1990 found that only 4 of 11 studies assessed behavior change. Of those studies, however, 2 reported a long-term effect on dating violence perpetration. The Safe Dates Program for middle and high school students, developed and evaluated by Foshee et al. (1996) was found to reduce perpetration of physical violence, serious physical violence, and sexual violence for intervention students relative to controls 4 years after the intervention (Foshee et al., 2004). Wolfe and colleagues' (2003) Youth Relationship Project followed 183 adolescents over a 16-month period, and found that the intervention reduced dating violence perpetration relative to control students who received the usual services available to them. Each of these studies were methodologically rigorous: both used experimental designs, reported excellent fidelity, included extended follow-up of participants (48 and 16 months), and had acceptable retention rates. Each included a structured curriculum, which was relatively lengthy compared to other dating violence prevention programs (Whitaker et al., 2006), and community-based components (e.g., training of community providers, community service). Neither study was designed to determine whether the curriculum or the community component was more important in changing behavior.

Dating violence prevention programs that include an individual-level curriculum and community-based activities are a recommended strategy for the primary prevention of IPV. We caution readers that this recommendation may not hold for programs that are substantially different in content from Safe Dates or the Youth Relationship Project and that partial implementation of either program (e.g., using only the curriculum portion) may yield reduced or no effectiveness. Thus we encourage those that intend to implement either of these programs to include all components of the intervention, as the authors have done (Foshee et al., 2004). There is insufficient evidence regarding the effectiveness of other types of dating violence prevention curricula, such as those whose focus is primarily educational or on attitude change.

11.2.2. Media Campaigns

Media campaigns are frequently used to prevent IPV and have taken various forms, such as posters, television and radio spots, and public service announcements. The goals of media campaigns are to increase awareness of IPV or to change attitudes associated with the use of violence in intimate relationships, and ultimately, to reduce the incidence and prevalence of IPV. Media campaigns can be targeted broadly to an entire population or can target specific subgroups of individuals. Because media campaigns are designed to change norms broadly, they can act as both primary and secondary prevention.

Media campaigns have been shown to be effective in reducing smoking among youth, increasing healthy eating habits, and changing attitudes associated with youth violence; however, much of the research suggests that to be most effective media campaigns should be used in conjunction with comprehensive interventions to change policy and social structures within a community (Meshack et al., 2004; Wakefield, Flay, Nichter, & Giovino, 2003). To date, there are few published evaluations regarding media campaigns for IPV prevention. One national campaign that was evaluated, There's No Excuse for Domestic Violence, was developed and implemented by the Family Violence Prevention Fund in July 1994. A random-digit dial survey showed that awareness of the campaign was related to greater perception of IPV as a social issue, greater action taken to reduce IPV, and beliefs that perpetrators of physical IPV should be arrested (Klein, Campbell, Soler, & Ghez, 1997). The evaluation study did not measure IPV incidence or prevalence rates over time, and thus it is not known whether the occurrence of IPV was reduced in the intervention communities. In February 2002, the Family Violence Prevention Fund launched a new national media campaign, Coaching Boys to Men, consisting of public service announcements that encourage men to talk with boys about violence against women and to model appropriate behavior. This campaign is in the process of being evaluated.

Because of limited outcome and impact data, there is insufficient evidence regarding the effectiveness of media campaigns. Evaluations of media campaigns are often inconclusive because of the difficulty in measuring exposure to the media campaign, interference from other media messages, and contamination that can occur if comparison participants are inadvertently exposed to the media campaign. In the absence of an evaluation, messages still should be pilot tested, and implementation procedures should be carefully planned to increase exposure and decrease contamination. Most important, they should be evaluated rigorously.

11.3.   SECONDARY PREVENTION PROGRAMS

11.3.1.   Couples Counseling/Marital Therapy

Couples counseling for couples with a history of IPV (also referred to as marital therapy or conjoint counseling) has been extremely controversial in the treatment and prevention of IPV. It has been widely argued that couples counseling is an inappropriate strategy; and, in fact, it is explicitly excluded by many state standards for batterer-treatment programs (Austin & Dankwort, 1999). The primary concerns are that female victims may be coerced into a treatment in which they cannot fully participate for fear of retribution and that involving victims in treatment implies some culpability on their part for the IPV, thereby partly exonerating the perpetrator. Recently, there has been some discussion that couples counseling might be appropriate under certain circumstances: situations in which there is low to moderate frequency and severity of IPV; when both partners agree to counseling and wish to remain an intact couple; when violence is perpetrated by both partners; and when there is little psychological abuse, intimidation, and fear (Bograd & Mederos, 1999; Gottman and Jacobson, 1998; Johnson, 1995; O'Leary, 2002; Stith, Rosen, McCollum, and Thomsen, 2004).

Recent studies have examined the efficacy of couples counseling among couples in which there was low to moderate partner violence. Most published studies of couples counseling have employed behavioral or cognitive-behavior treatment methods; other types of couples treatment exist, such as emotion-focused therapy, but are largely untested for treatment of IPV (Stith, Rosen, & McCollum, 2003). Brannen and Rubin (1996) compared couples counseling to gender-specific treatments and found reduced violence at posttest for those in couples counseling relative to gender-specific groups for men and women but found no difference at 6 months posttreatment. In a similar study, O'Leary, Heyman, and Neidig (1999) randomly assigned intact couples to either group conjoint therapy or gender-specific group treatment to reduce psychological and physical aggression. They found that both treatments yielded a similar reduction in violence in the year after treatment, no differences between the groups in levels of violence. Stith, Rosen, and colleagues (2004) compared individual couples counseling and couples group counseling to a no-treatment control. They found that group-format couples counseling was superior to counseling of individual couples and no-treatment control at reducing marital aggression at 6 months after treatment, and both forms of couples counseling were superior to no treatment at reducing recidivism 2 years after treatment (though only about half of the sample participated in the 2-year follow-up).

Couples counseling is a promising approach for secondary prevention of IPV. This recommendation includes the strong caveat that couples counseling for IPV is appropriate in the circumstances discussed above and by several authors (Bograd & Mederos, 1999; O'Leary, 2002; O'Leary et al., 1999; Stith et al., 2004).

11.3.2. Substance Abuse Counseling

The relationship between substance abuse and IPV has also been controversial. The controversy primarily concerns ensuring that substance use is not used as an excuse for the perpetration of IPV, and that the perpetrator takes full responsibility for his behavior. There are many studies that show a relationship between substance use and IPV, including a meta-analytic review (Stith et al., 2004). Studies of alcohol abusers find that IPV is common among them (Murphy & O'Farrell, 1994). Other research has shown that, within individuals, violent episodes co-occur with alcohol use (Fals-Stewart, 2003; Leonard & Quigley, 1999). Thus there appears to be a clear relationship between alcohol use and perpetration of IPV.

A few recent studies have examined the effect of substance abuse treatment on IPV. O'Farrell and colleagues conducted a series of naturalistic studies. In one study, male alcoholics treated with behavioral marital therapy showed significantly reduced episodes of IPV over 2 years; after 2 years, remitted alcoholics were no more violent toward their partners than matched controls (O'Farrell, Fals-Stewart, Murphy, Stephan, & Murphy, 2004; O'Farrell, Van Hutton, & Murphy, 1999). A different study using an individually based treatment for alcohol abuse found reduced IPV and equal levels of IPV between remitted alcoholics and matched controls at 1 year after treatment (O'Farrell, Murphy, Fals-Stewart, & Murphy, 2003). A recent study randomized participants to two forms of treatment: behavioral couples therapy and individually based treatment, both focused solely on drug abuse. Results at 1 year after treatment showed that (1) behavioral couples therapy resulted in significantly less IPV over time, but individually based treatment did not; and (2) IPV was significantly less likely among men who received behavioral couples therapy than those who received individually based treatment (Fals-Stewart, Kashdan, O'Farrell, & Birchler, 2002).

Behavioral couples therapy that focuses on reducing alcohol and drug abuse is a promising intervention for reducing IPV perpetration. There is insufficient evidence for the efficacy of individually based treatments for substance abuse on IPV. Again, issues of when couples counseling is appropriate and when it may be contraindicated must be considered.

11.3.3. Screening for IPV

Screening for IPV is an intervention implemented in a health care setting and involves health care practitioners asking structured questions to women to determine if they have been victims of IPV. Screening for IPV is based on a medical model of early detection, which assumes that if a condition can be detected and treated early (i.e., before symptoms arise) then morbidity and mortality from that condition can be reduced. Screening for IPV is recommended by several national organizations, such as the American Medical Association, American Academy of Pediatrics, and American Nurses Association, but has not been widely implemented.

Screening is virtually always linked with an intervention or referral for an intervention, making it difficult to determine the effect of screening per se. The evidence regarding the efficacy or effectiveness of interventions available for referral from the health care setting—primarily advocacy and shelters, which we discuss later—is limited (Wathen & MacMillan, 2003). Independent reviews by the U.S. Preventive Services Task Force (Nelson, Nygren, McInerney, & Klein, 2004) and the Canadian Task Force on Preventive Health Care (Wathen & MacMillan, 2003) to determine whether screening was effective concluded that there is insufficient data on the potential benefits and risks of screening to recommend its routine implementation. No studies have examined whether screening for IPV reduced revictimization compared to no screening. Two studies examined IPV victimization among pregnant women after screening (McFarlane, Soeken, & Wiist, 2000; Parker, McFarlane, Soeken, Silva, & Reed, 1999), and both found a decrease in IPV over time, but neither included a nonintervention comparison group. In a review of screening efforts based in emergency departments, Anglin and Sachs (2003) found no studies that evaluated the effectiveness of emergency department–based screening on the morbidity and mortality of IPV or on patient health status, resource use, or victimization from future violence.

There is insufficient evidence to suggest that screening for IPV reduces subsequent incidents of partner violence. Although neither the U.S. nor Canadian task force recommended screening, both suggested that clinicians should be alert to signs and symptoms of potential IPV and may wish to ask about exposure to IPV during diagnostic evaluations. In addition to a controlled trial examining the effect of screening plus intervention versus no screening, other questions should be addressed, including the optimal methods for screening (interview, survey, computer), what types of violence should be assessed (e.g., physical, sexual, psychological), and whether benefits vary by setting (e.g., primary care, emergency room, pediatric setting).

11.3.4.   Community-Based Services for Victims

Two types of community-based services for victims of IPV are shelters (or more broadly, housing programs) and advocacy. These services are almost exclusively for victimized women. Shelters and advocacy services grew from the service community rather than the research community; as a result, they are widely available, but data regarding their effect are limited.

11.3.4.1.   Shelters/Transitional Housing

Shelters for battered women and their children offer temporary shelter for 30–60 days in addition to services, such as support groups, legal assistance, and programs for children. To date, there are only a few published studies on the effect of a shelter stay on future violence. Results showed that for women who were actively attempting other strategies at the same time, a stay at a shelter greatly reduced the likelihood of further violence (Berk, Newton, & Berk, 1986). However, this study lacked a control group of women who had not stayed at a shelter. In fact, the authors suggest that in some cases, a shelter stay may lead to retaliatory violence from the perpetrator. In contrast, an examination of surveillance data by Dugan, Nagin, and Rosenfeld (1999) suggested no significant effect of shelter capacity on declining IPV homicide rates in the United States.

Transitional-housing programs provide women with housing for longer periods than do shelters, with many ranging from 1 to 2 years. Transitional-housing programs also provide additional services for women, such as counseling services, employment assistance, and permanent-housing assistance (National Council of Juvenile and Family Court Judges, 1998). Again, because a package of services is usually delivered, separating the effect of housing from other services is difficult. No controlled evaluations of transitional-housing programs have been conducted, but qualitative work indicates that these programs are of great value to women and their children. Women report that without transitional-housing they would likely become homeless, return to their violent partner, become incarcerated, or resort to prostitution (Sullivan, Melbin, & Cain, 2003).

There is insufficient evidence to judge the effectiveness of shelters and transitional-housing programs on IPV revictimization. Because shelter stays and transitional housing are often packaged with other services, it is important for policy makers and program managers to identify and provide the most optimal "package" of services that will maximize women's abilities to function independently and avoid future violence.

11.3.4.2. Advocacy

Advocacy services, offered through community-based agencies, have many goals, including social and emotional support, accessing services (e.g., housing and child care), and facilitating legal options to prevent revictimization (e.g., temporary restraining order). The goal of advocacy is both support and instruction regarding accessing needed resources and information so that victims will be able to advocate for themselves in the future.

Most of the data supporting advocacy is anecdotal and suggest that advocacy has positive psychological benefits for women (e.g., self-esteem, feelings of empowerment). However, one experimental study evaluated advocacy by randomly assigning 278 women who had recently left a shelter to either a 10-week advocacy intervention or services as usual. Women in both groups were followed for 2 years, with 94% of the sample retained. At the 2-year follow-up, 24% of women in the advocacy intervention group reported no physical IPV by the original assailant or any new partners compared to 11% in the services as usual group (Sullivan & Bybee, 1999).

Another slightly different form of advocacy is legal advocacy, which specifically helps victims of partner violence understand and use the legal system. Results from one study showed that women who had worked with legal advocates reported decreased IPV 6 weeks later, as well as higher emotional well-being compared to women who did not work with legal advocates (Bell & Goodman, 2001).

Based on these data, the provision of advocacy services to female victims represents a promising strategy for the prevention of IPV. It is important to note that we do not yet understand why advocacy is effective. That is, the relative importance of the various services advocacy offers and the supportive relationship between advocate and victim is not known. Likewise, it is necessary to consider for whom advocacy is effective. There is some evidence to suggest that although high levels of legal advocacy are associated with fewer IPV homicides for white married women there is a backlash effect such that these same levels are associated with more IPV homicides for black unmarried women (Dugan, Nagin, & Rosenfeld, 2003). Likewise, we do not know whether women respond differently to advocacy depending on the severity of their IPV victimization.

11.3.5.   Criminal and Civil Justice Responses

Policy strategies to prevent IPV typically include the criminal justice sector, including police/law enforcement, prosecutorial/judicial, and sentencing strategies. Like shelters and advocacy services, these interventions have been widely implemented but not rigorously evaluated (Buzawa & Buzawa, 2003). The lack of research is in part due to the difficulty in evaluating policy and structural changes and in part due to the fact that many criminal justice responses have been implemented simultaneously (e.g., mandatory arrest plus prosecution strategies), making it difficult to separate the effect of various interventions.

11.3.5.1.   Police Responses

The most well known police intervention for IPV is a mandatory arrest policy. This policy requires that police officers responding to a domestic violence call identify and arrest the primary aggressor in that situation. Mandatory arrest policies are widespread and have been implemented to remove the discretion to arrest from police officers and victims (Hirschel & Buzawa, 2002).

The trend to implement mandatory arrest policies was prompted by the Minneapolis Domestic Violence Experiment (MDVE) conducted by Sherman and Berk (1984). Results of that experiment showed that 10% of those arrested reassaulted their partner compared to 24% of those removed from the scene but not arrested. Replication of the MDVE was attempted in five jurisdictions, but the findings were not consistent with the original study (Berk, Campbell, Klap, & Western, 1992; Dunford, Huizinga, & Elliott, 1990; Hirschel & Hutchison, 1992; Pate & Hamilton, 1992; Sherman et al., 1992). Findings from four of the replications showed that employed offenders were less likely to recidivate after an arrest than unemployed offenders (Berk et al., 1992; Pate & Hamilton, 1992; Sherman et al., 1992). One explanation is that employed offenders may have more to lose from a rearrest than unemployed offenders, thus accounting for their lower recidivism.

With this mix of evidence, there are insufficient data available to draw conclusions about mandatory arrest policies. It is likely that mandatory arrest has a differential impact for offenders depending on their circumstances. The potential drawbacks to mandatory arrest policies must be considered. Mandatory arrest policies can lead to dual arrest and to retaliatory violence of the victim by the perpetrator, possibly deterring women from calling the police for help (Buzwa & Buzwa, 2003; Martin, 1997).

11.3.5.2.   Prosecutorial and Judicial Responses

The most well known prosecutorial intervention is the *no-drop policy*, which requires prosecution of a perpetrator once arrested and does not allow victims to withdraw violence charges. Although widespread, many jurisdictions have flexible no-drop policies, citing specific circumstances under which charges can be dropped (Buzawa & Buzawa, 2003).

A judicial intervention is the specialized domestic violence court, which is used to handle the growing caseload of IPV cases, to increase a coordinated response to the multiple issues often found in IPV cases (e.g., criminal, civil, child custody), and to ensure that better trained personnel handle sensitive cases of IPV. A second judicial response, and one that occurs in civil rather than criminal courts, is the issuance of a protective order. Protective orders are legally binding and prohibit the offender from contacting or engaging in further acts of violence against the petitioner. Protection orders can exclude the perpetrator from the shared residence; can prevent the perpetrator from harassing the petitioner by mail, phone, or in person; and can award temporary custody of minor children (Holt, Kernic, Lumley, Wolf, & Rivara, 2002).

Data on the effect of prosecutorial and judicial interventions are scarce. Only one study has examined the link between no-drop policies and revictimization, finding that, contrary to the policy, permitting victims to drop charges in cases that were victim initiated (as opposed to at the scene arrests by police) was associated with *fewer* reports of subsequent violence in the 6-month follow-up period compared to traditional processing (Ford, 1993). Similarly, only one study has evaluated the effectiveness of specialized domestic violence (DV) courts and found that postdisposition arrest rates were about 25% vs. 50% for those cases processed by the specialized DV courts compared to the general courts (Newmark, Rempel, Diffily, & Kane, 2004). However, there were limited data about the nature of those arrests, and domestic violence incidents could not be distinguished from other criminal incidents.

Between 23% and 50% of women who seek protection orders experience revictimization (Carlson, Harris, & Holden, 1999; Harrell & Smith, 1996; Klein, 1996), but few studies have examined the effect of protection orders on recidivism. One study, using a retrospective cohort design, found that permanent, but not temporary, protection orders were associated with a decrease in the risk of police-reported IPV in the 12 months after the index incident (Holt et al., 2002). Several studies have compared the experiences of women who filed protective orders with those who did not, and all reported no differences in rates of revictimization (Grau, Fagan, & Wexler, 1985; Harrell & Smith, 1996; Klein, 1996). Finally, some work has examined the combined effects of arrest and filing protective orders. Mears, Carlson, Holden, and Harris (2001) examined prevalence or time to revictimization among three groups of women who varied with respect to the presence of a protective order and the arrest of their partner and found no differences among the groups (no control group was included).

There are insufficient data to determine the efficacy or effectiveness of any prosecutorial or judicial interventions. In addition to the need for more data on the effectiveness of criminal and civil response to IPV, it is equally important to assess the potential for harm to participants from these interventions. For example, "strict" no-drop policies may place victims at risk for further violence by their partners (Ford, 2003). Specialized DV courts may also have negative effects: special needs of victims are ignored, women may lose custody of their children, and perpetrators escape sanctions through diversion to unproven treatment programs (Keilitz, 2004). Protective orders may provide women with a sense of control, which may in turn lead to reductions in subsequent violence (Fischer & Rose, 1995), but there is also the possibility of a backlash effect in which perpetrators may engage in retaliatory violence (Holt et al., 2002).

11.3.5.3. Sentencing Interventions

Many partner violence offenders are sentenced to *batterer-intervention programs* (BIPs) in lieu of jail time. BIPs are present in every state, and most states have standards for those programs that describe acceptable or required treatment modalities and content (Austin & Dankwort, 1999). The dominant approaches for BIPs are feminist psycho-educational models (e.g., the Duluth model), which address violence as part of a larger pattern of power and control in relationships, and cognitive-behavioral groups, which focus on the functional aspects of violence and involve training to learn alternatives to violence. Other less commonly employed approaches are anger management and psychodynamic approaches (Stosny, 1995). BIPs can last up to 52 weeks and are typically conducted in group settings.

There have been approximately 40 evaluation studies published on batterer-intervention programs, and a number of recent reviews. Most reviews agree that strong conclusions about the efficacy or effectiveness of BIPs are limited by a number of methodological weaknesses inherent to BIP evaluations: selection bias, program attrition, short follow-up periods, incomplete measurement of outcomes, and biased data sources (Gondolf, 2004). Babcock, Green, and Robie (2004) conducted a meta-analysis of the most rigorous BIP evaluations (22 total), and report an overall "small" effect of BIPs above and beyond sanctions from the criminal justice system. Based only on the experimental studies included ($n = 5$), Babcock et al. report a 5% increase in successful nonviolence for treated batterers; this translates into a 40% recidivism rate for untreated batterers and a 35% recidivism rate for treated batterers. The authors note that even the small effects of BIPs would result in the prevention of 42,000 reassaults each year. The BIP effect was no different for programs using feminist psycho-educational models from those using cognitive-behavioral models. Other recent research reviews have concluded that BIPs do appear to have some small effect (Bennett & Williams, 2001; Taylor & Davis, 1999), but their efficacy or effectiveness is not yet fully understood (Saunders & Hammill, 2003).

Based on the available data, we believe BIPs represent a promising strategy for reducing recidivism of reassault. Despite the amount of research conducted on BIPs (or perhaps because of it), there are many questions remaining about the size and nature of their influence on perpetrator behavior. Gondolf (2002; 2004) has argued that it is difficult to separate program effects due to BIPs from "system" effects attributable to the broader functioning of the criminal justice system of which BIPs are a part and that meta-analyses tend to decontextualize evaluations of BIPs. State-mandated standards for BIPs have potential negative consequences; several studies have suggested that a range of approaches may be needed for different types of batterers (Holtzworth-Munroe & Stuart, 1994; Saunders & Hammill, 2003), for men of different racial backgrounds (Gondolf & Williams, 2001), and for batterers with substance abuse or mental-health problems. Research is needed to better understand whether specific types of programs are effective in specific situations, and it is important that state policies regarding BIPs accommodate those new findings.

11.3.6.   Coordinated Community Responses/Community Intervention Projects

There has been a concerted effort to create integration or coordination among agencies that engage in IPV prevention. The goal of a coordinated community response (CCR) is to mobilize community leadership and resources, maximizing efficiency of resources, and to avoid duplicative services and contradictory messages (Hart, 1995). There are a number of different approaches for creating a CCR that have been described in the literature, including community partnering, community intervention, task forces or coordinating councils, training or technical assistance projects, and community organizing (Hart, 1995).

CCRs have been widely implemented in practice (Edelson, 1991; Goolkasian, 1986), but there are few data that speak to their effect. Most published studies have examined ongoing CCRs in an uncontrolled manner—for example, by examining recidivism rates of men arrested and prosecuted within a system that has implemented a CCR—and those studies generally support a more coordinated response. Studies have found arrest alone or arrest plus incarceration yield higher recidivism rates than arrest plus other types of criminal justice interventions, such as court-mandated treatment (Babcock & Steiner, 1999; Syers and Edelson, 1992; Shepard, Falk, & Elliot, 2002; Steinman, 1990). Two studies found lower recidivism among men who participated in a greater number of CCR components (Murphy, Winters, Fals-Stewart, O'Farrell, & Murphy, 1998; Tolman & Weisz, 1995). For example, Murphy et al. (1998) found that greater use of CCR component interventions (e.g., a guilty verdict for partner violence, probation, mandated counseling, attendance at counseling, and completing a batterers' counseling program) yielded an incremental effect on lowered recidivism. None of these cohort studies employed appropriate comparison groups. A recent report by Post, Klevens, Maxwell, Shelley, & Ingram (2005) compared 10 communities in which a CCR had been implemented to matched communities that had no CCR. A random-digit dial telephone survey of over 12,000 respondent found no difference in rates of partner violence, help-seeking behaviors, and service use or in attitudes and beliefs among CCR and control communities.

There are insufficient data at this time to determine the effectiveness of CCRs. The evaluation challenges regarding CCRs are significant. The CCR intervention strategy is expected to affect a number of systemic and community-level changes; but generally, those changes have not been measured and linked to outcomes (Roussos & Fawcett, 2000). Without doing this, it is unclear whether the effect of a CCR was due to the increased coordination of agencies or to specific changes made by various agencies. Tracking systems such as the Community Toolbox may be needed to properly measure community-level change and connect it to outcomes. The collection of appropriate community-level outcomes is another difficult challenge.

11.4. DISCUSSION

Research on the prevention of IPV is in an early stage. Many of the strategies and programs reviewed had no rigorous studies examining their effect, and even those with some support left many questions unanswered: For whom are those interventions efficacious or effective? What elements account for the effect on violence? Under what circumstances would they not be recommended? Community-based secondary prevention efforts, in particular, require stronger evaluation. Many of these programs (shelters/transitional housing, mandatory arrest, protective orders, BIPs) were developed from grassroots movements rather than research-based activities and have not been rigorously evaluated. Consequently, the most widely implemented interventions are often among the least well evaluated. Researchers and practitioners must work together to remedy this unfortunate disconnect; researchers must develop ways to evaluate widely implemented practices for both positive and negative effects, and practitioners must be open to evaluation designs and findings when modifying their efforts to prevent IPV. Likewise, when implementing state and local policies, programs, or services, it is important that policy makers and practitioners allocate sufficient staff and resources so as not to reduce the effect of the intervention (e.g., poorly enforced protective orders may increase women's risk of revictimization instead of decreasing it) (Dugan et al., 2003).

Table 11.2 shows IPV strategies characterized by prevention level and by social-ecological level. The interventions reviewed in this chapter are in boldface and recommendations are noted. New intervention approaches that need to be developed and evaluated are in italics. Table 11.2 highlights two critical needs in the field of IPV prevention: a greater range of primary prevention efforts and stronger evaluation of secondary prevention efforts.

Only two primary prevention strategies were identified—dating violence prevention programs and media campaigns—and only the former group has been rigorously evaluated. There are many more strategies that can be used for the primary prevention of IPV (Coker, 2004), including some strategies that were reviewed here as secondary prevention strategies. For example, couples counseling for violence and substance abuse counseling are promising interventions for couples exhibiting low to moderate levels of violence. These strategies may also be efficacious for couples who have not resorted to IPV, but who may be at risk for IPV. A notable omission from evaluated primary prevention strategies is the lack of family-based intervention strategies for the primary prevention of IPV. The few longitudinal studies examining the onset of IPV perpetration have implicated family factors in the development of IPV perpetration (Capaldi & Clark, 1998; Ehrensaft et al., 2003; Magdol, Moffit, Caspi, & Silva, 1998). Thus it seems likely that family processes should become a focal point of future primary prevention efforts for IPV, as they have for other teen risk behaviors (Kumpfer & Alvarado, 2003).

Regarding community-level primary prevention strategies, research in other areas such as youth violence has identified how changes to community-level variables

Table 11.2. Current and Proposed Intimate Partner Violence (IPV) Primary/Secondary Prevention Interventions by Social-Ecological Level[a]

Level	Primary Prevention	Secondary Prevention
Individual	• **Dating violence prevention programs (R)** • *Bullying prevention programs* • *Programs for children who have witnessed IPV*	• **Screening (IE)** • **Victim advocacy (P)** • **Shelters/transitional housing (P)** • **Temporary protective orders (IE)** • **Batterer intervention programs (P)**
Relational	• *Family-based interventions to promote positive communication, healthy relationships, and/or to prevent family violence* • *Couples counseling focused on violence* • *Couples counseling focused on substance abuse*	• **Couples counseling (P)** • **Alcohol abuse counseling (P)**
Community	• **Media campaigns (IE)** • *Community-level interventions to change community characteristics (e.g., social capital, social connectedness)*	• **Media campaigns (IE)** • **Mandatory arrest (IE)** • **No-drop policy (IE)** • **Specialized courts (IE)** • **Coordinated community response (IE)**

[a] *Boldface*, interventions reviewed in this chapter; *italics*, suggestions for future interventions; *IE*, insufficient evidence; *P*, promising; *R*, recommended.

can affect rates of youth violence perpetration and victimization. For example, the level of participation in community-based organizations can increase social cohesion among residents, which in turn promotes a community's capacity to manage and regulate crime. Communities with this type of capacity are said to be exhibiting high levels of collective efficacy (Sampson, 1997). There is initial evidence that collective efficacy relates to decreased lethal and nonlethal IPV (Browning, 2002), though results showing the strength of this relationship have been mixed (DeKeseredy, Schwartz, Alvi, & Tomaszewski, 2003; Miles-Doan, 1998). We suggest that advances in primary prevention of IPV may come from the development and implementation of community-level prevention strategies.

As research on prevention strategies accumulates, it is critical to remain cognizant that partner violence is not a unitary construct, that there are different motives for IPV, and that different circumstances support the perpetration of IPV. Thus no single intervention can be expected to work in all cases. More basic research is needed to examine risk and protective factors for different types of IPV, to better establish consensus about typologies of IPV and IPV perpetrators, and ultimately to publish consensus definitions about those typologies as has been done for definitions of *partner violence* and *sexual violence* (Saltzman et al., 1999). We also emphasize that there are other important outcomes that must be considered when evaluating prevention programs for IPV, specifically, physical and psychological health.

11.5. CONCLUSIONS

- The only recommended strategy is dating violence prevention, which uses an individual curriculum and community-based components. Promising prevention strategies include couples counseling when there is low to moderate violence, behavioral couples counseling for substance abuse, advocacy services for victims, and batterer-intervention programs.
- Stronger evaluation is needed for community-based secondary prevention efforts that have been widely implemented.
- New primary prevention strategies are needed, particularly for families and at the community level.
- There are few data to indicate the effectiveness of prevention interventions with different types of IPV or with different populations, and research must address these critical gaps.

REFERENCES

Anglin, D., & Sachs, C. (2003). Preventive care in the emergency department: Screening for domestic violence in the emergency department. *Academic Emergency Medicine, 10,* 1118–1127.

Archer, J. (2000). Sex differences in aggression between heterosexual partners: A meta-analytic review. *Psychological Bulletin, 26,* 651–680.

Austin, J. B., & Dankwort, J. (1999). Standards for batterer programs: A review and analysis. *Journal of Interpersonal Violence, 14* (2), 152–168.

Avery-Leaf, S., & Cascardi, M. (2002). Dating violence education: Prevention and early intervention strategies. In P. A. Schewe (Ed.), *Preventing violence in relationships: Interventions across the life span* (pp. 79–105). Washington, DC: American Psychological Association.

Babcock, J. C., Green, C. E., & Robie, C. (2004). Does batterers' treatment work? A meta-analytic review of domestic violence treatment. *Clinical Psychology Review, 23,* 1023–1053.

Babcock, J., & Steiner, R. (1999). The relationship between treatment, incarceration, and recidivism of battering: A program evaluation of Seattle's coordinated community response to domestic violence. *Journal of Family Psychology, 13*, 46–59.

Basile, K. C., Arias, I., Desai, S., & Thompson, M. P. (2004). The differential association of intimate partner physical, sexual, psychological, and stalking violence and posttraumatic stress symptoms in a nationally representative sample of women. *Journal of Traumatic Stress, 17*, 413–421.

Bell, M. E., & Goodman, L. A. (2001). Supporting battered women involved with the court system: An evaluation of a law school-based advocacy intervention. *Violence Against Women, 7* (12), 1377–1404.

Bennett, L., & Williams, O. (2001). Controversies and recent studies of batterer intervention program effectiveness. Retrieved June 30, 2003, from www.vaw.umn.edu/documents/vawnet/ar_bip/ar_bip.html.

Berk, R. A., Campbell, A., Klap, R., & Western, B. (1992). A Bayesian analysis of the Colorado Springs spouse abuse experiment. *Journal of Criminal Law & Criminology, 83* (1), 170–200.

Berk, R. A., Newton, P. J., & Berk, S. F. (1986). What a difference a day makes: An empirical study of the impact of shelters for battered women. *Journal of Marriage & the Family, 48* (3), 481–490.

Bograd, M., & Mederos, F. (1999). Battering and couples therapy: Universal screening and selection of treatment modality. *Journal of Marital & Family Therapy, 3*, 291–312.

Brannen, S. J., & Rubin, A. (1996). Comparing the effectiveness of gender-specific and couples groups in a court-mandated spouse abuse treatment program. *Research on Social Work Practice, 6*, 405–424.

Browning, C. R. (2002). The span of collective efficacy: Extending social disorganization theory to partner violence. *Journal of Marriage & Family, 64*, 833–850.

Buzawa, E. S., & Buzawa, C. G. (2003). *Domestic violence: The criminal justice response* (3rd ed). Thousand Oaks, CA: Sage.

Capaldi, D. M., & Clark, S. (1998). Prospective family predictors of aggression toward female partners for at-risk young men. *Developmental Psychology, 34*, 1175–1188.

Carlson, M. J., Harris, S. D., & Holden, G. W. (1999). Protective orders and domestic violence: Risk factors for re-abuse. *Journal of Family Violence, 14*, 205–226.

Coker, A. L. (2004). Primary prevention of intimate partner violence for women's health: A response to Plichta. *Journal of Interpersonal Violence, 19* (11), 1324–1334.

Coker, A. L., Smith, P. H., Bethea, L., King, M. R., & McKeown, R. E. (2000). Physical health consequences of physical and psychological intimate partner violence. *Archives of Family Medicine, 9*, 451–457.

DeKeseredy, W. S., Schwartz, M. D., Alvi, S., & Tomaszewski, E. A. (2003). Perceived collective efficacy and women's victimization in public housing. *Criminal Justice, 3* (1), 5–27.

Dugan, L., Nagin, D. S., & Rosenfeld, R. (1999). Explaining the decline in intimate partner homicide: The effects of changing domesticity, women's status, and domestic violence resources. *Homicide Studies, 3* (3), 187–214.

Dugan, L., Nagin, D. S., & Rosenfeld, R. (2003). Exposure reduction or retaliation? The effects of domestic violence resources on intimate partner homicide. *Law & Society Review, 37* (1), 169–198.

Dunford, F. W., Huizinga, D., & Elliott, D. S. (1990). The role of arrest in domestic assault: The Omaha experiment. *Criminology, 28*, 183–206.

Edelson, J. (1991). Coordinated community responses to woman battering. In M. Steinman (Ed.), *Woman battering: Policy responses* (pp. 203–219). Cincinnati, OH: Anderson Press.

Ehrensaft, M. K., Cohen, P., Brown, J., Smailes, E., Chen, H., & Johnson, J. G. (2003). Intergenerational transmission of partner violence: A 20-year prospective study. *Journal of Consulting and Clinical Psychology, 71*, 741–753.

Fals-Stewart, W. (2003). The occurrence of partner physical aggression on days of alcohol consumption: A longitudinal diary study. *Journal of Consulting and Clinical Psychology, 1*, 41–52.

Fals-Stewart, W., Kashdan, T. B., O'Farrell, T. J., & Birchler, G. R. (2002). Behavioral couples therapy for drug-abusing patients: Effects on partner violence. *Journal of Substance Abuse Treatment, 22*, 87–96.

Fischer, K., & Rose, M. (1995). When "enough is enough": Battered women's decision-making around court orders of protection. *Crime & Delinquency, 41* (4), 414–430.

Ford, D. A. (1993). *The Indianapolis Domestic Violence Prosecution Experiment* (Final report submitted to the National Institute of Justice). Indianapolis: Indiana University-Purdue University, Department of Sociology.

Ford, D. A. (2003). Coercing victim participation in domestic violence prosecutions. *Journal of Interpersonal Violence, 18* (6), 669–684.

Foshee, V. A., Linder, G. F., Bauman, K. E., Langwick, S. A., Arriaga, X. B., Heath, J. L., McMahon, P. M., & Bangdiwala, S. (1996). The Safe Dates Project: Theoretical basis, evaluation, design, and selected baseline findings. *American Journal of Preventive Medicine, 12* (Supplement 5), 29–47.

Foshee, V., Bauman, K., Ennett, S., Linder, G., Benefield, T., & Suchindran, C. (2004). Assessing the long-term effects of the safe dates program and a booster in preventing and reducing adolescent dating violence victimization and perpetration. *American Journal of Public Health, 94*, 619–624.

Gondolf, E. W. (2002). *Batterer intervention systems: Issues, outcomes, and recommendations.* Thousand Oaks, CA: Sage.

Gondolf, E. W. (2004). Evaluating batterer counseling programs: A difficult task showing some effects and implications. *Aggression & Violent Behavior, 9*, 605–631.

Gondolf, E., & Williams, O. (2001). Culturally focused batterer counseling for African American men. *Trauma, Violence, & Abuse, 2* (4), 283–295.

Goolkasian, G. A. (1986). *Confronting domestic violence: A guide for criminal justice agencies.* Washington, DC: National Institute of Justice.

Gottman, J., & Jacobson, N. (1998). *When men batter women: New insights into ending abusive relationships.* New York: Simon & Schuster.

Grau, J., Fagan, J., & Wexler, S. (1985). Restraining orders for battered women: Issues of access and efficacy. In C. Schweber & C. Feinman (Eds.), *Criminal justice politics and women: The aftermath of legally mandated change* (pp. 13–28). New York: Haworth.

Harrell, A., & Smith, B. (1996). Effects of restraining orders on domestic violence victims. In E. S. Buzawa & C. G. Buzawa (Eds.), *Do arrests and restraining orders work?* (pp. 214–242). Thousand Oaks, CA: Sage.

Hart, B. J. (1995). Coordinated community approaches to domestic violence. Paper presented at the Violence Against Women Research, Strategic Planning Workshop, National Institute of Justice, Washington, DC.

Hickman, L. J., Jaycox, L. H., & Aranoff, J. (2004) Dating violence among adolescents: Prevalence, gender distribution, and prevention program effectiveness. *Trauma, Violence, & Abuse, 5*, 123–142.

Hirschel, D., & Buzawa, E. (2002). Understanding the context of dual arrest with directions for future research. *Violence Against Women, 8* (12), 1449–1473.

Hirschel, J. D., & Hutchison, I. W. (1992). Female spouse abuse and the police response: The Charlotte, North Carolina experiment. *Journal of Criminal Law & Criminology, 83* (1): 73–119.

Holt, V. L., Kernic, M. A., Lumley, T., Wolf, M. E., & Rivara, F. P. (2002). Civil protection orders and risk of subsequent police-reported violence. *Journal of the American Medical Association, 288* (5), 589–594.

Holtzworth-Munroe, A., & Stuart, G. L. (1994). Typologies of male batterers: Three subtypes and the differences among them. *Psychological Bulletin, 116*, 476–497.

Johnson, M. P. (1995). Patriarchal terrorism and common couple violence: Two forms of violence against women. *Journal of Marriage & the Family, 57*, 283–294.

Keilitz, S. (2004). Specialization of domestic violence case management in the courts: A national survey (NCJ 199724). Washington, DC: National Institute of Justice.

Klein, A. R. (1996). Re-abuse in a population of court-restrained male batterers after two years: Development of a predictive model. In E. S. Buzawa & C. G. Buzawa (Eds.), *Do arrests and restraining orders work?* (pp. 192–213). Thousand Oaks, CA: Sage.

Klein, E., Campbell, J., Soler, E., & Ghez, M. (1997). *Ending domestic violence: Changing public perceptions/halting the epidemic.* Thousand Oaks, CA: Sage.

Kumpfer, K. L., & Alvarado, R. (2003). Family-strengthening approaches for the prevention of youth problem behavior. *American Psychologist, 58*, 457–465.

Leonard, K. E., & Quigley, B. M. (1999). Drinking and marital aggression in newlyweds: An event-based analysis of drinking and the occurrence of husband marital aggression. *Journal of Studies on Alcohol, 60* (4), 537–545.

Magdol, L., Moffitt, T. E., Caspi, A., & Silva, P. A. (1998). Developmental antecedents of partner abuse: A prospective-longitudinal study. *Journal of Abnormal Psychology, 107*, 375–389.

Martin, M. (1997). Double your trouble: Dual arrest in family violence. *Journal of Family Violence, 12*, 139–157.

McFarlane, J., Soeken, K., & Wiist, W. (2000). An evaluation of interventions to decrease intimate partner violence to pregnant women. *Public Health Nursing, 17*, 443–451.

Mears, D. P., Carlson, M. J., Holden, G. W., & Harris, S. D. (2001). Reducing domestic violence revictimization: The effects of individual and contextual factors and type of legal intervention. *Journal of Interpersonal Violence, 16* (12), 1260–1283.

Meshack, A. F., Hu, S., Pallonen, U. E., McAlister, A. L., Gottlieb, N., & Huang, P. (2004). Texas Tobacco Prevention Pilot Initiative: Processes and effects. *Health Education Research, 19* (6), 657–668.

Miles-Doan, R. (1998). Violence between spouses and intimates: Does neighborhood context matter? *Social Forces, 77* (2), 623–645.

Murphy, C. M., & O'Farrell, T. J. (1994). Factors associated with marital aggression in male alcoholics. *Journal of Family Psychology, 8,* 321–335.

Murphy, C. M., Winters, J., Fals-Stewart, W., O'Farrell, T. J., & Murphy, M. (1998). Alcohol consumption and intimate partner violence by alcoholic men: Comparing violence and nonviolent couples. *Psychology of Addictive Behaviors, 19,* 35–42.

National Center for Injury Prevention and Control. (2003). *Cost of intimate partner violence against women in the United States.* Atlanta GA: Centers for Disease Control and Prevention.

National Council of Juvenile and Family Court Judges. (1998). *Family violence: Emerging programs for battered women and their children.* Reno, NV: Author.

Nelson, H. D., Nygren, P., McInerney, Y., & Klein, J., (2004). Screening women and elderly adults for family and intimate partner violence: A review of the evidence for the U. S. Preventive Services Task Force. *Annals of Internal Medicine, 140,* 387–396.

Newmark, L., Rempel, M., Diffily, K., & Kane, K. M. (2004). *Specialized felony domestic violence courts: Lessons on implementation and impacts from the Kings County experience* (NCJ 199723). Washington, DC: National Institute of Justice.

O'Farrell, T. J., Fals-Stewart, W., Murphy, C. M., Stephan, S. H., & Murphy, M. (2004). Partner violence before and after couples-based alcoholism treatment for male alcoholic patirnets: The role of treatment involvement and abstinence. *Journal of Consulting and Clinical Psychology, 72,* 202–217.

O'Farrell, T. J., Murphy, M., Fals-Stewart, W., & Murphy, C. M. (2003). Partner violence before and after individually based alcoholism treatment for male alcoholic patients. *Journal of Consulting and Clinical Psychology, 71,* 92–102.

O'Farrell, T. J., Van Hutton, V., & Murphy, C. M. (1999). Domestic violence before and after alcoholism treatment: A two-year longitudinal study. *Journal of Studies on Alcohol, 60,* 317–321.

O'Leary, K. D. (2002). Conjoint therapy for partners who engage in physically aggressive behavior: Rationale and research. *Journal of Aggression, Maltreatment, & Trauma, 5,* 145–164.

O'Leary, K. D., Heyman, R. E., & Neidig, P. H. (1999). Treatment of wife abuse: A comparison of gender-specific and conjoint approaches. *Behavior Therapy, 30,* 475–505.

Parker, B., McFarlane, J., Soeken, K., Silva, C., & Reed, S. (1999). Testing an intervention to prevent further abuse to pregnant women. *Research in Nursing & Health, 22,* 59–66.

Pate, A. M., & Hamilton, E. E. (1992). Formal and informal deterrents to domestic violence: The Dade County Spouse Assault Experiment. *American Sociological Review, 58,* 691–697.

Post, L. A., Klevens, J., Maxwell, C., Shelley, G., & Ingram E. (2005). *The impact of coordinated communities' responses on communities' attitudes and rates of intimate partner violence* Atlanta, GA: Centers for Disease Control and Prevention.

Roussos, S. T., & Fawcett, S. B. (2000). A review of collaborative partnerships as a strategy for improving community health. *Annual Review of Public Health, 21,* 369–402.

Saltzman, L. E., Fanslow, J. L., McMahon, P. M., & Shelley, G. A. (1999). Intimate partner violence surveillance: Uniform definitions and recommended data elements. Atlanta, GA: Centers for Disease Control and Prevention.

Sampson, R. J. (1997). The embeddedness of child and adolescent development: A community-level perspective on urban violence. In J. McCord (Ed.), *Violence and childhood in the inner city* (pp. 31–77). Cambridge, UK: Cambridge University Press.

Saunders, D. G. (1996). Feminist-cognitive-behavioral and process-psychodynamic treatments for men who batter: Interaction of abuser traits and treatment model. *Violence & Victims, 11,* 393–414.

Saunders, D. G., & Hamill, R. M. (2003). Violence against women: Synthesis of research on offender interventions. Retrieved March 27, 2006, from www.ncjrs.org/pdffiles1/grants/201222.pd.

Shepard, M. F., Falk, D. R., & Elliott, B. A. (2002). Enhancing coordinated community responses to reduce recidivism in cases of domestic violence. *Journal of Interpersonal Violence, 17,* 551–569.

Sherman, L. W., & Berk, R. A. (1984). The specific deterrent effects of arrest for domestic assault. *American Sociological Review, 49,* 261–272.

Sherman, L. W., Schmidt, J. D., Rogan, D. P., Smith, D. A., Gartin, P. R., Cohn, E. G., Collins, D. J., & Bacich, A. R. (1992). The variable effects of arrest on criminal careers: The Milwaukee Domestic Violence Experiment. *Journal of Criminal Law & Criminology, 83* (1), 137–169.

Steinman, M. (1990). Lowering recidivism among men who batter women. *Journal of Police Science & Administration, 7,* 124–132.

Stith, S. M., Rosen, K. H., & McCollum, E. M. (2003). Effectiveness of couples treatment for spouse abuse. *Journal of Marital & Family Therapy, 29,* 407–426.

Stith, S. M., Rosen, K. H., McCollum, E. E., & Thomsen, C. J. (2004). Treating intimate partner violence within intact couple relationships: Outcomes of multi-couple vs. individual couple therapy. *Journal of Marital & Family Therapy, 30,* 305–318.

Stith, S. M., Smith, D. B., Penn, C. E., Ward, D. B., & Tritt, D. (2004). Intimate partner physical abuse perpetration and victimization risk factors: A meta-analytic review. *Aggression & Violent Behavior, 10*, 65–98.

Stosny, S. (1995). *Treating attachment abuse: A compassionate approach.* New York: Springer.

Straus, M. A., Gelles, R. J., & Steinmetz, S. (1980). *Behind closed doors: Violence in the American family.* Andover Hill, MD: Anchor.

Sullivan, C. M., & Bybee, D. I. (1999). Reducing violence using community-based advocacy for women with abusive partners. *Journal of Consulting and Clinical Psychology, 67* (1), 43–53.

Sullivan, C. M., Melbin, A., & Cain, D. (2003). Transitional housing policy and practices: Battered women's and service providers' perspectives. Manuscript submitted to VAWnet.

Syers, M., & Edelson, J. L. (1992). The combined effects of coordinated criminal justice intervening in women abuse. *Journal of Interpersonal Violence, 7*, 490–502.

Taylor, R. C., & Davis, B. G. (1999). Does batterer treatment reduce violence? A synthesis of the literature. *Women & Criminal Justice, 10*, 69–93.

Tjaden, P., & Thoennes, N. (1998). *Prevalence, incidence, and consequences of violence against women: Findings from the National Violence Against Women Survey.* Washington, DC: U.S. Department of Justice.

Tolman, R. M. & Weisz, A. (1995). Coordinated community intervention for domestic violence: The effects of arrest and prosecution on recidivism of woman abuse perpetrators. *Crime & Delinquency, 41*, 481–495.

Wakefield, M., Flay, B., Nichter, M., & Giovino, G. (2003). Effects of anti-smoking advertising on youth smoking: A review. *Journal of Health Communication, 8* (3), 229–247.

Wathen, C. N., & MacMillan, H. L. (2003). Interventions for violence against women: Scientific review. *Journal of the American Medical Association, 289*, 589–600.

Whitaker, D. J., Morrison, S., Lindquist, C., Hawkins, S. R., O'Neil, J. A., Nesius, A. M., Mathew, A., & Reese, L. (2006). A critical review of interventions for the primary prevention of partner violence. *Aggression & Violent Behavior, 11*, 151–166.

Wolfe, D. A., Wekerle, C., Scott, K., Straatman, A., Grasley, C., & Reitzel-Jaffe, D. (2003). Dating violence prevention with at-risk youth: A controlled outcome evaluation. *Journal of Consulting and Clinical Psychology, 71* (2), 279–291.

Chapter 12

Interventions to Prevent Sexual Violence

Paul A. Schewe

12.1. INTRODUCTION

Historically, the majority of rape-prevention efforts have been directed at female college populations, primarily teaching avoidance and self-defense skills (Parrot, 1990). Little was known about adolescent dating and even less about sexual violence in adolescence. As knowledge of adolescent sexual assault advanced, primary prevention efforts expanded, and more programs began to target younger audiences. Developmentally, it makes sense to educate children about appropriate and inappropriate sexual behavior at the same time that their sexual identities are forming and their attitudes, beliefs, and behaviors toward romantic partners are beginning to develop. However, despite the data on adolescent sexual development suggesting that attitudes legitimizing sexual coercion may begin as early as age 12 years (Burkhart & Fromuth, 1991) and despite the fact the women aged 12–18 years experience a greater rate of sexual assault than any other age group (Bachman & Saltzman, 1995), the majority of research in the area of rape prevention has been conducted with college students (Brecklin & Forde, 2001; Schewe, 2002). Although most researchers in the field of sexual assault prevention work with college-age populations, the majority of prevention programs delivered by rape crisis centers and domestic violence agencies target students younger than 18 years of age (Schewe, 2004). This gap between research and practice must be addressed. Furthermore, nearly all sexual assault interventions and research have been directed at the level of the individual. More work and research needs to be directed at preventing violence at multiple levels of the social ecology.

This chapter explores the research on sexual assault prevention, focusing on data from adolescent populations when possible, in an effort to define the state of the art in sexual assault prevention efforts for adolescents and young adults. The chapter focuses on primary prevention—that is, efforts to prevent first occurrences of sexual assault perpetration or victimization. This chapter will not address sexual abuse committed against children by an older perpetrator because these situations are more appropriately addressed with the prevention of child abuse. The prevention programs discussed in this chapter primarily address any nonconsenting sexual behavior committed against an acquaintance, a dating partner, or a stranger. These nonconsenting behaviors are commonly referred to as rape, sexual assault, sexual abuse, or sexual harassment.

12.2. PREVALENCE OF SEXUAL AGGRESSION

12.2.1. Middle School

Data from middle school students indicate that between 28% and 45% of students have experienced some form of sexual harassment by a peer or group of peers (Cascardi, Avery-Leaf, & O'Brien, 1998; Connolly, McMaster, Craig, & Pepler, 1997). Represented by these data are students from a Canadian urban community of primarily European descent and a U.S. urban community of predominantly African American students. Only one published study reports rates of sexual aggression among middle school students, with 1–5% of students reporting perpetration of sexual aggression and 7–15% reporting sexual victimization (Foshee, Linder, Bauman, & Langwick, 1996).

12.2.2. High School

Data from high school students indicate that the rate of sexual violence in a multiethnic, economically diverse sample was 15.7% (Bergman, 1992). Females consistently report higher rates of sexual victimization than do males; one study found that 17.8% of high school females reported experiencing forced sexual activity, compared to 0.3% of males (Molidor & Tolman, 1998). Similarly, Bennett and Fineran (1998) found that 16% of high school girls reported being the victim of sexual violence, whereas only 1% said that they had perpetrated sexual violence; for boys, the rates were 6% and 4%, respectively. Finally, in a survey of 830 high school boys from across Illinois, Schewe (2004) found that 12% reported that they would be "very likely" or "likely" to force a woman to have sex with them if they could be assured that they would not be punished. Only 47% of the boys indicated they were "not at all likely" to force sex on a woman under those circumstances.

12.2.3. College

Survey research among American college women indicates that as many as half report being victims of some form of sexual abuse, and 27% report being victims of rape (15%) or attempted rape (12%) (Koss, 1988). Gavey (1991) found a similar rate (25.3%) using Koss's survey in New Zealand. Moreover, 25% of men in Koss's survey indicated that they had behaved sexually with a woman against her will. Finally, Denmare, Briere, and Lips (1988) found that 22% of undergraduate males reported at least some future likelihood of raping.

12.3.   THE CONSEQUENCES OF SEXUAL ASSAULT

Victims of rape often manifest long-term symptoms of chronic headaches, fatigue, sleep disturbance, recurrent nausea, decreased appetite, eating disorders, menstrual pain, sexual dysfunction, and suicide attempts (Resnick, Acierno, & Kilpatrick, 1997). Victims of date rape are 11 times more likely to be clinically depressed, and 6 times more likely to experience social phobia than are non-victims. Psychological problems are still evident in cases as long as 15 years after the assault (Kilpatrick, Best, Saunders, & Veronen, 1988). In a longitudinal study, sexual assault was found to increase the odds of substance abuse by a factor of 2.5 (Kilpatrick, Acierno, Resnick, Saunders, & Best, 1997). The adult pregnancy rate associated with rape is estimated to be 5%, and estimates of the occurrence of sexually transmitted diseases resulting from rape range from 3.6% to 30% (Resnick et al., 1997). A study examining the use of health services over a 5-year period by female members of a health maintenance program found that the number of visits to physicians by rape victims increased 56% in the year after the crime, compared to a 2% use increase by nonvictims (Koss, Koss, & Woodruff, 1991). The tangible and intangible cost of each rape in the United States in 1996 is estimated to be $94,466, which totals to over more than $26 billion each year (Post, Mezey, Maxwill, & Wibert, 2002).

12.4.   SIGNIFICANT THEORIES PERTAINING TO SEXUAL AGGRESSION IN ADOLESCENCE

12.4.1.   Feminist Theory

Feminist theory (Dobash & Dobash, 1992; Yllo, 1993) identifies a patriarchal social structure as the root of relationship violence, with male as perpetrator and female as victim, except in same-sex relationships. This model posits a gender-specific explanation of relationship violence within the context of gender-role socialization, societal inequalities, and power and control. Thus a feminist approach targets attitudes and beliefs as the key to preventing intimate partner violence, specifically, individuals' attitudes toward interpersonal violence, adherence to traditional gender roles, and the behavioral expression of power and control.

12.4.2.   A Sociobiological Approach

Finkelhor et al. (1986) proposed a model to account for child sexual abuse that could be adapted to account for adolescent sexual assault. He proposed that four components must be present before sexual offenses can occur. The first component can be termed *motivation to sexually offend*, which includes deviant arousal (sexual arousal to aggression or sexual violence) or the unavailability of more appropriate sources of sexual satisfaction. The second component entails overcoming internal inhibitions. A variety of personal and social factors, such as feelings of guilt or fear of criminal sanctions, ordinarily work together to inhibit sexual offending. Perceptions of social tolerance for the behavior and low probability of negative sanctions as well as distorted ideas or myths about rape and drug or alcohol abuse all work against the normal mechanisms that inhibit sexual offending. The third factor involves overcoming external inhibitions. Bystanders and witnesses will generally not tolerate sexually offensive behavior. Offenders overcome external inhibitions by isolating their victims either by design or accident (Finkelhor et al., 1986). Last, the offender must overcome the target's resistance. An offender may overcome the victim's resistance through persuasion or coercion, by taking advantage of the victim's relative powerlessness, or by using threats of violence or other sanctions (Finkelhor et al., 1986; Walker, Bonner, & Kaufman, 1988).

12.4.3. Cognitive-Behavioral Theory

A cognitive-behavioral explanation of sexual assault is evident in most explicit and implicit theories of rape. Cognitive distortions justifying rape are the most common immediate precursor to rape (Scully & Marolla, 1985). Perhaps consequently, cognitive distortions justifying rape (rape myths) are targeted more often than any other construct in programs designed to prevent rape (Schewe, 2002). On the behavioral side, repeated pairings of sex and violence might account for the development of deviant arousal to violence, whereas a lack of skills (communication skills, anger management skills, ability to cope with rejection, etc.) might prevent adolescents from developing healthy sexual relationships. One example of how sex and violence are paired occurs in the stereotypical horror movie shower scene in which a naked actress is violently attacked. For adolescent boys, this is a near perfect pairing of sexual arousal and violence.

12.5. PROMISING PRACTICES

Currently there are few evidence-based sexual assault prevention curricula. Typically, packaged curricula offered for sale have little to no evidence of their effectiveness, and programs that have been evaluated have generally not been developed into packaged curricula. The two exceptions to this are the Safe Dates curriculum and a collection of six curricula recently published by the Illinois Coalition against Sexual Assault (ICASA). The Safe Dates intervention includes a 10-session curriculum, a play, and a poster contest and has demonstrated long-term effectiveness in reducing adolescents' self-reports of victimization and perpetration of dating and sexual violence (Foshee et al., 2004). Furthermore, a prevention educator in Illinois implementing the Safe Dates Program achieved greater improvements in students' attitudes, beliefs, and behavioral intentions concerning dating violence than 17 other teen dating violence prevention programs (Schewe, 2004). ICASA recently published 6 curricula, ranging from one to five sessions after a statewide evaluation of their 29 sexual assault prevention programs. These 6 curricula produced the best outcomes for students in terms of improvements in rape-related attitudes, beliefs, and behavioral intentions compared to the 23 other interventions (Schewe, 2004). Because of the scarcity of published curricula with documented effectiveness addressing sexual assault, this chapter explores the constructs that have been targeted in educational rape-prevention programs and evaluates evidence for the effectiveness of these intervention strategies (Table 12.1).

Table 12.1. Summary of Effectiveness of Sexual Assault Prevention Strategies[a]

Strategy	Gender Primarily Targeted	Reducing Sexual Assault Perpetration	Reducing Sexual Assault Victimization	Changing Knowledge, Attitudes, Beliefs, or Behavioral Intentions
Intervention strategies				
Bystander interventions	Both	NE	NE	4
Addressing rape myths	Both	NE	NE	4
Teaching self-defense skills	Females	NE	4	4
Communication training	Both	NE	NE	4
Teaching victim empathy	Males	NE	NE	3
Avoiding high-risk situations	Females	NE	NE	3
Addressing negative consequences for perpetrators	Males	NE	NE	3
Addressing social norms	Both	NE	NE	NE
Rape-awareness programs	Both	NE	NE	2
Education about self-defense	Females	NE	2	2
Other considerations				
More sessions		NE	NE	5
Shorter sessions		NE	NE	4
Culturally relevant programs		NE	NE	4
Single-gender audience		NE	NE	4
Targeting younger students		NE	NE	4
Male–female co-presenters		NE	NE	3
Interactive presentations		NE	NE	3
Exploiting cognitive dissonance		NE	NE	NE
Confrontation		NE	NE	1

[a] The scale is as follows: *5*, effective (supported by two or more well-designed studies or systematic review); *4*, promising (supported by a preponderance of the evidence); *3*, insufficient (insufficient or mixed evidence); *2*, not effective (no effect found in two or more studies or systematic review); *1*, harmful (negative effect supported by two or more studies or systematic review); *NE*, no Evidence.

12.5.1.   Problems with Measuring Outcomes

Unfortunately, the problems associated with measuring outcomes of rape-prevention programs (Schewe & O'Donohue, 1993a) have not yet been solved. Clearly the most obvious measure of the effectiveness of rape-prevention programs would be a decrease in the incidence of rape. However, because so few sexual assault victims seek help from formal institutions and such a small percentage of rapes result in criminal convictions, tracking the incidence of rape from official sources is implausible. Also, while self-reports of sexual assault have been very useful in establishing prevalence and incidence statistics, the use of self-reports after intervention is problematic because an individual's definition or perception of what constitutes sexual assault is likely to change after sexual assault education. Individuals' reports of sexual assault and related behaviors might increase or decrease after intervention, regardless of any real changes in sexual assault experiences. Self-reports of perpetration have the added problem that after education, individuals may realize that past behaviors could be considered criminal, and this new understanding might suppress reporting. Evidence supporting these speculations comes from studies that have found that reports of lifetime victimization and/or perpetration *decrease* after intervention (Foshee el al., 2000; Schewe,

1999). Clearly, such changes in reporting would likely differ between treatment and control groups.

Without reliable incidence data, most evaluations of sexual assault prevention programs instead measure intermediate outcomes—changes in knowledge, attitudes, beliefs, behaviors, or behavioral intentions that are theoretically or rationally linked to the outcome of interest (a decrease in sexual assault). These measures suffer in that none of them has strong empirical links to changes in actual behavior.

12.5.2.   Interventions with Preponderance of Evidence

12.5.2.1.   *Bystander Interventions*

One of the more recently developed strategies for educating young people about sexual assault takes a "bystander" approach to prevention. With this strategy, audience members are addressed not as potential perpetrators or victims of sexual assault but as bystanders. This approach teaches students how to support a friend or loved one who discloses sexual assault and instructs students how to confront friends who express sexist attitudes and how they can potentially intervene with friends in risky situations (i.e., at a party where a friend has had too much to drink). The implied goal of these rape-prevention programs, changing participants' attitudes, beliefs, and behaviors regarding sexual assault, is often left unstated. One rape-prevention program using this approach documented positive changes in rape myths and likelihood of raping among college fraternity members (Foubert, 2000). Similarly, across 29 different rape-prevention programs for high school students in Illinois, the content area most associated with positive outcomes for students was discussing how to help a friend who had been assaulted (Schewe, 2004).

Addressing students as potential bystanders to sexual assault has a number of benefits for prevention educators. The approach can be used with males and females in mixed-gender classrooms with less risk of being interpreted as victim blaming or male bashing than other approaches (e.g., discussions of high-risk situations, gender stereotypes, communication skills.). In addition, it can make use of much of the other information commonly presented in sexual assault prevention programs (i.e., prevalence statistics establish the likelihood that someday someone you love will be sexually assaulted, and information about the consequences and aftermath of rape provides motivation to learn how to help a friend who has been victimized and can increase empathy for victims of sexual assault). Evidence for the success of this approach and the fact that it can be implemented or incorporated into existing interventions makes this an approach that prevention educators should strongly consider.

12.5.2.2.   *Rape Myths*

A review of recent literature reveals that rape myth acceptance is the most common construct addressed in rape-prevention programming; it is important to note that rape myth acceptance scales were the most frequently used measure of program outcomes (Schewe, 2002). A variety of irrational beliefs are associated with rape and sexual offending (Burt, 1980; Hildebran & Pithers, 1989; Muehlenhard & Linton, 1987), making rape myths an ideal target for prevention programming. For example, Pithers, Kashima, Cumming, Beal, and Buell (1988) analyzed the case records of 64 incarcerated rapists and found that cognitive distortions justifying rape (rape myths) were the second most frequent immediate precursor to rape (anger was the first). In published evaluations of rape-prevention programs over the last 15 years, rape myths were frequently targeted in "successful" intervention programs and were rarely targeted in "unsuccessful" programs (Schewe, 2002). Again, success was largely defined as changes in students' belief in rape myths. In a comprehensive study that evaluated 29 sexual assault prevention programs simultaneously, linear regression revealed that providing information about rape myths was positively and significantly associated with students' change scores on the Illinois Rape Myth Acceptance Scale (Schewe, 2004).

Effective interventions targeting rape myths have been as minimal as the presentation of brief written material (Malamuth & Check, 1984) to as thorough as a 2-hour workshop targeting only empathy and rape myths (Lee, 1987). One warning is that a rape myths intervention (a presentation of false beliefs about rape along with corrective information) should not be confused with the presentation of factual information alone. Factual information such as legal definitions of rape, descriptions of victims and offenders, and descriptions of rape trauma syndrome have been found to have no effect on students' attitudes about rape or their empathy for victims of rape (Borden, Karr, & Caldwell-Colbert, 1988; Lenihan, Rawlins, Eberly, Buckley, & Masters, 1992; Schewe & O'Donohue, 1993b).

12.5.2.3. Teaching Self-Defense Skills

Teaching women self-defense strategies appears to be an effective tool in helping students avoid rape. An evaluation of a "model mugging" course found that 46 of 48 women assaulted after taking the course fought back sufficiently to avoid harm (Peri, 1991). Other studies cite beneficial psychological consequences for women taking self-defense classes compared to a no-treatment control group (Cohen, Kidder, & Harvey, 1978). Furthermore, there is fairly strong evidence concerning the types of strategies that are effective in deterring an attacker. Ullman and Knight (1993) examined police reports and court testimonies of 274 women who were either raped or avoided rape by subsequently incarcerated violent stranger rapists. They found that women who fought back forcefully were more likely to avoid rape, that women who screamed or fled when confronted with weapons experienced less severe sexual abuse, and that increased physical injury was associated with pleading, crying, reasoning, and the women's use of drugs or alcohol. Furthermore, when the sequence of attack–resistance–injury has been taken into account, studies show that fighting leads to less completed rape and *no* increase or decrease in physical injury (Quinsey & Upfold, 1985; Ullman & Knight, 1992; Ullman, 1998). The most important implication of this research is that women should be encouraged (if they are able and so choose) to resist rape with active strategies of fleeing, screaming, and fighting known to be associated with decreased rape completion.

When teaching self-defense or discussing effective rape-avoidance strategies, it is important to address social barriers that may prevent women from using effective defense strategies. For example, students might be too embarrassed to yell or scream or may be afraid of losing a friend if they fight back or may be so shocked that someone they trust is attacking them that they are unable to react. Also, participants should be warned that although active resistance strategies will generally be most effective, in some instances fighting back could result in greater physical injury to the victim. Participants should, therefore, be instructed that the decision to fight back is extremely personal, and its effectiveness will vary from situation to situation. Finally, educating women about effective self-defense strategies in the absence of teaching actual self-defense skills is questionable.

12.5.2.4. *Communication Training, Assertiveness, Limit Setting*

Miscommunication has been implicated as a cause of date rape for many years. Results of one study involving prison inmates suggest that rapists are particularly poor at interpreting negative cues from women in first date situations when compared to incarcerated nonrapists (Lipton, McDonel, & McFall, 1987). Muehlenhard and Linton (1987) postulate that men interpret women's behavior more sexually than do women, and that this misunderstanding can lead to sexual offending. Muehlenhard and Andrews (1985) studied men's reactions to a woman's stating directly that she did not want to do anything more than kiss. The researchers found that this direct form of limit setting decreased men's ratings of how much the woman wanted to have sex, men's ratings of how likely they would be to try sexual behaviors beyond kissing, men's ratings of how much she led the man on, and men's ratings of how justified the man was to engage in petting after the woman said no. The construct of communication skills has been included along with other interventions in at least three different rape-prevention programs that have been evaluated and published. Each of these programs has indicated some level of success in changing knowledge and attitudes, although communication skills were not evaluated specifically as an outcome measure (Foubert & McEwen, 1998; Gilbert, Heesacker, & Gannon, 1991; Proto-Campise, Belknap, & Woodlredge, 1998). In addition, addressing healthy relationship skills, a construct that might include communication skills and problem-solving skills, was positively associated with successful outcomes in Schewe's (2004) evaluation of 29 sexual assault prevention programs.

12.6. POSSIBLE PRACTICES

This section discusses interventions that have demonstrated mixed evidence of their effectiveness.

12.6.1. Victim Empathy

Victim empathy is a cognitive-emotional recognition of a rape victim's trauma (Hildebran & Pithers, 1989). Programs that target victim empathy attempt to help students develop an understanding of the experiences of a rape victim and typically involve both an understanding of the victim's experience of the actual rape as well as the aftermath of rape (shame, guilt, depression, pregnancy, and social sanctions—what has been called by some as the "second assault" (Williams & Holmes, 1981). The idea behind these interventions is that students who understand the horrible experience of rape would never inflict that type of pain on anyone and would be more likely to help/believe a person who reports that he or she has been raped. Examination of the evaluation literature reveals mixed support for including victim empathy in rape-prevention programs. Of the 10 programs that targeted victim empathy, 8 reported positive effects on student attitudes. One of the few prevention programs to demonstrate long-term positive effects included victim empathy as a key component (Foubert, 2000). The two exceptions provide useful information for developers of prevention curricula. In Berg, Lonsway, and Fitzgerald's (1999) study of 54 college males, they found that men who were asked to empathize with a female rape victim reported a greater likelihood of sexual aggression than men who were asked to empathize with an adolescent male who was victimized by another adolescent male. In a similar study, Ellis, O'Sullivan, and Sowards (1992) found that when mixed-gender groups of undergraduates were asked to consider a situation in which a close friend told them that she was raped, women became more rejecting of rape myths, but men became *less* rejecting of them. Review of the other empathy programs reveals that having males empathize with other male victims of rape was a key part of many of the more successful programs (Schewe, 2002). However, in Schewe's (2004) outcome evaluation of 29 rape-prevention programs for high school students, victim empathy was *inversely* related to student outcomes as measured by the Illinois Rape Myth Acceptance Scale (Payne, Lonsway, & Fitzgerald, 1999). Unfortunately, details about how educators addressed victim empathy were not supplied.

Typical victim empathy interventions involve having participants listen to survivors' stories of rape, engage in written exercises describing a victim's experiences, or imagine themselves as a victim of rape. Whenever males are in the audience, empathy-inducing exercises should absolutely include at least one scenario in which the victim is a male. To reflect the reality of male rape, the perpetrator should also be male and the perpetrator should have a heterosexual orientation.

12.6.2. Avoidance of High-Risk Situations

Early research identifying high-risk situations for sexual assault (e.g., use of alcohol, hitchhiking, attending parties, dating in isolated locations, being involved with older men) (Muehlenhard & Linton, 1987; Ullman, 1997) suggested that educating women to avoid these situations could be an important part of efforts to reduce the incidence of rape among program participants. One program addressed this construct and was able to successfully increase women's perceptions of their vulnerability to rape and increase their intentions to avoid risk-taking behaviors (Gray, Lesser, Quinn, & Bounds, 1990). Hanson and Gidycz's (1993) risk-reduction program was successful in decreasing both women's involvement in situational factors associated with rape and victimization among women who did not have a history of sexual victimization. However, in Schewe's (2004) statewide outcome evaluation, teaching students to avoid high-risk situations was inversely associated with change scores on the Illinois Rape Myth Acceptance Scale (Payne et al., 1999).

There are two major cautions for educators attempting to incorporate information regarding high-risk situations into their curricula. One is that these programs should not be used for male or mixed-gender audiences. In the course of a program that highlights women's awareness of high-risk situations and perceptions of vulnerability, women in the audience may learn that date rape occurs very frequently, that most rapes go unreported to police, and that they should avoid alcohol and isolated dating locations. Men in the same audience may learn that rape is a common experience; that if they do commit rape, the chances of being caught are slim; and that if they get a woman intoxicated and take her to an isolated location, their chances of being caught are even slimmer. Given the differences in the information that men and women need concerning rape, it is important that coordinators of programs that attempt to target both sexes are very careful when selecting information to present. A second caution is that information regarding high-risk situations might unintentionally increase victim blaming. Educators implementing such programs have the difficult job of teaching women about situations in which sexual assault is more likely to occur while instilling the belief that rape is never the survivors' fault, regardless of her prior behavior.

12.6.3.   Negative Consequences for Perpetrators

Perceived rewards and costs and low probability of punishment can be viewed as contributory factors of rape (Bandura, 1973; Scully & Marolla, 1985). Decision-making theory asserts that when deciding which course of action to take, people weigh the costs and benefits of their actions along with the probabilities of potential outcomes. Breslin, Riggs, O'Leary, and Arias (1990) found that male undergraduates who committed acts of dating violence anticipated fewer negative consequences than nonaggressive students. Scully and Marolla (1985) used information from interviews of 114 incarcerated rapists to suggest that most rapists viewed rape as a rewarding, low-risk act.

Decision theories suggest that information that changes men's perceptions of rape so they begin to view it as less rewarding than consensual sex, in both the short term and the long term; more costly than consensual sex (e.g., imprisonment, guilt, loss of job); and more likely to lead to negative consequences (e.g., high probability of getting caught or feeling guilt) might be beneficial in preventing attempted rapes. However, out of the 33 rape-prevention programs reviewed by Schewe (2002), only 3 addressed the negative consequences of raping for men. Of these, 2 evidenced positive outcomes, and the other, a program highlighting victim empathy and the negative consequences of rape, was less effective than program's targeting rape myths (Intons-Peterson, Roskos-Ewoldsen, Thomas, Shirley, & Blut, 1989; Schewe & O'Donohue, 1996; Schewe & Shizas, 2000). In addition, in Schewe's (2004) statewide evaluation, programs that included discussions of the negative consequences of committing rape were less likely to demonstrate positive outcomes for students.

12.6.4.   Changing Social Norms

Originally applied to substance abuse prevention, interventions to correct misperceptions about social norms have recently been applied to sexual assault prevention (Fabiano, Perkins, Berkowitz, Linkenbach, & Stark, 2003). This approach involves surveying students regarding risk and protective behaviors to identify misperceptions. For example, if male students are asked if it is important to get consent before sexual intimacy, 90% may report that consent is important; but the same students may also believe that only 40% of other men feel that consent is important. The correct information can then be fed back to students. The intended outcome is that with accurate information students will identify the protective behavior as normative, and social support for the protective behavior may increase. Social norms campaigns can similarly target risk behaviors (e.g., binge drinking in college students) by demonstrating that those behaviors, contrary to popular belief, are outside the norm. Although social norms campaigns have been effectively applied to substance abuse on college campuses, the effectiveness of the approach for addressing sexual assault has not yet been tested.

This approach may be particularly useful for engaging men as allies in prevention efforts by aligning them with the majority who do not support rape and sexually abusive behaviors. Instead of driving a wedge between men and women by defining male culture as being synonymous with rape culture, prevention educators should try to support the positive qualities of the majority of men. Traditional educational programs can be revised to include data from a social norms survey; social marketing strategies, which have the potential to reach thousands of students, can be developed in collaboration with or independent of educational workshops (Fabiano et al., 2003).

12.7.   UNSUPPORTED PRACTICES

This section discusses interventions that have demonstrated no effect or negative effects supported by two or more studies or systematic review.

12.7.1.   Knowledge/Rape-Awareness Programs

The type of information covered by rape-awareness interventions include the definitions of *rape* and legal terms, presentation of statistics regarding the prevalence of rape, discussion of the ways that society condones or perpetuates rape, descriptions of typical perpetrators and victims, descriptions of the rape trauma syndrome, and information on local resources for victims of rape. These programs appear to operate on the premise that the more students know about rape, the less likely it is that they will become victims or perpetrators. However, perhaps the clearest message that comes from the evaluation literature is that these programs rarely work. When these programs do report success, often the success is based on increased knowledge or changed attitudes among females, with little or no change among male participants, the population for whom change is most essential (Schewe, 2002). In Schewe's (2004) statewide evaluation of sexual assault prevention programs, programs that emphasized statistics and sexual assault definitions were less likely than other programs to document positive changes among students.

12.7.2.   Education about Self-Defense

Two prevention programs included a discussion of self-defense strategies without teaching actual self-defense skills (Hanson & Gidycz, 1993; Women against Rape, 1980). Both programs were effective in either decreasing the incidence of victimization or increasing confidence in the use of self-defense strategies and willingness to confront a perpetrator, but only for women without a history of sexual assault. However, two subsequent evaluations of educational sexual assault prevention programs focusing on psychological barriers to resistance found no reduction in sexual assault risk at follow-up, regardless of sexual assault history (Breitenbecher & Gidycz, 1998; Breitenbecher & Scarce, 2001).

12.8.   OTHER CONSIDERATIONS

12.8.1.   Promising Practices

12.8.1.1.   *More Sessions*

Practical limitations often only allow a single session, and the majority of sexual assault prevention programs described in journal articles and implemented in the field are single-session interventions (Schewe, 2002, 2004). However, as a general rule, more sessions are better than fewer sessions. Heppner, Neville, Smith, Kivlighan, and Gershuny (1999) evaluated a three-session rape-prevention program and found the strongest predictor of whether male participants would change and stay changed over a 5-month period was how many of the sessions they attended. Similarly, across 29 rape-prevention programs for high school students, the number of sessions (range 1–10) was positively and significantly related to positive outcomes (Schewe, 2004). Some curricula developers have overcome some of the practical barriers to multiple sessions by designing their programs to meet state guidelines for health education. In this way, the Safe-T for Teens program has replaced the existing health education classes in several middle schools; its 30-hour curriculum emphasizes healthy relationship skills and sexual abuse prevention.

12.8.1.2. Shorter Sessions

The attention spans of adolescents and young adults place a limit on the length of sexual assault interventions. The results of Schewe's (2004) evaluation of sexual assault prevention programs revealed that shorter programs were more effective than longer programs (range 40–90 minutes). Note that the effect sizes of interventions dropped off rapidly after 60 minutes. This result was more pronounced for male students than for female students.

12.8.1.3. Specifically Targeting the Race/Ethnicity of the Audience

Heppner et al.'s (1999) study is the only one to date that has tested the effects of including culturally relevant material in a prevention program. This study compared the effects of a "color-blind" intervention to one that subtly but purposefully integrated African American content and process into the intervention. The results indicate that "Black students in the culturally relevant treatment condition were more cognitively engaged in the intervention than their peers in the traditional treatment condition" (Heppner et al., 1999, p. 16). Cultural relevance meant having a Black group facilitator, including incidence and prevalence figures for both Black and White populations, specifically targeting race-related rape myths and facts, and presenting culture-specific information concerning the recovery processes of Black and White women.

12.8.1.4. Single-Gender Audience

As noted above, some of the information included in rape-prevention programs is more appropriate for one gender or the other. Many authors have cited strong arguments for addressing single-gender audiences in rape-prevention programs (Berkowitz, 1992; Lonsway, 1996; Schewe & O'Donohue, 1993a). A recent meta-analysis found that males in mixed-gender prevention programs experienced less attitude change than males in single-gender groups (Brecklin & Forde, 2000). Kline (1993) found greater positive changes for males in a single-gender group than for males in a co-ed group. Furthermore, both males and females in the single-gender groups reported a more positive group experience than those in the mixed-gender groups. When possible, single-gender curricula should be developed. However, because of practical constraints (schools often are not willing or able to split up classrooms), mixed-gender curricula should be developed that avoid blaming men and blaming victims and do not unintentionally teach males how to rape and get away with it.

12.8.1.5.   Intervening with Younger Students

While advocates and researchers have argued for the need to intervene with younger students for some time, Schewe's (2004) statewide evaluation of sexual assault prevention programs was the first research to provide empirical data. The results of his study indicate that across interventions, younger students changed more than older students (range 9th–12th grades).

12.8.2.   Possible Practices

12.8.2.1.   Male-Female Co-presenters

Both educators and researchers have held a variety of beliefs about the gender of the presenter as it relates to the audience. Some believe that male presenters will have the greatest effect on male audiences, whereas females will have the greatest effect on female audiences. Others believe the exact opposite. Still others believe that a male and female team of presenters works best for all audiences because of the team's ability to model healthy male–female relationships. Jones and Muehlenhard (1990) specifically addressed the gender of the presenters in their experimental design and found that the gender of presenters (male, female, or male and female team) had no effect on the outcome of a prevention program to a mixed-gender college audience. However, Schewe's (2004) statewide evaluation of 29 sexual assault prevention programs found that a male and female team of prevention educators had a larger effect on high school students than male-only and female-only educators. Furthermore, results indicated that male educators had a much larger effect on the female students than on the male students in their classrooms.

12.8.2.2.   Using Multiple, Interactive Presentation Methods

To maximize learning among students, educators should use several presentation methods. Students' memory for information will be enhanced when they hear it, see it, write it, read it, speak it, and do it. Heppner, Humphrey, Hillenbrand-Gunn, & DeBord (1995) compared a standard video and lecture presentation to an interactive drama and found that students in the interactive drama program were more motivated to hear the message, were more able to recognize consent and coercion, and were more likely to demonstrate behavioral changes. Generalizing from this study and from the literature on persuasion and attitude change, interactive presentations should be more effective than lecture only. Educators should engage students in discussions that draw on the students' own experiences and should use role-playing to help students understand the perspective of another person and to practice skills. Written exercises also help cement memories and reinforce what was learned. Homework assignments that involve parents can give them the opportunity to reinforce what their child learned at school. Videotapes might also be useful. In several interventions, videos alone were as effective as alternate treatments or video plus discussion and were more effective than discussion alone (Anderson et al., 1998; Harrison, Downes, & Williams, 1991; Mann, Hecht, & Valentine, 1988). Schewe's (2004) evaluation of sexual assault prevention programs showed mixed results for interactive formats; games, quizzes, handouts, and survivor presentations were all positively associated with positive outcomes, whereas lectures, videos, and drama were inversely related to success. Prevention educators from some of the more successful programs in Illinois anecdotally recommended using short clips from recently produced videos rather than using an entire video or using older videos. No recommendations were offered regarding dramatic presentations.

12.8.2.3. *Exploiting Cognitive Dissonance*

The cognitive dissonance literature informs us that changing behavior can be an effective way of changing attitudes. It suggests that students who engage in antirape activities should show a positive shift in their attitudes concerning rape. Rape-prevention programming can take advantage of this knowledge by having students engage in activities that are the opposite of supporting rape. Such activities might include participating in antirape discussions, making antirape posters or artwork, performing in a dramatic presentation, or convincing a hypothetical person not to use force in sexual relations.

12.8.3. Unsupported Practices

The one study that specifically examined a "confrontational" format in a rape-prevention program found that confrontation resulted in a greater tolerance for rape among men (Fischer, 1986). Heppner, Good, et al. (1995) found that one third of the men reacted to a sexual assault prevention program in a bored or negative manner. In Heppner's next two studies, the researchers worked to reduce male defensiveness by letting men know that they are leaders in their schools and that they can be part of the solution and by supporting men who got training.

12.9.   LIMITATIONS OF THIS REVIEW

One limitation of this review is that it was based mostly on reports of rape-prevention evaluations that have been published in scientific journals. One bias in these journals is that studies with negative outcomes are less likely to be published. For researchers and rape advocates developing curricula, the lessons that can be learned from unsuccessful programs are at least as important, and may be more important, than the lessons learned from programs documenting success.

12.10.   CONCLUSIONS

Although our knowledge of how to prevent rape is still in its infancy, the number of people dedicated to eradicating rape and improving the quality of rape-prevention programs continues to expand. This chapter presented a list of lessons learned from the hard work of advocates, educators, and researchers. The most effective sexual assault prevention programs will take a bystander approach and will address rape myths while teaching communication skills. Self-defense training is also indicated for women. Educational interventions will be most effective when they include multiple, short sessions (i.e., less than 1 hour) that are culturally relevant and target younger students in single-gender audiences by a male and female team of co-facilitators.

At this time, there remain many agencies providing school-based prevention services with little solid evidence of effectiveness. To progress as a field, more research regarding effective interventions is necessary both at the individual level and at broader levels of the ecosystem. Research that will most benefit prevention educators in the field are studies that evaluate multiple interventions, use a wide variety of outcome measures, and include long-term follow-up. At the same time, more basic research needs to be conducted to identify differences in individual characteristics and life experiences between sexually aggressive men and nonsexually aggressive men and to link proximal outcomes (i.e., changes in knowledge, attitudes, beliefs, and behaviors) to distal outcomes of reduced sexual aggression.

While the decision to commit rape remains a very private, individual choice and interventions specifically aimed at changing individuals may always be necessary, more efforts need to focus on interventions aimed at the family, community, and societal level (Table 12.2 presents a matrix of potential activities at various levels of the social ecology). Also, by focusing on promoting positive behaviors (increasing communication skills and teaching conflict-resolution and social problem-solving skills) instead of focusing on risk factors (correcting rape myths, avoiding high-risk situations, changing perceptions of negative consequences), sexual assault prevention advocates may find it easier to collaborate with other advocates working to prevent other problem behaviors, such as teen suicide, alcohol and drug abuse, delinquency, dating violence, and teen pregnancy.

Table 12.2. Multilevel Prevention of Sexual Violence[a,b]

Activities	Sample Interventions within Settings[c]
Change individual's knowledge, attitudes, beliefs, behaviors, and skills	• Provide universal rape-prevention education and parent education through schools and workplaces • Insert character development into training for young athletes and sexual assault education for high school, college, and pro athletes
Promote community education	• United Way parent education through multiple agencies
Educate providers	• Train teachers, staff, and administrators, along with students • Teach coaches to be mentors
Foster coalitions and networks	• Organize family well-being committees at places of worship • Organize athletes against sexual assault
Change organizational practices	• Create gender-inclusive classes • Develop bullying, sexual harassment, and order of protection policies at schools and workplaces • Infuse violence against women into curricula at all levels • Change training programs • Promote family-friendly holidays, proactive policies • Get women involved in running sports organizations, promote greater inclusion (e.g., eliminate tryouts), alter definitions of success • Integrate prevention programs into mandatory coursework, such as health education
Influence policy and legislation	• Revise juvenile sex offender laws • Change educational reporting requirements • Expand the Family Leave Act • Enact school and workplace sexual harassment laws • Expand the Violence Against Women Act

[a]Adapted from the work of Baguato, Bowen, Browning, Bubar, Cohen, Domas, Faweett, Hargreaves, Kegler, McNamee, Moos, Prothrow-Stith, Schewe, Shea, and Sollivan who served on a Centers for Disease Control and Prevention expert advisory panel on multilevel prevention of intimate partner and sexual violence, May 2005.
[b]Additional dimensions to address within each setting are cultural/ethnic groups; sexual orientation; universal, selected, and indicated interventions; and the age and developmental stage of the audience.
[c]Possible settings include family, neighborhoods, schools, justice, government, arts/culture, media, health care, sports, and workplace.

REFERENCES

Anderson, L. A., Stoelb, M. P., Duggan, P., Heiger, B., Kling, K. H., & Payne, J. P. (1998). The effectiveness of two types of rape prevention programs in changing the rape-supportive attitudes of college students. *Journal of College Student Development, 39*, 131–142.

Bachman, R., & Saltzman, L. E. (1995). Violence against women: Estimates from the redesigned survey. Bureau of Justice Statistics, Washington, D.C.: U.S. Department of Justice, Office of Justice Programs.

Bandura, A. (1973). *Aggression: A social learning analysis.* Englewood Cliffs, NJ: Prentice Hall.

Bennett, L., & Fineran, S. (1998). Sexual and severe physical violence among high school students: Power beliefs, gender, and relationship. *American Journal of Orthopsychiatry, 68* (4), 645–652.

Berg, D. R., Lonsway, K. A., & Fitzgerald, L. F. (1999). Rape prevention education for men: The effectiveness of empathy-induction techniques. *Journal of College Student Development, 40* (3), 219–234.

Bergman, L. (1992). Dating violence among high school students. *Social Work, 37*, 21–27.

Berkowitz, A. (1992). College men as perpetrators of acquaintance rape and sexual assault: A review of recent research. *Journal of American College Health, 40*, 175–181.

Borden, L. A., Karr, S. K., & Caldwell-Colbert, A. (1988). Effects of a university rape prevention program on attitudes and empathy toward rape. *Journal of College Student Development, 29* (2), 132–136.

Brecklin, L R., & Forde, D. R. (2000). A meta-analysis of rape education programs. *Violence & Victims, 16*, 303–321.

Breitenbecher, K. H., & Gidycz, C. A. (1998). An empirical evaluation of a program designed to reduce the risk of multiple sexual victimization. *Journal of Interpersonal Violence, 13*, 472–488.

Breitenbecher, K. H., & Scarce, M. (2001). An evaluation of the effectiveness of a sexual assault education program focusing on psychological barriers to resistance. *Journal of Interpersonal Violence, 16*, 387–407.

Breslin, F. C., Riggs, D. S., O'Leary, K. D., & Arias, I. (1990). Family precursors: Expected and actual consequences of dating aggression. *Journal of Interpersonal Violence, 5* (2), 247–258.

Burt, M. (1980). Cultural myths and supports for rape. *Journal of Personality & Social Psychology, 38* (2), 217–230.

Burkhart, B., & Fromuth, M. E. (1991). Individual psychological and social psychological understandings of sexual coercion. In Grauerholz, E. & Koralewski, M. (Eds). *Sexual coercion: A sourcebook on its nature, causes, & prevention.* (pp. 76–89). Lexington, MA: Lexington Books.

Cascardi, M., Avery-Leaf, S., & O'Brien, M. K. (1998). *Dating violence among middle school students in an low income urban community.* Paper presented at Grantee Meeting, Centers for Disease Control and Prevention, Atlanta, GA.

Cohen, E. S., Kidder, L., & Harvey, J. (1978). Crime prevention versus victimization: The psychology of two different reactions. *Victimology, 3*, 285–296.

Connolly, J. A., McMaster, L., Craig, W., & Pepler, D. (1997). *Dating, puberty, & sexualized aggression in early adolescence.* Paper presented at the annual meeting of the Association for the Advancement of Behavior Therapy, Miami, FL.

Denmare, D., Briere, J., & Lips, H. M. (1988). Violent pornography and self-reported likelihood of sexual aggression. *Journal of Research in Personality, 22*, 140–153.

Dobash, R. E., & Dobash, R. P. (1992). *Violence against wives: A case against patriarchy.* New York: Free Press.

Ellis, A.L., O'Sullivan, C. S., & Sowards, B. (1992). The impact of contemplated exposure to a survivor of rape on attitudes toward rape. *Journal of Applied Social Psychology, 22*, 889–895.

Fabiano, P. M., Perkins, W., Berkowitz, A., Linkenbach, J., & Stark, C. (2003). Engaging men as social justice allies in ending violence against women: Evidence for a social norms approach. *Journal of American College Health, 52* (3), 105–112.

Finkelhor D., Araji, S., Baron, L., Browne, A., Peters, S., & Wyatt, G. (Eds.), (1986). *A sourcebook on child sexual abuse,* Beverly Hills, CA.: Sage Publications.

Fischer, G. J. (1986). College student attitudes toward forcible date rape: Changes after taking a human sexuality course. *Journal of Sex Education & Therapy, 12*, 42–46.

Foshee, V. A., Bauman, K. E., Ennett, S. T., Linder, G. F., Benefield, T., & Suchindran, C. (2004). Assessing the long-term effects of the Safe Dates Program and a booster in preventing and reducing adolescent dating violence victimization and perpetration. *American Journal of Public Health, 94* (4), 619–624.

Foshee, V. A., Bauman, K. E., Greene, W. F., Koch, G. G., Linder, G. F., & MacDougall, J. E. (2000). The Safe Dates Program: 1-year follow-up results. *American Journal of Public Health, 90* (10), 1619–1622.

Foshee, V. A., Linder, G. F., Bauman, K. E., & Langwick, S. A. (1996). The Safe Dates Project: Theoretical basis, evaluation design, and selected baseline findings. *American Journal of Preventive Medicine, 12*, 39–46.

Foubert, J. D. (2000).The longitudinal effects of a rape-prevention program on fraternity men's attitudes, behavioral intent, and behavior. *Journal of American College Health, 48* (4), 158–163.

Foubert, J. D., & McEwen, M. K. (1998). An all-male rape prevention peer education program: Decreasing fraternity men's behavioral intent to rape. *Journal of College Student Development, 39* (6), 548–555.

Gavey, N. J. (1991). Sexual victimization among Auckland University students: How much and who does it? *New Zealand Journal of Psychology, 20* (2), 63–70.

Gilbert, B., Heesacker, M., & Gannon, L. (1991). Changing the sexual aggression-supportive attitudes of men: A psychoeducational intervention. *Journal of Counseling Psychology, 38* (2), 197–203.

Gray, M., Lesser, D., Quinn, E., & Bounds, C. (1990). Effects of rape education on perception of vulnerability and on reducing risk-taking behavior. *Journal of College Student Development, 31* (2), 217–223.

Hanson, K. A., & Gidycz, C. A. (1993). Evaluation of a sexual assault prevention program. *Journal of Consulting & Clinical Psychology, 61*, 1046–1052.

Harrison, P. J., Downes, J., & Williams, M. D. (1991). Date and acquaintance rape: Perceptions and attitude change strategies. *Journal of College Student Development, 32* (2), 131–139.

Heppner, M. J., Good, G. E., Hillenbrand-Gunn, T. L., Hawkins, A. K., Hacquard, L. L., Nichols, R. K., DeBord, K. A., & Brock, K. J. (1995). Examining sex differences in altering attitudes about rape: A test of the elaboration likelihood model. *Journal of Counseling & Development, 73*, 640–647.

Heppner, M. J., Humphrey, C., Hillenbrand-Gunn, T. L., & DeBord, K. A. (1995). The differential effects of rape prevention programming on attitudes, behavior, and knowledge. *Journal of Counseling Psychology, 42*, 508–518.

Heppner, M. J., Neville, H. A., Smith K., Kivlighan, D. M., & Gershuny, B. S. (1999). Examining immediate and long-term efficacy of rape prevention programming with racially diverse college men. *Journal of Counseling Psychology, 46* (1), 16–26.

Hildebran, D., & Pithers, W. (1989). Enhancing offender empathy for sexual-abuse victims. In D. Laws (Ed.), *Relapse prevention with sex offenders* (pp. 236–243). New York: Guilford Press.

Intons-Peterson, M. J., Roskos-Ewoldsen, B., Thomas, L., Shirley, M., & Blut, K. (1989). Will educational materials reduce negative effects of exposure to sexual violence? *Journal of Social & Clinical Psychology, 8*, 256–275.

Jones, J., & Muehlenhard, C. (1990). *Using education to prevent rape on college campuses.* Paper presented at the annual meeting of the Society for the Scientific Study of Sex, Minneapolis, MN.

Kline, R. J. (1993). The effects of a structured-group rape-prevention program on selected male personality correlates of abuse toward women. Unpublished doctoral dissertation. Bethlehem, PA: Lehigh University.

Kilpatrick, D. G., Acierno, R., Resnick, H. S., Saunders, B. E., & Best, C. L. (1997). A 2-year longitudinal analysis of the relationships between violent assault and substance use in women. *Journal of Consulting and Clinical Psychology, 65* (5): 834–847.

Kilpatrick, D. G., Best, C. L., Saunders, B. E., & Veronen, L. J. (1988). Rape in marriage and in dating relationships: How bad is it for mental health? *Annals of New York Academy of Sciences, 528*, 335–344.

Koss, M. (1988). Hidden rape: Sexual aggression and victimization in a national sample of students in higher education. In A. Burgess (Ed.), *Rape & sexual assault II* (pp. 3–25). New York: Garland.

Koss, M. P., Koss, P. G., & Woodruff, W. J. (1991). Deleterious effects of criminal victimization on women's health and medical utilization. *Archives of Internal Medicine, 151*, 342–347.

Lenihan, G., Rawlins, M., Eberly, C. G., Buckley, B., & Masters, B. (1992). Gender differences in rape supportive attitudes before and after a date rape education intervention. *Journal of College Student Development, 33*, 331–338.

Lonsway, K. A. (1996). Preventing acquaintance rape through education: What do we know? *Psychology of Women Quarterly, 20*, 229–265.

Lee, L. (1987). Rape prevention: Experimental training for men. *Journal of Counseling & Development, 66*, 100–101.

Lipton, D. N., McDonel, E. C., & McFall, R. M. (1987). Heterosocial perception in rapists. *Journal of Consulting and Clinical Psychology, 55*, 17–21.

Malamuth, N. M., & Check, J. V. P. (1984). Debriefing effectiveness following exposure to pornographic rape depictions. *Journal of Sex Research, 20*, 1–13.

Mann, C. A., Hecht, M. L., & Valentine, K. B. (1988). Performance in a social context: Date rape versus date right. *Central States Speech Journal, 3/4*, 269–280.

Molidor, C., & Tolman, R. M. (1998). Gender and contextual factors in adolescent dating violence. *Violence Against Women, 4* (2), 180–194.

Muehlenhard, C. L., & Andrews, S. L. (1985). *Sexual aggression in dating situations: Do factors that cause men to regard it as more justifiable also make it more probable?* Paper presented at the annual meeting of the Association for the Advancement of Behavior Therapy, Washington, DC.

Muehlenhard, C. L., & Linton, M. A. (1987). Date rape and sexual aggression in dating situations: Incidence and risk factors. *Journal of Counseling Psychology, 34*, 186–196.

Payne, D. L., Lonsway, K. A., & Fitzgerald, L. F. (1999). Rape myth acceptance: Exploration of its structure and its measurement using the Illinois Rape Myth Acceptance Scale. *Journal of Research in Personality, 33* (1), 27–68.

Parrot, A. (1990). *Do rape education programs influence rape patterns among New York State college students?* Paper presented at the 1990 annual meeting of the Society for the Scientific Study of Sex, Minneapolis, MN.

Peri, C. (1991, March). Below the belt: Women in the martial arts. *Newsletter of the National Women's Martial Arts Federations*, 6–14.

Pithers, W. D., Kashima, K., Cumming, G. F., Beal, L. S., & Buell, M. (1988). Relapse prevention of sexual aggression. In R. Prentky & V. Quinsey (Eds.). *Human sexual aggression: Current perspectives* (pp. 244–260). New York: New York Academy of Sciences.

Post, L. A., Mezey, N. J., Maxwill, C., & Wibert, W. N. (2002). The rape tax: Tangible and intangible costs of sexual violence. *Journal of Interpersonal Violence, 17* (7), 773–782.

Proto-Campise, L., Belknap, J., & Wooldredge, J. (1998). High school students' adherence to rape myths and the effectiveness of high school rape-awareness programs. *Violence Against Women, 4*, 308–328.

Quinsey, V. L., & Upfold, D. (1985). Rape completion and victim injury as a function of female resistance strategy. *Canadian Journal of Behavioural Science, 17*, 40–50.

Resnick, H. S., Acierno, R., & Kilpatrick, D. G. (1997). Health impact of interpersonal violence 2: Medical and mental health outcomes. *Behavioral Medicine, 23*, 65–78.

Schewe, P. A. (1999). The Centers for Disease Control and Prevention funded STAR Project. Unpublished raw data.

Schewe, P. A. (2002). Guidelines for developing rape prevention and risk reduction interventions for adolescents and young adults: Lessons from evaluation research. In P. Schewe (Ed.), *Preventing intimate partner violence: Developmentally appropriate interventions across the life span (pp. 107–136)*. Washington, DC: American Psychological Association.

Schewe, P. A. (April 2004). *Best practices for school-based sexual assault & teen dating violence prevention programs*. Paper presented at the 2004 Illinois Prevention First Conference, Rosemont, IL.

Schewe, P. A., & O'Donohue, W. T. (1993a). Rape prevention: Methodological problems and new directions. *Clinical Psychology Review, 13*, 667–682.

Schewe, P. A., & O'Donohue, W. T. (1993b). Sexual abuse prevention with high risk males: The roles of victim empathy and rape myths. *Violence & Victims, 8* (4), 339–351.

Schewe, P. A., & O'Donohue, W. T. (1996). Rape prevention with high risk males: Short-term outcome of two interventions. *Archives of Sexual Behavior, 25* (5), 455–471.

Schewe, P. A., & Shizas, N. (May 2000). *Rape prevention with college age males: Short-term outcomes of a videotaped intervention vs. a peer-mediated group discussion*. Paper presented at the National Sexual Violence Prevention Conference, Dallas, TX.

Scully, D., & Marolla, J. (1985). "Riding the bull at Gilley's": Convicted rapists describe the rewards of rape. *Social Problems, 32* (3), 251–263.

Ullman, S. E. (1997). Review and critique of empirical studies of rape avoidance. *Criminal Justice & Behavior, 24* (2), 177–204.

Ullman, S. E. (1998). Does offender violence escalate when rape victims fight back? *Journal of Interpersonal Violence, 13*, 179–192.

Ullman, S. E., & Knight, R. A. (1993). The efficacy of women's resistance strategies in rape situations. *Psychology of Women Quarterly, 17*, 23–38.

Ullman, S. E., & Knight, R. A. (1992). Fighting back: Women's resistance to rape. *Journal of Interpersonal Violence, 7*, 31–43.

Walker, C. E., Bonner, B. L., & Kaufman, K. L. (1988). *The physically & sexually abused child: Evaluation & treatment*. New York: Pergamon Press.

Williams, J. E., & Holmes, K. A. (1981). *The second assault: Rape & public attitudes*. Westport, CT: Greenwood Press.

Women against Rape. (1980). A rape prevention program in an urban area: Community action strategies to stop rape. *Signs, 5*, 238–241.

Yllo, K. (1993). Through a feminist lens. In R. J. Gelles & D. R. Loseke (Eds.), *Current controversies in family violence (pp. 47–62)*. Newbury Park, CA: Sage.

Chapter 13

Interventions to Prevent Elder Mistreatment

**Karl A. Pillemer, Katrin U. Mueller-Johnson,
Steven E. Mock, J. Jill Suitor, and Mark S. Lachs**

13.1. BACKGROUND AND INTRODUCTION

Over the past two decades, increasing attention has been paid to mistreatment of older persons by researchers, policy makers, and the general public. In this chapter, we review issues related to the prevention of elder abuse and neglect. We begin by discussing the state of existing research and estimates of the extent of the problem. We provide a discussion of risk factors, because prevention programs necessarily need to take probable risk factors into account. We then review types of interventions that have been used to prevent elder abuse. As will be discussed, there is a paucity of reliable research on elder abuse in general and almost no scientifically acceptable research on the effectiveness of various prevention strategies for elder mistreatment. For this reason, we focus on identifying promising program examples and on suggestions for future research. Further, several preventive options are controversial in the field of elder abuse and, therefore, require rigorous evaluation.

13.1.1. Definitions

A recent panel convened by the U.S. National Academy of Sciences (National Research Council, 2002) has proposed a useful scientific vocabulary for elder mistreatment, which we follow in this chapter. Elder abuse is defined as: "(a) intentional actions that cause harm or create a serious risk of harm (whether or not harm is intended), to a vulnerable elder by a caregiver or other person who stands in a trust relationship to the elder, or (b) failure by a caregiver to satisfy the elder's basic needs or to protect the elder from harm." This definition encompasses two key ideas: that the older individual has suffered injury, deprivation, or unnecessary danger and that a specific other person (or persons) is responsible for causing or failing to prevent it.

Within the overarching framework of elder abuse, there is now general agreement on the scope of actions that fall under this rubric. Researchers, practitioners, and most legal statutes recognize the following types of abuse: (1) physical abuse, which includes acts carried out with the intention to cause physical pain or injury; (2) psychological abuse, defined as acts carried out with the intention of causing emotional pain or injury; (3) sexual assault; (4) material exploitation, involving the misappropriation of the elder's money or property, and (5) neglect, or the failure of a designated caregiver to meet the needs of a dependent older person. For the purposes of this chapter, we focus primarily on physical abuse, because of its clear relationship to the potential for injury. However, a number of studies and prevention programs focus on one or more additional types of abuse, and we have included them in our discussion.

13.1.2. Problems in the Research Base

Before summarizing the available findings, it is important to review briefly the problems in using existing research to understand risk factors for elder mistreatment and the potential effectiveness of prevention programs. The first major limitation of previous research is an unclear definition of the object of study. Most studies are weakened by their undifferentiated treatment of various types of abuse and neglect. Second, different criteria have been used to determine the population at risk of elder mistreatment. Some researchers have included people younger than 60 years of age in their studies, whereas most others have chosen 60 or 65 years as the entry point. A number of investigators have restricted their studies to caregivers to elderly people, frail elders, or to people sharing a residence, while others have included all categories of older people.

Third, few studies that have purported to address risk factors have in fact included comparison groups in their designs. For this reason, the generalizations made by the researchers are necessarily suspect. Fourth, studies have employed widely differing methods, including random sample surveys, interviews with patients in medical practices or caregivers in support programs, and reviews of agency records. Fifth, a number of studies have not employed reliable and valid measurement of the indicators of risk.

Sixth, with one exception (Lachs, Berkman, Fulmer, & Horwitz, 1994; Lachs, Williams, O'Brien, Hurst, & Horowitz, 1997), prospective studies of elder abuse do not exist. As Lachs et al. (1994) point out, retrospective research designs contain several potential biases, including recall bias, the respondent reinterpreting key facts or feelings from a later vantage point; information bias, the respondent (especially if cognitively impaired) may not be able to recall or provide valid information about exposure to maltreatment; and the failure of retrospective studies to take into account the timing and duration of events and their progression over time.

Finally, and most pertinent to this chapter, there is little hard evidence regarding the effects of interventions of any kind, including preventive interventions. A review of the elder abuse literature for the period 1980–1996 by the National Academy of Sciences Committee on Family Violence Interventions (Chalk & King, 1998) produced reports on approximately a dozen elder abuse programs. Seven of these were evaluation studies that included outcome measures, but only two met the scientific standard for inclusion in the evidentiary base for the committee's report. Both of the latter were small-scale projects: one assigned advocates to elder victims to help them navigate the criminal justice system; the second offered stress-management and self-esteem training to potential victims. The others lacked random assignment or the sample size was too small for meaningful comparisons. Unfortunately, the intervening years have uncovered only a few additional intervention studies that used scientifically acceptable methods (discussed later in this chapter).

13.1.3. Extent of Elder Abuse

To justify expending resources for prevention programs, the question of the size and scope of a problem must be addressed: Is elder abuse sufficiently extensive to justify investment in prevention programs? Evidence is available from four large-scale population surveys that have been conducted to date. Pillemer and Finkelhor (1988), in a probability sample of noninstitutionalized elders in the Boston, Massachusetts, metropolitan area, found an overall prevalence rate of 3.2%. A national random sample survey of elderly persons in Canada used similar methods and uncovered a rate of 4% reporting having experienced maltreatment since turning 65 (Podnieks, 1992). The difference in rate may be explained by the fact that the U.S. survey assessed physical abuse, psychological abuse, and neglect, whereas the Canadian survey included material abuse in addition to these categories. A Dutch study (Comijs, Penninx, Knipscheer, & van Tilberg, 1999), which included these four types of abuse, found a 1-year prevalence rate of 5.8%. Researchers in Scandinavia conducted a telephone survey of national samples from Denmark and Sweden but used more inclusive definitions of elder abuse (including theft). This study found a prevalence of 8%, but the higher rate is driven by the inclusion of theft as a type of abuse (Tornstam, 1989).

These results suggest that the extent of elder abuse is sufficiently large that social service and health professionals who serve older adults are likely to encounter it on a routine basis. Indeed, elder abuse is prevalent enough to be encountered in daily clinical practice with regularity. For example, using the prevalence rates just described, a clinician seeing between 20 and 40 older adults a day could encounter at least one clinical or subclinical victim of elder abuse daily (Lachs & Pillemer, 2004). Further, as our discussion of risk factors below shows, some subpopulations that are overrepresented in the elder service system (such as people with dementia) have higher risk of abuse. Thus prevention programs appear to be well justified for this population.

13.1.4. Risk Factors for Elder Mistreatment

The development of effective prevention programs is predicated on an understanding of risk factors for mistreatment. Because of the problems in the research base discussed earlier, it must be acknowledged that any statements about relative risk among the elderly must be viewed with caution. However, the small number of studies using acceptable research designs does reveal some patterns of potential risk factors, as follows (Lachs & Pillemer, 2004).

13.1.4.1. *Living Arrangement*

Both clinical accounts and limited empirical research suggest that a shared living situation is a major risk factor for elder mistreatment; older people who live alone are at the lowest risk (Lachs et al., 1997; Paveza et al., 1992; Pillemer & Finkelhor,

1988; Pillemer & Suitor, 1992). A shared residence increases the opportunities for contact, and thus conflict and mistreatment. Further, tensions that might be relieved by simply leaving the immediate situation can escalate into maltreatment (Wolf and Pillemer, 1989).

13.1.4.2. Social Isolation

Social isolation has been found to be characteristic of families in which other forms of domestic violence occur. Research on elder abuse provides support for this view. In Lachs et al.'s (1994) prospective, community-based study of risk factors for elder abuse, having a "poor social network" significantly increased risk of mistreatment. Findings from a number of other studies indicate that victims and abusive relatives have lower levels of social support (Compton, Flanagan, & Gregg, 1997; Grafstrom, Nordberg, & Windblad, 1993; Phillips, 1983; Wolf & Pillemer, 1989).

13.1.4.3. Dementia

There is evidence suggesting that dementia places elderly persons at greater risk of mistreatment. Several studies have attempted to determine prevalence rates of elder mistreatment in samples of dementia caregivers; these rates can then be compared to rates in general population surveys. Coyne, Reichman, & Berbig (1993) found that 11.9% of the dementia caregivers in their sample reported having committed physical abuse. Paveza et al. (1992) found a rate of severe physical violence toward care recipients of 5.4%, which is close to Pillemer and Suitor's (1992) finding of 5% in a similar sample. Homer and Gilleard (1990) found physical abuse occurring in 14% of caregivers to Alzheimer's disease (AD) patients in a respite care program. Given the prevalence findings of rates of physical abuse in the 1–3% range, dementia patients would appear to be at greater risk of such mistreatment. It should be noted that it is possible that caregivers may be more likely to report mistreatment than older persons themselves, leading to an inflation of the rates among demented individuals. However, in a longitudinal panel study that did not relay on caregiver interviews, Lachs et al. (1997) found that dementia predicted identification as an abuse victim.

13.1.4.4. Psychological Problems and Substance Abuse

A history of mental illness has been found to characterize elder abusers (Pillemer & Finkelhor, 1989; Reis & Nahmiash, 1998; Wolf & Pillemer, 1988). Several studies have specifically pointed to depression as characteristic of perpetrators of elder mistreatment (Coyne et al., 1993; Fulmer, 1991; Homer & Gilleard, 1990; Paveza et al., 1992; Reay Campbell & Browne, 2002; Williamson & Shaffer, 2001). Substance misuse on the part of family members also is related to elder abuse. Indeed, studies of elder mistreatment suggest that alcohol abuse on the part of perpetrators is a disproportionately common occurrence (Anetzberger, Korbin, & Austin, 1994; Bristowe & Collins, 1989; Greenberg, McKibben, & Raymond, 1990; Homer & Gilleard, 1990; Reay Campbell & Browne, 2002; Wolf & Pillemer, 1989).

13.1.4.5. Abuser Dependency

Related to the previous risk factor, findings from research on elder mistreatment suggested that perpetrators tend to be dependent on the individual they are mistreating (Anetzberger, 1987; Greenberg et al., 1990; Pillemer, 1986, 2004; Pillemer & Finkelhor, 1989; Wolf & Pillemer, 1989; Wolf, Strugnell, & Godkin, 1982).

13.1.4.6.   Health and Functional Status

The role of victim health and functional status as a risk factor in elder abuse is complex. Although anecdotal and clinical reports have long suggested that the frailty of elderly persons in itself is a risk factor for abuse, studies have generally failed to find a direct relationship between elder abuse and victims' poor health or functional impairment (Bristowe & Collins, 1989; Cooney & Mortimer, 1995; Paveza et al., 1992; Phillips 1983) or excessive dependency on the abuser (Bristowe & Collins, 1989; Homer & Gilleard, 1990; Phillips, 1983; Pillemer, 1985; Pillemer & Finkelhor, 1989; Pillemer & Suitor, 1992; Reis & Nahmiash, 1997; Wolf & Pillemer, 1989). Nonetheless, it is likely that increased frailty in the elder does play at least some role in abuse. Rather than increasing risk in and of itself, greater impairment may diminish the individual's ability to defend himself or herself or to escape the situation. Further, impairment may increase social isolation, and thus raise risk for elder abuse. It seems reasonable to consider physical health problems as a predisposing factor in elder maltreatment, which may increase vulnerability in the presence of risk other factors.

A variety of other potential risk factors are discussed in the literature, but reliable scientific evidence regarding them is lacking. Potential but unsubstantiated factors include caregiver stress and burden and the intergenerational transmission of violent behavior (i.e., abuse experienced as a child). Relative risk that results from race, gender, or relationship to the abuser (spouse or adult child) is inconclusive.

13.2.   ELDER ABUSE PREVENTION PROGRAMS: THE STATE OF THE ART

In the remainder of this chapter, we discuss a variety of interventions that may have the potential to prevent elder abuse. We do so with the caution, however, that not only are evaluation data typically lacking on the options but well-documented practical experience is also limited in most cases. The analysis here must, therefore, be seen as speculative. Indeed, as we discuss in the concluding section, rigorously conducted intervention studies are greatly needed to determine the most effective elder abuse prevention strategies.

13.2.1.   Screening

A considerable literature exists on screening programs for elder abuse. The premise behind such programs is that predicting the possibility of abusive practices allows for intervention before maltreatment occurs. Screening programs often use interviews and/or direct observation of older persons (and sometimes family members) to identify potentially abusive situations. A few elder abuse screening instruments have been validated in preliminary ways (Fulmer, Guadano, Dyer, & Connolly, 2004; Reis & Nahmiash, 1998; Schofield & Mishra, 2003). The intuitive appeal of screening instruments and programs is clear: elder abuse victims may "suffer in silence" until the problem is brought to light by a health or social service professional.

In general, existing screening protocols suffer from methodological problems in their construction and validation, which derive largely from the special nature of elder abuse and its difference from medical problems typically addressed by screening. Specifically, in the traditional medical model of screening, an individual who wishes early detection of a prevalent disease (e.g., diabetes, high blood pressure) presents asymptomatically for a minimally invasive test. Further, typically a definitive gold standard test exists to confirm or refute the findings of a positive screening test. This situation, however, has limited applicability to elder abuse (Lachs & Pillemer, 2004). Victims may be frail and socially isolated, cognitively impaired, and not receptive to additional investigation or treatment. They may be accompanied to the screening venue (e.g., a doctor's office) by the abuser. Unlike the "worried well" individual who wishes detection of an early disease, the elder abuse victim may actively seek to hide its manifestations from a screening professional.

Even more compellingly, there is no universally agreed-on gold standard test as to what constitutes definitive elder abuse, so verification of the screen is difficult. Thus the potential for both false positives and false negatives exists to a much greater degree than with screening for other types of problems. For example, injuries could be a sign of elder abuse but are more often sustained through falls or other accidents. Weight loss might result from the intentional withholding of food or care but is equally or more likely caused by other factors such as cancer or chronic disease.

In sum, given the state of the art, wide-scale screening does not appear to have significant potential for elder abuse prevention at present. The threat to both sensitivity and specificity are great—that is, screening instruments' accuracy in identifying high-risk subjects on the one hand, and in correctly exempting low-risk subjects on the other. A compelling reason for caution thus exists. If screening is carried out with unvalidated instruments, the reliability of which is unknown, then risks to older people may result. In particular, if the screen incorrectly identifies an older person as being at risk, he or she may be subject to an invasive investigation and to possible stigmatization as an "abused elder." Thus, although early identification of elder abuse victims is clearly desirable, it is prudent to await more definitive research findings before promoting screening programs on a wide scale.

Given these caveats, how should we proceed in this area? Fulmer and O'Malley (1987) proposed a reasonable solution that has been supported by more recent discussions. They suggest that the best role for screening instruments is to heighten professional awareness of the possibility of elder abuse and to alert clinicians to signs and symptoms that might otherwise be missed. Lachs and Pillemer (2004) concur that the best policy at this time, rather than overreliance on a specific screening strategy or clinical algorithm, is education to raise awareness of elder abuse in clinicians. Incorporation of training on the general detection of elder abuse (rather than reliance on a specific screening instrument) into medical and other relevant professional education should be a high priority.

13.2.2. Mandatory Reporting

Most states have laws that specifically mandate the reporting of elder abuse, although the statutes differ considerably in terms of definitions of mistreatment, population covered, sanctions for not reporting, and other aspects. Mandatory reporting is seen by proponents as having an important tertiary prevention component. That is, by bringing cases of elder abuse to the attention of an agency, services can be initiated that prevent revictimization. Further, it is claimed that mandatory reporting laws serve to increase public awareness of the problem of elder abuse and prompt service providers to be on the lookout for suspected maltreatment. In contrast, opponents argue that there is no evidence that mandatory reporting is effective. Critics note that states have failed to provide sufficient funds for services to victims and abusers, and limited staff must attempt to handle a large number of referrals in response to the law. Others claim that reporting interferes with the relationship and confidentiality between the professionals and clients.

Under mandatory reporting legislation, professionals are faced with a dilemma: either to violate the law or break trust with a client and possibly jeopardize a therapeutic relationship. Critics maintain that by extending a child abuse model to the elderly, a set of assumptions has been adopted that are not applicable to older people. Specifically, they infantilize the elder's position in society, foster negative stereotypes of the aged, and limit the older people's abilities to control their own lives. At a minimum, mandatory reporting must be accompanied by a substantial commitment of resources to the designated reporting agency. To date, no scientific evidence exists on which to evaluate the costs and benefits of mandatory reporting.

13.2.3. Adult Protective Services

All states offer some form of protective services for elder abuse victims, although there is again significant variation from state to state. If a state protective services program operates under an *adult* protective service statute, it is generally limited to "incapacitated" adults, leaving other agencies such as the police, legal services, and the criminal justice system to handle situations involving more competent and physically able persons. On the other hand, programs authorized under *elder* abuse legislation usually apply to any older individual who is at risk of abuse, neglect, or exploitation. Some states restrict their cases to people living in their own homes; others include group and institutional settings as well.

It is possible that adult protective services may constitute a form of tertiary prevention, helping abused older people escape further victimization and its consequences. However, although adult protective services have gained greater visibility and credibility in the past decade, it is a controversial area of service. Some critics see such programs as an intrusion on the civil liberties of the elderly. They also argue that states define abuse too broadly and allow an intrusion into families with merely the normal range of human problems. States have responded to such criticisms by emphasizing that the client's right to self-determination is one of the basic principles of protective services (Wolf & Pillemer, 1989).

Despite the fact that hundreds of thousands of cases have been investigated and millions of dollars spent by protective services, evaluation data are sorely lacking. This is somewhat troubling in light of the only two studies that have attempted to examine the effect of elder protective services. Both studies found a negative effect of protective services intervention for older persons; protective service clients are more likely to be placed in nursing homes than nonclients and to experience greater mortality (Blenkner, 1971; Lachs, Williams, O'Brien, & Pillemer, 2002; Lachs, Williams, O'Brien, Pillemer, & Charlson, 1998). Because of the possibility of this type of unanticipated negative effect, evaluation of the effect of elder protective services is greatly needed.

13.2.4. Education of Professionals

Over the past two decades, a wide variety of educational and training programs has been developed, targeted at virtually every profession that encounters older people, including physicians (Ahmad & Lachs, 2002; Lachs & Pillemer, 2004), nurses (Bond, 2004; Richardson, Kitchen, & Livingston, 2002), and social workers (Richardson et al., 2002; Wilke & Vinton, 2003). In theory, such programs may help professionals detect elder abuse by increasing their awareness of potential signs and symptoms. Little evidence exists as to whether such programs are effective in raising professional awareness, although two studies indicate that professional education did increase knowledge about elder abuse compared to control groups (Anetzberger et al., 2000; Richardson et al., 2002). No studies have been conducted regarding whether education of professionals leads to outcomes of any kind for victims, including prevention.

13.2.5. Caregiver Support Interventions

Another approach to elder abuse prevention has been based on the assumption that dependency of the victim and resulting caregiver stress is a major cause of maltreatment. Prevention programs based on this paradigm have taken several forms. Some communities and agencies have emphasized health and social services for the elderly that are not specific to abuse. In many cases, services to relieve the burden of caregiving, such as housekeeping and meal preparation, respite care, support groups, and day care are promoted as abuse-prevention strategies.

Such programs are undoubtedly useful for the primary purpose for which they are intended: improving older persons' functioning and reducing caregiver burden and distress. In fact, preliminary evidence from two recent studies suggests that an intervention targeted toward abusive caregivers may help prevent revictimization (Nahmiash & Reis, 2000; Reay Campbell & Browne, 2002). However, the research discussed earlier indicates that caregiver stress and elder dependency are causal factors in only a small number of cases (in the absence of other risk factors such as mental illness or substance abuse on the part of the caregiver). Therefore, caregiver stress—oriented interventions may have preventive potential in only a limited subset of cases.

13.2.6. Education of Potential Victims

Adult protective services and other intervention programs report the lack of self-referral from victims, who are often ashamed to admit family problems and are unaware that services may exist to help them. Public-awareness campaigns directed toward older people may encourage victims to report abuse in its early stages (or to seek help before a tense family situation erupts into abuse) and thus serve a preventive function. A currently ongoing public awareness campaign in Vermont, for instance, includes the placement of flyers with information about elder abuse in prescription bags in pharmacies and stickers on Meals on Wheels containers and distributes brochures to senior centers, congregate meal sites, and doctors' offices (Vermont Center for Crime Victim Services, 2003).

Potential abusers could also be targeted for information, encouraging them to seek help if they fear becoming abusive (or are actually engaging in abusive behaviors). Television and radio spots, newspaper ads, and posters are some of the avenues currently used in such campaigns to reach the public, including potential abusers (California Attorney General's Crime and Violence Prevention Center, 2003, Vermont Center for Crime Victim Services, 2003). Although such programs appear promising, no evaluation data as yet exist.

13.2.7.   Legal and Victim Advocacy Services

The findings that many elders are abused by a dependent relative suggest that maltreated older persons may benefit from interventions found to be effective with victims of partner abuse. Options for the elderly that relate to the partner abuse model include social support for the older person, employing the use of self-help groups that contribute to consciousness-raising, "safe houses" or emergency shelters, and legal action. Although individual examples of these programs exist, no evaluation data regarding their effectiveness are available.

One type of intervention derived from the partner abuse model is law enforcement involvement in cases of elder mistreatment. A single controlled study has been conducted, with unexpected results. Davis and Medina-Ariza (2001) used a randomized controlled experiment to evaluate a program that involved home visits by a team of a police officer and a domestic violence counselor to known elder abuse victims, in an effort to reduce revictimization. Those individuals who received a home visit, however, reported more physical abuse at follow-up than did the controls. The authors speculated that the increase in violence after the home visits could have occurred because the home visits angered the perpetrators; but because the perpetrators in the study were not interviewed, this point had to remain conjecture. Clearly, such programs require careful additional evaluation before they can be promoted as prevention strategies.

13.3.   CONCLUSIONS AND RECOMMENDATIONS

We have reviewed a variety of preventive options for elder mistreatment in this chapter. A helpful way to organize potential elder mistreatment prevention programs uses a paradigm that identifies universal, selective, and indicated measures (Gordon, 1983; Mrazek and Haggerty, 1994). Universal preventive measures are used for the general public and for all members of potentially affected groups—in this case, older people. Table 13.1 organizes selected elder abuse prevention options using this prevention model. In the case of elder abuse, universal prevention can refer to efforts to increase societal awareness and educate the public about elder mistreatment. Selective prevention is targeted at at-risk populations, either those at risk of becoming victims of elder mistreatment or those at risk of engaging in mistreating behavior. It seeks to prevent mistreatment by directly addressing risk factors, such as caregiver stress, and thus reducing the likelihood that abuse will occur. Indicated prevention is targeted at particularly high-risk individuals. Indicated prevention could take the form of an adult protective service investigation, the separation of the mistreater and the mistreated, or legal proceedings.

As Table 13.1 makes clear, reliable evaluation data clearly do not exist to suggest the relative effectiveness of elder abuse prevention programs; indeed, this field of study is in its infancy. However, the extent of the problem and its potentially serious consequences clearly justify the development of prevention strategies. The

Table 13.1. Summary of Elder Abuse Prevention Options

Prevention Level	Intervention Types	Evaluation Status
Universal prevention	• Public awareness campaigns (TV and radio ads, flyers, posters, community presentations)	• No evaluation data
	• Professional awareness (educational materials and workshops for professionals working with older adults)	• Higher rates of awareness of mistreatment
Selective prevention	Directed at potential victim • Screening	• No evaluation data
	Directed at person at risk of becoming abuser • Caregiver support interventions (e.g., stress management, respite care)	• Effective in providing support (e.g., reducing stress)
	• Caregiver training about dementia	• No evaluation data
	• Interventions targeted at other known risk factors for elder mistreatment, such as mental-health and substance abuse treatment, job-skills training, creation of affordable housing	• Interventions not yet developed, but theoretically promising
Indicated prevention	Directed at potential victim • Screening	• No evaluation data
	• Mandatory reporting	• No evaluation data
	• Adult protective services	• Some adverse effects, more evaluation data needed
	• Home visitation by police and social worker	• Adverse effects
	• Social support and self-help groups	• No evaluation data
	• Safe houses and emergency shelters	• No evaluation data
	Directed at person at risk of becoming abuser • Mental-health and substance abuse treatment	• No evaluation data
	• Anger-management training and counseling	• Reduction in anger
	• Caregiver support interventions	• Reduction of revictimization
	• Home visitation by police and social worker	• Adverse effects

following are several recommendations to advance the field of elder abuse prevention, which we believe will help remedy the gaps we have noted in our analysis.

13.3.1. Scientifically Credible Prevention Research Is Greatly Needed

Although knowledge regarding probable risk factors has increased over the past two decades, development and evaluation of prevention programs has lagged woefully behind. Indeed, only a handful of studies exist that have attempted any form of comparison group design, and these studies suffer from methodological concerns that limit generalizability. It is fair to say that we know little more of value regarding elder abuse prevention now than when the problem was "discovered" as a social problem in the 1970s. Professionals who work with older persons struggle against a weak knowledge base and a lack of practical experience in elder abuse prevention.

Of particular concern is the possibility that several widely used approaches to prevention and treatment of elder abuse may have unexpected negative consequences in some cases. Although data are by no means sufficient on this topic, in this chapter we reviewed concerns regarding screening, mandatory reporting, adult protective services, and law-enforcement options. This evidence, although from a limited number of studies, constitutes perhaps the most compelling argument for additional research—the need to ensure that programs intended to prevent abuse do not in fact have negative effects on those persons they are designed to help.

13.3.2.   Multicomponent Interventions Are Needed

It is clear from the review presented here that elder abuse is a complex phenomenon that has multiple causes. Taken together, the research suggests that physical elder abuse is most likely in situations in which several characteristics are present: (a) a shared living situation, (2) an older person with some degree of physical vulnerability, (3) a family member who has psychological and/or substance abuse problems, (4) a family member who is to some degree dependent on the victim, and (5) a context of relative social isolation. Each of these risk factors could be addressed individually, but it is likely that a multicomponent prevention intervention addressing some or all of these factors will be more effective.

13.3.3.   Target Intervention Programs toward Abusers

The risk factor research indicates that prevention programs aimed at abusers may be effective. Indeed, the studies reviewed in this chapter strongly suggest moving from an emphasis on victim characteristics as causes of elder abuse to a focus on perpetrators (Pillemer, 2004). The provision of counseling for the abusive (or potentially abusive) relative could be explored, and the effectiveness of mental health treatment for abusers could be tested to determine if it prevents revictimization. A further prevention program could be targeted toward reducing the relative's dependence on the older person; this might involve aiding the relative in establishing an independent living situation or finding employment (to reduce financial dependency).

13.3.4.   Translation of Validated Prevention Programs from Other Fields Should Be Tested for Elder Abuse

To a surprising degree, there has been little translation of successful strategies from other forms of family violence to elder abuse. One of the frequently used universal prevention program for intimate partner violence is public-awareness campaigns, which recently have been adopted for elder abuse prevention, such as in Vermont and California. Evaluations of domestic violence awareness campaigns have shown that they can be effective (Wolfe & Jaffe, 1999). Although evaluation data for the public awareness campaigns targeted at elder abuse are not available at this time, they are feasible and merit testing.

However, direct translation of strategies from other forms of family violence may not be straightforward. As discussed above, one project was modeled on programs that had been successfully employed in reducing younger partner violence (Davis & Medina-Ariza, 2001). This study, which is the only project to include a rigorous randomized controlled design with victims of elder abuse, resulted in more reported incidents of abuse than the control group (Davis & Medina-Ariza, 2001). As the program had been effective with the partner violence sample in the same local area, the negative result in the elder abuse sample was entirely unexpected. This example shows that translating what works in family violence prevention to the field of elder abuse, although a promising avenue to advance knowledge, can be a highly complicated process.

13.3.5. The Development of Prevention Programs Specifically for Dementia Caregivers Is Warranted

Evidence was reviewed in this chapter regarding the special risk for violence in dementia caregiving relationships. Specifically, severe behavior problems on the part of dementia patients, and in particular physical violence, are related to verbal and physical aggression by caregivers. This pattern of what appears to be retaliative violence appears to hold across settings; a study of abuse by staff in nursing homes found violence by residents to be a major risk factor (Pillemer & Moore, 1989). Several programs exist to reduce behavioral symptoms among dementia patients; these strategies should be systematically evaluated for the elder abuse prevention potential. Promising intervention programs for caregivers in general (Anetzberger et al., 2000; Scogin et al., 1992) would benefit greatly from evaluation studies that in addition to measures of the reduction in caregiver stress and anger also included measures of abusive behavior (e.g., from caregiver self-reports or care-recipient reports).

13.3.6. Summary

The available evidence suggests the following points:

- The elder mistreatment research literature does not as yet provide consistent guidelines for prevention programs. Promotion of research on this topic that uses scientifically acceptable designs is critically important to improve prevention practice. Longitudinal studies, case-comparison designs, and carefully controlled intervention studies are particularly needed.
- Elder mistreatment is estimated to affect 2–5% of the older population, suggesting that the magnitude of the problem justifies the development of prevention programs.
- Risk factors for elder mistreatment include living with other persons; social isolation; the presence of dementia; psychological problems, substance abuse, and dependency on the part of perpetrators; and poor health and functional status of victims. Additional research to specify risk factors is greatly needed.
- Commonly used prevention programs—such as screening instruments, mandatory reporting, and adult protective services—have little demonstrated effectiveness for elder mistreatment and may have unanticipated negative consequences. These programs require careful evaluation of both positive and negative outcomes.
- Potentially promising interventions include education of potential victims and professionals and support for caregivers of dementia patients. Extensive effort is needed to create new and innovative prevention programs.

REFERENCES

Ahmad, M., & Lachs, M. S. (2002). Elder abuse and neglect: What physicians can and should do. *Cleveland Clinic Journal of Medicine, 69* (10), 801–808.

Anetzberger, G. (1987). *The etiology of elder abuse by adult offspring.* Springfield, IL: Thomas.

Anetzberger, G. J., Korbin, J. E., & Austin, C. (1994). Alcoholism and elder abuse. *Journal of Interpersonal Violence, 9* (2), 184–193.

Anetzberger, G. J., Palmisano, B. R., Sanders, M., Bass, D., Dayton, C., Eckert, S., & Schimer, M. R. (2000). Model intervention for elder abuse and dementia. *Gerontologist, 40* (4), 492–497.

Blenkner, M. (1971). A research and demonstration of protective services. *Social Casework, 52,* 483–497.

Bristowe, E., & Collins, J. B. (1989). Family mediated abuse of noninstitutionalized frail elderly men and women living in British Columbia. *Journal of Elder Abuse and Neglect, 1* (1), 45–64.

Bond, C. (2004). Education and a multi-agency approach are key to addressing elder abuse. *Professional Nurse, 20* (4), 39–41.

California Attorney General's Crime and Violence Prevention Center. (2003). Elder and dependent adult abuse media campaign. Retrieved April 17, 2005, from safestate.org/index-print.cfm?navid=195.

Chalk, R., & King, P. (1998). Assessing family violence interventions. *American Journal of Preventive Medicine, 14* (4), 289–292.

Comijs, H. C., Penninx, B. W., Knipscheer, K. P., & van Tilberg, W. (1999). Psychological distress in victims of elder abuse: The effects of social support and coping. *Journals of Gerontology, 54B* (4), 240–245.

Compton, S. A., Flanagan, P., & Gregg, W. (1997). Elder abuse in people with dementia in Northern Ireland: Prevalence and predictors in cases referred to a psychiatry of old age service. *International Journal of Geriatric Psychiatry, 12* (6), 632–635.

Cooney, C., & Mortimer, A. (1995). Elder abuse and dementia: A pilot study. *International Journal of Social Psychiatry, 41* (4), 276–283.

Coyne, C., Reichman, W. E., & Berbig, L. J. (1993). The relationship between dementia and elder abuse. *American Journal of Psychiatry, 15* (4), 643–646.

Davis, R. C., & Medina-Ariza, J. (2001). *Results from an elder abuse prevention experiment in New York City* (Research in Brief). Washington, DC: National Institute of Justice.

Fulmer, T. (1991). Elder mistreatment: Progress in community detection and intervention. *Family & Community Health, 14* (2), 26–34.

Fulmer, T., Guadano, L., Dyer, C., & Connolly, M. T. (2004). Progress in elder abuse assessment instruments. *Journal of the American Geriatrics Society, 52,* 297–304.

Fulmer, T., & O'Malley, T. A. (1987). *Inadequate care of the elderly: A healthcare perspective on abuse and neglect.* New York: Springer.

Gordon, R. (1983). An operational classification of disease prevention. *Public Health Reports, 98,* 107–109.

Grafstrom, M., Nordberg, A., & Winblad, B. (1993). Abuse is in the eye of the beholder. *Scandinavian Journal of Social Medicine, 21* (4), 247–255.

Greenberg, J. R., McKibben, M., & Raymond, J. A. (1990). Dependent adult children and elder abuse. *Journal of Elder Abuse and Neglect, 2,* 73–86.

Homer, A. C., & Gilleard, C. (1990). Abuse of elderly people by their careers. *British Medical Journal, 301* (6765), 1359–1362.

Lachs, M. S., Berkman, L., Fulmer, T., & Horwitz, R. I. (1994). A prospective community-based pilot study of risk factors for the investigation of elder mistreatment. *Journal of the American Geriatrics Society, 42* (2), 169–173.

Lachs, M. S., & Pillemer, K. (2004). Elder abuse. *Lancet, 364* (9441), 1263–1273.

Lachs, M. S., Williams, C., O'Brien, S., Hurst, L., & Horowitz, R. (1997). Risk factors for reported elder abuse and neglect: A nine-year observational cohort study. *Gerontologist, 37,* 469–474.

Lachs, M. S., Williams, C. S., O'Brien, S., & Pillemer, K. (2002). Adult protective service use and nursing home placement. *Gerontologist, 42,* 734–739.

Lachs, M. S., Williams, C. S., O'Brien, S., Pillemer, K., & Charlson, M. E. (1998). The mortality of elder mistreatment. *Journal of the American Medical Association, 280,* 428–432.

Mrazek, P. J., & Haggerty, R. J. (Eds.). (1994). *Reducing risks for mental disorders: Frontiers for preventive intervention research.* Washington, DC: Committee on Prevention of Mental Disorders, Institute of Medicine.

Nahmiash, D., & Reis, M. (2000). Most successful intervention strategies for abused older adults. *Journal of Elder Abuse and Neglect, 12* (3–4), 53–70.

National Research Council. (2002). *Elder mistreatment: Abuse, neglect, and exploitation in an aging America.* Washington, DC: The National Academy Press.

Paveza, G. J., Cohen, D., Eisdorfer, C., Freels, S., Semla, T., Ashford, J. W., Gorelick, P., Hirschman, R., Luchins, D., & Levy, P. (1992). Severe family violence and Alzheimer's disease: Prevalence and risk factors. *Gerontologist, 32* (4), 493–497.

Phillips, R. L. (1983). Abuse and neglect of the frail elderly at home: An exploration of theoretical relationships. *Journal of Advanced Nursing, 8,* 379–392.

Pillemer, K. (1985). The dangers of dependency: New findings on domestic violence against the elderly. *Social Problems, 33* (2), 146–158.

Pillemer, K. A. (1986). Risk factors in elder abuse: Results from a case-control study. In K. A. Pillemer & R. S. Wolf (Eds.), *Elder abuse: Conflict in the family* (pp. 239–263). Dover, MA: Auburn House.

Pillemer, K. (2004). Elder abuse is caused by the deviance and dependence of abusive caregivers. In D. Loseke, R. Gelles, & M. Cavanaugh (Eds.), *Current controversies on family violence* (2nd ed). (pp. 207–220). Newbury Park, CA: Sage.

Pillemer, K., & Finkelhor, D. (1988). The prevalence of elder abuse: A random sample survey. *Gerontologist, 28* (1), 51–57.

Pillemer, K., & Finkelhor, D. (1989). Causes of elder abuse: Caregiver stress versus problem relatives. *American Journal of Orthopsychiatry, 59,* 179–187.

Pillemer, K., & Moore, D. W. (1989). Abuse of patients in nursing homes: Findings from a survey of staff. *Gerontologist, 29,* 314–320.

Pillemer, K., & Suitor, J. J. (1992). Violence and violent feelings: What causes them among family givers? *Journal of Gerontology, 47,* 165–172.

Podnieks, E. (1992). National survey on abuse of the elderly in Canada. *Journal of Elder Abuse and Neglect, 41,* 5–58.

Reay Campbell, II, A. M., & Browne, K. D. (2002). The effectiveness of psychological interventions with individuals who physically abuse or neglect their elderly dependents. *Journal of Interpersonal Violence, 17* (4), 416–431.

Reis, M., & Nahmiash, D. (1997). Abuse of seniors: Personality, stress, and other indicators. *Journal of Mental Health and Aging, 3,* 337–356.

Reis, M., & Nahmiash, D. (1998). Validation of the indicators of abuse (IOA) screen. *Gerontologist, 38* (4), 471–480.

Richardson, B., Kitchen, G., & Livingston, G. (2002). The effect of education on knowledge and management of elder abuse: A randomized controlled trial. *Age and Ageing, 31,* 335–341.

Schofield, M. J., & Mishra, G. D. (2003). Validity of self-report screening scale for elder abuse: Woman's Health Australia Study. *Gerontologist, 43* (1), 110–120.

Scogin, F., Stephens, J., Bynum, L., Baumhover, C., Beall, C., & Grote, N. P. (1992). Emotional correlates of caregiving. *Journal of Elder Abuse and Neglect, 4,* 59–69.

Tornstam, L. (1989). Abuse of the elderly in Denmark and Sweden: Results from a population study. *Journal of Elder Abuse and Neglect, 1* (1), 35–44.

Vermont Center for Crime Victim Services. (2003). Respect our elders. Center for Crime Victim Services launches public education campaign. Retrieved April 17, 2005, from www.ccvs.state.vt.us/pub_ed/lauch.html.

Wilke, D. J., & Vinton, L. (2003). Domestic violence and aging: Teaching about their intersection. *Journal of Social Work Education, 39* (2), 225–235.

Williamson, G. M., & Shaffer, D. R. (2001). Relationship quality and potentially harmful behaviors by spousal caregivers: How we were then, how we are now. *Psychology & Aging, 16* (2), 217–226.

Wolf, R. S., & Pillemer, K. (1988). Intervention, outcome, and elder abuse. In D. Finkelhor & G. T. Hotaling (Eds.), *Coping with family violence: Research and policy perspectives* (pp. 257–274). Thousand Oaks, CA: Sage.

Wolf, R. S., & Pillemer, K. (1989). *Helping elderly victims: The reality of elder abuse.* New York: Columbia University Press.

Wolf, R. S., Strugnell C. P., & Godkin, M. A. (1982). Preliminary findings from three model projects on elderly abuse. Worcester: Centre on Aging, University of Massachusetts Medical Centre.

Wolfe, D. A., & Jaffe, P. G. (1999). Emerging strategies in the prevention of domestic violence. *The Future of Children, 9* (3), 133–144.

Part III

Cross-Cutting Intervention Issues

Chapter **14**

Changing the Built Environment to Prevent Injury

Catherine E. Staunton, Howard Frumpkin, and Andrew L. Dannenberg

14.1. INTRODUCTION

The "built environment" is the part of the environment designed and constructed by humans; it includes buildings, neighborhoods, sporting facilities, roadways, and vehicles. It is thus a logical but often overlooked fact that the built environment can be modified to help prevent both unintentional injuries, such as young children falling from balconies, and violent injuries, such as injuries incurred during an armed robbery.

Improved safety codes in the United States have made fire-related injuries in public places very rare. In 1911, fire broke out on the ninth floor of the Triangle Shirt Waist Factory in Manhattan. The main exit was engulfed with flames and alternative exits were either locked or had doors that opened inward. The fire escape collapsed under the weight of fleeing employees, and 146 people died. This tragedy resulted in some of the first fire codes affecting the built environment: multiple fire escape routes, outward opening doors, and sprinkler systems for higher floors (Von Drehle, 2003). The deadly 1942 Coconut Grove Night Club fire resulted in new laws requiring emergency lighting systems and flame-retardant decorations in public buildings and prohibiting the use of revolving doors as principal exits (Moulton, 1943). And the fatal 1980, MGM Grand Hotel fire led to the adoption of retroactive fire safety improvements (including sprinklers) in older, publicly occupied buildings (Nolan, 2001).

Injury prevention strategies that decrease injury risk through environmental design are among the most successful interventions and the focus of this chapter. Although built environment modifications may be expensive initially, once in place they protect many people over many years.

This chapter examines built environment features that prevent injuries associated with transportation, sports and recreation, the home environment, and violence. It analyzes current surveillance of built environment factors, reviews efficacy studies of environmental modifications, and examines the role of legislation and enforcement. The chapter also looks at new built environmental designs that may reduce injury and promote health.

14.2.   TRANSPORTATION-RELATED INJURY AND THE BUILT ENVIRONMENT

Motor-vehicle-related transportation accounts for more than 90% of the transportation-related fatalities (Centers for Disease Control and Prevention [CDC], 2005a). Modifications to enhance the safety of motor vehicles (MV) and roadways have been among the most successful strategies to reduce transportation-related injuries; nonetheless, motor vehicles continue to be a leading cause of injury and death in the United States and worldwide (Peden et al., 2004). Transportation safety has focused primarily on MV occupants, even though public transit offers much safer modes. In addition, MVs are responsible for most pedestrian and bicyclist injury-related deaths. There are many environmental modifications that effectively decrease pedestrian and bicyclist injury potential and, in turn, allow for safer active transportation and improved health on many levels.

14.2.1.   Injury Prevention Through Motor Vehicle and Roadway Design

Since 1925, the annual death rate per million vehicle miles traveled has decreased over 90% (National Safety Council [NSC], 2003), largely because of modifications in driver behavior, vehicle crashworthiness, road design, and changes in the built environment making it safer for all to travel (CDC, 1999; Dellinger, Sleet, & Jones, 2006). The U.S. Highway Safety Act and the National Traffic and Motor Vehicle Safety Act of 1966, set safety and regulatory standards for motor vehicle and roadway safety, leading to changes in vehicle and highway design. Resulting MV safety features included head rests, energy-absorbing steering wheels, shatter-resistant windshields, and safety belts (Transportation Research Board [TRB], 1990; Waller, 2002). MV safety modifications have continued to improve to the present day, including lap and shoulder belts for all passengers, front and side air bags, reinforced side and roof beams, center-mounted brake lights, increased interior padding, tire pressure monitoring systems, and daytime running lights (Elvik, & Vaa, 2004; Jagger, 1992; National Highway Traffic Safety Administration [NHTSA], 2005).

The 1966 act also improved roadways and led to redesigned horizontal curves, the use of painted lanes and reflectors, divided interstate highways with on and off ramps, the use of breakaway sign and utility poles, improved lighting, addition of barriers separating oncoming traffic lanes, and guard rails (Houk, Millar, Rosenberg, & Waxweiler, 1992). More recent roadway modifications include enhanced pavement markings, skid-resistant pavement, turning lanes, eliminating shoulder dropoffs, and impact attenuators that yield on contact (TRB, 2003). Modifications to urban intersections that have reduced crashes and injuries include improved visibility, more conspicuous stop signs, red light cameras, and small roundabouts (Retting, Ferguson, & Hakkert, 2003; Retting, Persaud, Garder, & Lord, 2001; Retting, Weinstein, & Solomon, 2003).

Despite these successes, MV travel has notable shortcomings. Even with improved safety features, MV injuries in the United States remain the leading cause of death for children and young adults and a leading injury cause of death for all ages (CDC, 2005b) (see Chapter 4). Worldwide, there are an estimated 1.2 million deaths and a minimum of 20 million injuries caused by MVs each year (Peden et al., 2004). More than 85% of road traffic injuries occur in middle- and low-income countries; in these countries, over half of MV crash-related deaths involve pedestrians (Nantulya & Reich, 2002).

Even though new vehicle and roadway design features have generally decreased the risk of injuries, there are some new vehicle and roadway designs that have increased injury risk. The U.S. vehicle fleet is rapidly changing from predominantly passenger vehicles to light truck vehicles (LTVs): sport utility vehicles (SUVs), light trucks, and vans (Federal Highway Administration [FHWA], 2001). Because these vehicles are prone to roll over in crashes, LTVs do not provide more safety for occupants than the average passenger vehicle (Bureau of Transportation Statistics [BTS], 2004; Farmer & Lund, 2002). However, because of poor visibility, LTVs are more likely than passenger vehicles to hit pedestrians and much more likely to severely injure or kill the pedestrians they hit (Brison, Wicklund, & Mueller, 1988; Roudsari et al., 2004). Also, crashes involving a passenger vehicle and an LTV pose a much higher risk of death to passenger vehicle occupants than crashes involving two passenger vehicles (Insurance Institute for Highway Safety [IIHS], 1999). Airbags, once touted to be the passive solution to the occupant injury problem, have proven effective in decreasing adult injuries but unfortunately have also resulted in increased injuries to children and occasionally to small-statured adults sitting in the front passenger compartment (Smith & Cummings, 2006; Newgard & Lewis, 2005; Evans, 2004).

Roadway design has in some instances indirectly contributed to increased injury risk. The extensive system of well-built roadways in the United States has helped fuel sprawling suburban development. Sprawling development means longer commutes and thus more MV-related injuries; sprawl is directly related to increased occupant and pedestrian fatalities (Ewing, Schieber, & Zegeer, 2003). In fact, the risk of dying in a MV crash in the suburbs is higher than the risk of dying from stranger homicide in central cities, an ironic fact because many people move from cities to suburbs in search of safer neighborhoods (Lucy, 2003).

14.2.2. Building Transportation Systems Focused on Public Transit, Pedestrians, and Cyclists

Travel by public transit is much safer than by car. Private vehicle occupants have a 29-fold higher risk than bus passengers and an 11-fold higher risk than train passengers of fatal injury per mile traveled (BTS, 2004; NSC, 2003). The special case of school travel has been well studied. Fatality rates among children traveling to school on school buses are 0.3 per 100 million trips, 1.6 for those in cars driven by adults, and 13.2 for those in cars driven by teens (TRB, 2002). Currently in the United States, over 85% of trips are made by private vehicle and less than 2% by public transit (FHWA, 2001); if fewer people drove and more trips were made by public transit, overall injuries would likely decrease dramatically.

Walking, biking, and public transit are important forms of transportation for several public health reasons. Use of public transit is also associated with substantial walking to and from the transit stops (Besser & Dannenberg, 2005). Walking and biking for transportation are an excellent form of physical activity. MVs are a leading cause of air pollution (and greenhouse gases); increased walking, biking, and public transit would improve air quality (U.S. Environmental Protection Agency [EPA], 2004). Walking, biking, and public transit are important forms of transportation for people who cannot afford private vehicles and for people who cannot drive, such as children, those with some types of handicaps, and some elderly persons. Last, walking increases social capital and improves mental health (Leyden, 2003; Salmon, 2001).

Despite these benefits of active transport, less than 10% of all trips in the United States are made by walking and biking. One of the leading barriers to walking and biking in the United States is traffic danger (Zegeer et al., 2000; CDC, 2005b). Even though pedestrian danger is frequently avoided by driving, the risk of fatal injury in the United States per distance traveled is sevenfold higher for walking and fivefold higher for biking than for driving (Pucher & Dijkstra, 2003). In the United States these high injury rates may be exacerbated by the fact that less than 1% of federal transportation funds are spent on pedestrian and bicycle facilities and safety (Ernst, 2004).

Although walking and biking are relatively dangerous in the United States and probably even more dangerous in many middle- and low-income countries, it is possible to build communities that promote safe walking and biking. Looking at pedestrian deaths per distance traveled, pedestrians in Germany are threefold and pedestrians in the Netherlands are fivefold safer than U.S. pedestrians. This improved safety arises from an extensive effort to design and build transportation systems that focus on safe walking and biking while restricting MV use and vehicle speeds (Pucher & Dijkstra, 2003).

14.2.3. Built Environments That Enhance Pedestrian Safety

Built environment modifications, if carefully planned, are effective in preventing pedestrian injuries (Retting, Ferguson, & McCartt, 2003). Separating pedestrians from MVs is effective in decreasing collisions and injury. These strategies include installation of traffic signals, in-pavement flashing lights, four-way stops, pedestrian overpasses, fences to inhibit street access, and sidewalks (Retting et al., 2003). On the other hand, crosswalks without traffic signals increase risk for elderly pedestrians (Koepsell et al., 2002), and crosswalks without traffic signals located on busy streets and/or on streets with more than two lanes increase risk for all pedestrians (Zegeer, Stewart, Huang, & Lagerwey, 2001).

Engineering measures designed to increase visibility and conspicuity of pedestrians, such as increased roadway illumination and relocating bus stops to the far side of intersections, also decrease injury risk. Of the engineering measures to manage vehicle speed, small roundabouts on residential roads and four-way stops at intersections are effective (Fig. 14.1) (Retting et al., 2003). Speed humps can decrease overall child pedestrian injuries in a neighborhood setting (Tester, Rutherford, Wald, & Rutherford, 2004). Because a MV is less likely to collide with a person walking or biking in areas with heavier pedestrian and bicycle traffic (Jacobsen, 2003; Leden, 2002), pedestrian and bicycle safety measures may have a dual effect in that safety modifications may increase pedestrian traffic which in turn further decreases pedestrian risk.

Three promising designs that need further evidence-based research to assess effectiveness are routing traffic away from residential settings, creating off-road trails for pedestrians and bikes, and developing area-wide traffic calming (neighborhood-based, design intervention strategies such as reducing speed by narrowing street width and installing speed humps) (Bunn et al., 2003). Although much is known about building environments that enhance pedestrian safety, there is much less known about creating safe environments for bicycles. Further research in this area is needed.

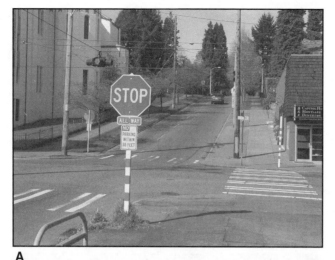

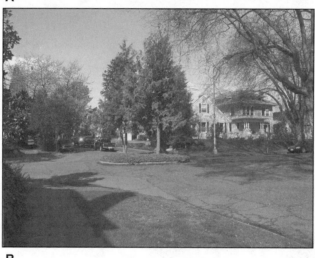

Figure 14.1. Intersections with four-way stops (**A**) and small traffic circles (**B**) slow traffic speeds and decrease the risk of pedestrian injuries.

In summary, the built environment and transportation safety are closely linked. Motor vehicle and roadway environmental modifications have been very successful at decreasing the risk of motor vehicle related injuries and death. Pedestrians and cyclists are particularly vulnerable to injury in MV crashes. Increased focus on building and retrofitting communities to promote safe walking, biking, and public transit will help reduce transportation related injuries, promote physical and mental health, improve air quality, and increase social equity.

14.3.   SPORTS AND RECREATION INJURY PREVENTION

14.3.1.   Playground Safety by Design

Built environment aspects related to sports and recreational injuries have been closely studied in only a few areas, such as playgrounds. The study of playground injury prevention provides an excellent example of how the built environment can be redesigned to reduce injuries. Before the 1970s, hazards existed in many playgrounds. For example, towering metal slides with small sidewalls and no handrails situated on hard-packed earth and slippery monkey bars anchored into asphalt slabs lead to frequent falls and serious injuries. Hard wooden swing seats were just the right height to strike a child's face or head, resulting in lacerations and skull fractures (Illingworth, Brennan, Jay, Al-Rawi, & Collick, 1975). As early as 1978, injury surveillance by the U.S. Consumer Product Safety Commission (CPSC) revealed that playgrounds were a leading location for pediatric injuries, including head injuries, fractures, lacerations, and abrasions in the United States (Rivers, Boyd, & Baderman, 1978). Response to this public health issue has not been to discourage playground use or to dress kids in protective playground gear, such as helmets and elbow pads. Instead, the approach has been to use evidence-based injury data to design safer playground environments in which injuries are rare (Fig. 14.2).

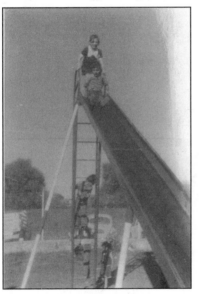

A

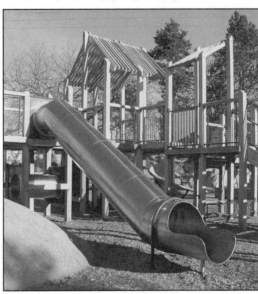

B

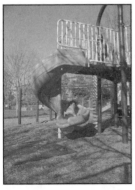

C

Figure 14.2. A slide from the early 1970s (**A**) poses a higher risk of fall-related injuries than newer slide designs (**B** and **C**). (Panel A reprinted by permission from L. S. Ryan.)

MacKay's (2003, p.194) editorial concisely summarizes more than 25 years of peer-reviewed articles on playground injuries and efforts to create safer environments:

> We know that the most common cause of playground injuries are falls from equipment (for example, climbers, monkey bars, slides). However, injury also results when children are struck by moving objects or strangled either through head entrapment or as the result of clothing caught in equipment. Of non-fatal injuries involving playground equipment, the most serious relate to the height of equipment (swings, slides, and climbers). . . . Height of equipment also has direct implications for type and depth of surfacing underlying playground equipment.

Norton, Nixon, and Sibert's (2004) review of effectiveness of playground safety interventions found that serious head injuries are now rare on playgrounds. Swings that used to be considered one of the most dangerous pieces of equipment are now one of the safest. Limiting maximum heights to 1.5 m decreases injuries 50–75%, and impact-absorbing surfaces decrease injuries 50–83%.

Almost three decades of epidemiologic data and collaboration between public health practitioners, safety engineers, and playground manufacturers has culminated in detailed recommendations from the CPSC and other agencies on building and maintaining safe playgrounds. Although equipment standards vary internationally, playgrounds adhering to these guidelines have markedly decreased injury rates (MacKay, 2003). In many ways, playground injury prevention can be considered a built environment success story.

Unfortunately, more than 200,000 children with playground-related injuries are still being treated in U.S. hospital emergency departments annually; almost half of these injuries are severe (Tinsworth & McDonald, 2001). Probably the leading cause of this ongoing morbidity is that many playgrounds do not meet current guidelines; the most frequent deviation from guidelines is inadequate surfacing depth (MacKay, 2003). Playgrounds in poor neighborhoods may be particularly vulnerable to guideline breaches (Suecoff, Avner, Chou, & Crain, 1999). Enforcement of guidelines varies greatly in different locations. In the United States, some states have laws that require playgrounds to follow standards, but other states have no such policies (NSC, 2002). California law mandates that safety standards and guidelines be followed and requires inspections to document adherence (Kelter, 2001).

Last, although detailed studies of the relationship between playground engineering and injury are now available, playground design has not been studied in a larger public health context. Public health practitioners know a lot about designing and building playgrounds that minimize injury but have less familiarity with designing and building playgrounds that attract children; create social capital in neighborhoods; and promote the development of a child's imagination, agility, and strength while increasing physical activity levels (Moore, Goltsman, & Iacofano, 1992).

14.3.2.   The Built Environment and Sports Injury

Although there are thousands of peer-reviewed articles on recreational and sports related-injuries, few of these analyze environmental factors. Environmental factors contributing to sports injury are rarely noted in surveillance. One reason for this discrepancy is that most injury data are collected in health care settings, such as emergency departments, where demographic and injury related information are most readily available. Relevant environmental data are not always obvious and are more difficult to collect.

Although environmental design factors have not been closely studied in most areas of sports and recreation, there are several notable examples of built environment changes significantly lowering injury rates. Padded soccer goal posts securely anchored to the ground decrease injuries associated with player–goal post collisions (Janda, Bir, Wild, Olsen, & Hensinger, 1995) and injuries caused by heavy soccer goals toppling forward onto players (CDC, 1994). One study of recreational soft ball league injuries found that 71% of injuries were related to sliding; installation of break-away bases (vs. stationary bases) decreased sliding injuries by 96% (Janda, Hankin, & Wojtys, 1986). Analysis of hockey rink size found the larger international size ice surfaces to have significantly fewer collisions and injuries during competitive hockey games than the smaller and therefore more crowded North American ice surfaces (Wennberg, 2004).

Although many sports and recreational injuries are not related to the built environment, design and maintenance features undoubtedly play a role in some of these injuries. Unlike most studies, Cheng et al. (2000) looked closely for design and maintenance factors involved in injuries. The U.S. trauma center–based study analyzed 2563 sports related injuries in urban youth and found 16% of visits and 20% of hospitalizations were related to environmental factors amenable to preventive strategies. These cases included injuries from striking basketball backboards and poles; collisions with goal posts, walls, fences, cars, and bleachers; falls onto glass, metal, sticks, and stones; being struck by football helmets; and falls onto bicycle center bars and handle bars. These examples highlight the need for more detailed sports and recreational injury surveillance with an increased focus on equipment, field conditions, and the other contributing environmental circumstances (see Chapter 7).

14.3.3. Prevention of Water-Related Injuries by Environmental Design

Drowning is a leading cause of injury death in the United States (CDC, 2005a), and the risk of drowning in low- and middle-income countries is 4.5-fold higher than it is in high-income countries (Peden, MeGee, & Sharma, 2002). Creating effective strategies for addressing water-related injuries is particularly challenging because demographic risk factors are diverse and because injuries occur in a variety of settings (the home, pools, open water, and irrigation ditches). Fishing docks situated near overhead power lines, diving platforms, motor boat propellers, and sailboat booms all increase the risk of injuries (Chalmers & Morrison, 2003). Tailoring the built environment to decrease water-related injury has not been a major public health focus, except for residential swimming pool fencing.

Prevention of child drowning by pool fencing is probably the single most effective strategy for reducing unintentional drowning. Fencing is most effective if it surrounds a pool on all four sides; is of sufficient height and design to resist climbing attempts; and has a secure, self-closing and self-latching gate (Thompson & Rivara, 2000). Although this built environment solution prevents at least three quarters of all childhood pool drownings (Thompson & Rivara, 2000), implementing appropriate fencing regulations has proven difficult. Legislation and inspections to ensure safe pool fencing in Australia lagged 25 years behind the proven benefit of such interventions (Scott, 2003). Now, Australia has uniform legislation for pool fencing, but many states in the United States do not (National SAFE KIDS Campaign, 2004). Although pools are a leading site of drowning in 1- to 4-year-old children in developed countries, the majority of drownings in the United States and around the world do not occur in pools (CDC, 2005a). Other solutions are needed (see Chapter 5).

Most water-related injury surveillance contains very limited environmental information. The recently formulated *Recommended Guidelines for Uniform Reporting of Data from Drowning* suggested 42 core and supplemental questions to collect information on the victim, the scene, emergency department and hospital courses, and patient disposition. Of these questions, only one relates to the built environment: "Location of drowning" (Idris et al., 2003).

Important questions about the relationship between the built environment and water injuries still remain. These include: Do wading pools, fountains, and garden pools pose a significant drowning risk and, if so, which design features are associated with risk? Which toilet designs pose a risk of toddler drowning? Do poolside shepherd's hooks, life rings, or telephones decrease swimming injuries? What factors in bathtub design minimize infant and elderly drowning risk? What are the prominent road and vehicle characteristics leading to drownings in a car? Do warning labels on 5-gallon buckets decrease toddler drownings? Would impact-absorbing surfaces installed around or in pools decrease injuries? Does signage advocating for personal flotation devices prevent injuries? How can drainage ditches be built to minimize toddler access? In what circumstances would fencing of natural bodies of water be cost effective?

In summary, sports and recreational injury prevention by environmental design have some notable successes, but these successes have been limited by lack of legislation and enforcement that is often necessary to effectively incorporate safer designs. Overall, the interventions related to the built environment in sports and recreational injuries have not been suitably studied. Further research in this area is warranted.

14.4.   HOME INJURIES AND ENVIRONMENTAL MODIFICATIONS

In the United States, about one third of all unintentional injuries occur in the home environment, accounting for over 30,000 fatal injuries and 13 million non-fatal injuries per year (NSC, 2003). Most of these injuries occur in young children, the elderly, and the poor (NSC, 2003). Falls and burns are particularly amenable to prevention through environmental modification.

14.4.1.   Design Modifications and Fall-Related Injuries

Falls are the leading cause of fatal and nonfatal unintentional injury in the home setting, accounting for about 8000 deaths per year (NSC, 2003). Although fall-related injuries in children have been steadily declining over the last several decades (American Academy of Pediatrics [AAP], 2001), fall-related injuries in the elderly have slowly been rising, probably due to the increasing proportion of elderly in the United States (NSC, 2003).

Several simple environmental modifications have played important roles in reducing pediatric injuries caused by home falls. Bergner, Mayer, and Harris (1971) noted that 12% of all pediatric fatal injuries in New York City were the result of home falls; the most common scenarios were young children falling from windows in multistory dwellings and older children falling from roofs and fire escapes. A pilot program combining education and free window guards led to a 35% reduction in window-related fall injuries. In 1976, the New York City Board of Health passed a law requiring the owners of multistory buildings to provide window guards for units housing children. This mandatory program was followed by a 96% reduction in local hospital admissions for window-related falls (AAP, 2001). Further research has found windows positioned low to the floor to be particularly hazardous (Istre et al., 2003). Window stops that restrict openings to 4 inches are an alternative to window guards. It is important that window guards or stops be *operable* (can be opened quickly by an adult) and not *fixed* to allow egress in case of fire. Despite the proven effectiveness of window guards, some areas have been slow to include them in building codes (AAP, 2001).

Spacing of railings has been found to be important in reducing falls from balconies, decks, porches, and roofs. Most children 5 years old and younger can slip through a 6-inch space. However, children 1 year and older cannot slip through a 4-inch opening (Fig. 14.3). Railings with vertical bars spaced 4 inches or closer effectively prevent pediatric falls. Building codes in much of the United States now require new construction to comply with 4-inch spacing. However, retrofitting of older buildings is often not required (AAP, 2001; Istre et al., 2003).

Home falls are a leading cause of mortality and morbidity in people over 65 years of age. The home environment is identified as a contributing factor in most incidents (Sattin, Rodriguez, DeVito, & Wingo, 1998) and stairs pose a particular fall risk (Cayless, 2001). Most homes in which elderly people live have at least one environmental hazard that might cause a fall, such as loose throw rugs, poorly maintained stairways, poor lighting, and lack of stair railings (Gill, Williams, Robison, & Tinetti, 1999). However, measures aimed solely at eliminating environmental fall hazards have not proven effective, except in elderly persons with a prior fall history (Gillespie et al., 2003; Stevens & Olson, 2000) (see Chapter 3).

There are several possible reasons why environmental modifications alone have not proven to be effective. First, risk factors for falls in the elderly are multifaceted and include increasing age, lack of recent physical activity, functional limitations, and psychoactive medications in addition to environmental factors (Stevens & Olson, 2000). Second, studies looking at environmental modifications have often had relatively few participants or short follow-up resulting in statistical power that may have been too low to detect an effective intervention (Lyons et al., 2003). Last, most home modifications studied to date are changes that can be quickly and inexpensively implemented. Prevention of fall-related injuries in the elderly may require more complicated interventions such as improved stairway design, padded flooring, and even impact-absorbing bathroom surfaces. Most surveillance systems that capture data on falls in the elderly collect little or no information on contributing environmental factors (Cayless, 2001; Home Safety Council [HSC], 2004). Detailed case-control studies to elucidate the causes of slips and trips leading to falls, to define the surfaces and objects landed on, and to document the location and height of falls would help determine the environmental factors most closely associated with fall-related injuries in the elderly.

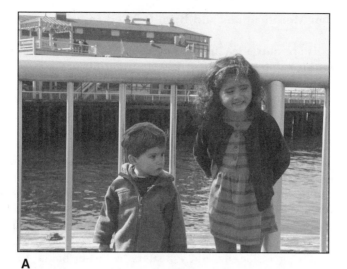

A

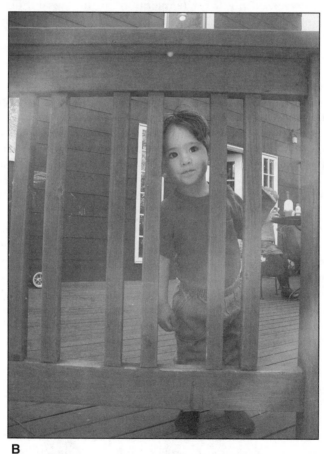

B

Figure 14.3. A. The 5-year-old girl and her 1-year-old brother could squeeze through the balusters, here with 6-inch spacing. **B.** Balusters with a maximum spacing of 4 inches safely contain even the 1-year-old child.

14.4.2.   Design Modifications and Burn-Related Injuries

Residential burns are also a leading cause of fatal and nonfatal injury, resulting in about 2,200 deaths and more than 250,000 injuries in the United States annually (HSC, 2004; NSC, 2003). Of all burn-related injuries, 90% of the fatalities and 57% of nonfatal injuries occurred in the home (HSC, 2004). Although residential fires are responsible for most burn-related fatalities, scalds and thermal and electrical burns also contribute to home burn injury, mortality, and morbidity rates (see Chapter 6).

Many successful interventions to decrease burn injuries have involved environmental modifications. Feldman, Schaller, Feldman, & McMillon (1978) noted that many scald burns were caused by hot tap water. A survey of Seattle area homes revealed the average hot water at the tap to be 142°F. Full-thickness burns result from a 2-second exposure to 150°F water but do not occur at 130°F water until exposure reaches 30 seconds (Moritz & Henriques, 1947). Legislation in Washington State requiring residential water heaters to be set below 130°F has been associated with decreased hot water temperature at the tap and decreased scald burns (Erdmann, Feldman, Rivara, Heimbach, & Wall, 1991). Yet, many areas in the United States do not regulate tap water temperatures; and hot tap water remains a major cause of scald burns.

Other successful strategies for reducing burn injuries may include child-resistant lighters; roll-up cords for electric coffee pots; design of kitchens to shorten the distance between the stove and sink; and the design of pots, pans, and kettles to reduce the probability of tipping and spilling, and cooker safeguards (a guardrail around the edge of the stove) that may prevent toddlers from reaching pots of hot food). Many of these interventions are promising but await further outcome evaluation. Self-extinguishing cigarettes, which could markedly decrease the number of residential fires, have been developed, yet opposition from the cigarette industry has prevented widespread legislation that would require their manufacture and use (Warda, Tenenbein, & Moffatt, 1999).

Smoke detectors are a highly effective and inexpensive way to reduce residential fire injuries by providing early warning; 97% of households recently reported having at least one smoke detector and 80% reported one on each level of their home (Runyan et al., 2005). Unfortunately, less than 20% of households regularly check smoke detectors to see if they are functioning appropriately. Although no evidenced-based public health literature is yet available, it is hoped that some of the newer smoke detectors now on the market powered by household electricity or long-lasting lithium batteries will decrease the incidence of nonfunctional alarms.

Automatic sprinkler systems may prove to be the most effective approach to preventing residential fire injuries because they require less maintenance than smoke detectors, substantially reduce property damage, and give high-risk populations (e.g., young children, the elderly and alcohol-intoxicated people) more time to exit the building. Preliminary testing suggests that sprinkler systems may be extremely effective in preventing fire-related injuries (Cote, 1984; Smith, 1994). Further research into maintenance issues and cost effectiveness of widespread residential sprinkler systems is needed.

The home environment can be modified in a number of ways to reduce injury risk. There is a need for more detailed surveillance and scientifically rigorous investigations to identify effective home safety modifications and devices. Legislation and enforcement may be especially important in home injuries because these injuries are particularly common among children and other vulnerable populations, such as low-income families who frequently rent housing in old and poorly maintained buildings (Cubbin, LeClere, & Smith, 2000; Shenassa, Stubbendick, & Brown, 2004).

14.5.   VIOLENCE PREVENTION THROUGH COMMUNITY DESIGN

This section examines environmental modifications aimed at decreasing intentional injuries—that is, violent injuries. Violence is an important public health concern because homicide, suicide, rape, and other assaults are common and exact huge emotional and financial tolls (Mair & Mair, 2003). Suicide and homicide are the second and third leading causes of injury death, respectively, in the United States (CDC, 2005a). Although the criminal justice system has traditionally focused on apprehending and incarcerating offenders, for the last several decades, some criminologists have studied the relationship between the built environment and crime. Jacobs (1961) was the first modern author to call attention to the fact that some places could promote safety whereas others could encourage criminal behavior. Over the following three decades, a number of authors built on this premise, giving rise to a variety of theories about the relationship between the built environment and crime. In 1991, Crowe developed a now widely used approach to crime prevention through environmental design (CPTED) that incorporates three basic environmental design concepts: natural surveillance, access control, and territoriality.

Natural surveillance assumes that crimes are less likely to occur when a potential criminal is being observed. Built environment features that increase watchful observation decrease crime. Examples of such features are windows with clear views of the street, reception desks located in office lobbies, store cash registers in areas of high visibility, balconies and porches, bright outside lighting, and neighborhoods with frequent pedestrian activity. Access control consists of environmental features that limit access to and escape routes from potential crime targets. For example, day-care centers might have only one entrance that opens from the outside, and that entrance might require electronic identification. Additional emergency exits are locked on the outside and sound an alarm when opened from the inside. Locks, fencing, and alarm systems are other examples of access control. Territoriality is the capacity to distinguish clearly between public and private space, which in turn helps establish individuals who belong in that space vs. trespassers. For example, a café with storefront landscaping and sidewalk seating claims ownership of its front yard, and in doing so discourages loitering. Maintenance is considered an important component of establishing territoriality. Signs of property damage and neglect, such as broken windows, graffiti, litter, burned-out light bulbs, and peeling paint, signal lack of owner interest and thus may invite crime. Although not part of the CPTED principles, limiting the number of alcohol retail stores in a given area is an environmental feature known to decrease violence (Zhu, Gorman, & Horel, 2004).

CPTED interventions have been used in a number of settings, including work places and retail establishments, schools, public transit, jails, new communities, and projects to revitalize inner city areas (Mair & Mair, 2003; Zhu et al., 2004). Statisticians and public health epidemiologists have important roles to play in evaluating the relationship between the built environment and crime, which has not previously undergone evidence-based evaluation. Although most studies in this field have focused primarily on decreasing overall crime, not just violent crimes, some interventions have specifically targeted violence. Examples of three strategies aimed at decreasing violence by environmental modifications are summarized below. The first example examines an attempt to decrease work place homicide, the second suggests possible design strategies to decrease school violence and bullying, and the third strategy focuses on potential interventions to decrease sexual violence in refugee camps.

Loomis, Marshall, Wolf, Runyan, and Butts (2002) investigated the effectiveness of environmental and administrative measures to prevent workplace homicide in a population-based, case-control study. Workplaces with bright exterior lighting, security alarms, a cash drop box, and workplaces having at least five environmental measures (e.g., barriers between employees and the public, video cameras, and mirrors) were half as likely to experience a homicide as places without these measures. Workplaces where employees never worked nights alone and those having at least five administrative measures (e.g., locked entrances, employee ID badges, and warning signs) were associated with a significant reduction in homicide risk (Mair & Mair, 2003).

Schneider (2006) summarizes the variety and frequency of violent crimes in schools and notes that most crimes occur between students in locations where staff observation is limited. He then offers a broad array of possible design solutions aimed primarily at increasing surveillance: A main school office with large windows that sits adjacent to the front entrance provides surveillance of approaching visitors and of the main hallway (Fig. 14.4). Placement of student lockers in thoroughfares avoids isolation, while spreading out lockers decreases conflicts caused by crowding. Open stairway designs avoid entrapment. Convex mirrors can improve visibility in crowds and around corners. Wrought-iron fencing works well to define school territory, control access, and limit graffiti.

Third, Dugan, Fowler, and Bolton (2000) suggest potential environmental changes to reduce sexual violence against women and children in refugee camps by incorporating design features that reduce opportunities for sexual violence to occur. For example, placing the women's bathrooms in highly visible, central locations rather than on the edge of a camp, and installing lighting to aid in surveillance are possible measures to prevent sexual assaults. Placing women, rather then unsupervised men, in charge of food distribution limits male access to women's quarters and eliminates the risk that women might be forced to exchange sexual favors for food. Other environmental measures recommended for preventing sexual violence in refugee camps include housing single women, mothers with children, and unaccompanied children in accommodations separate from men and installing perimeter fencing to prevent trespassers from entering the camp.

Design features will likely prove an important tool in reducing unintentional injuries. The field of CPTED holds promise for reducing violent injury and other crimes. However, to date very few of these modifications have been analyzed in a scientifically rigorous manner; further evidence based evaluations using epidemiologic and statistical tools is greatly needed. Public health specialists have an important role to play in advancing this field (Branche & Stevens, 2003).

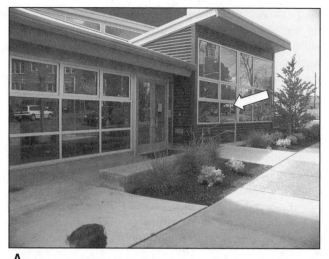

A

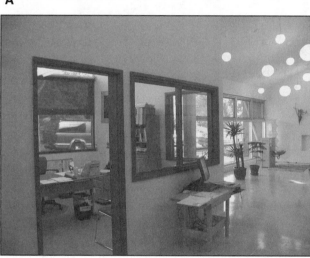

B

Figure 14.4. A. From the outside, this school office *(arrow)* has a clear view of the main entrance, providing surveillance of people arriving at the school. **B.** On the inside, the school office has a view of the main lobby, providing surveillance of activities within the school. Although not shown here, the main lobby and office also have clear views into several classrooms and the kitchen, which are located around the lobby's perimeters. In addition, an open stairway and upstairs' balcony visually connect the office and lobby to the main hallway on the second floor.

14.6.   CONCLUSIONS

In reviewing the current literature on the relationship between environmental design and injury prevention, the following key points emerge:

- Because the built environment is designed and constructed by people, it can be modified to prevent injuries.
- Injury prevention strategies that decrease risk by environmental design are among the most successful interventions.

- Most injury surveillance systems collect very limited information on contributing built environmental factors. More detailed surveillance will pave the way for identifying and redesigning environmental factors associated with injuries.
- Once environmental factors are identified, collaboration with engineers, architects, and manufacturers can often produce safety-focused design modifications.
- Ideally, new designs will consider overall health effects in addition to injury prevention.
- It is important to conduct evidence-based evaluations to confirm or rebut the effectiveness of new design modifications.
- For environmental interventions with proven injury prevention effectiveness, cost-effectiveness analysis is useful.
- Although education can be helpful, legislation and enforcement are often essential to implement widespread use of injury-preventing designs and safety devices.

REFERENCES

American Academy of Pediatrics. (2001). Falls from heights: Windows, roofs, and balconies. *Pediatrics, 107* (5), 1188–1191.

Bergner, L., Mayer, S., & Harris, D. (1971). Falls from heights: A childhood epidemic in an urban area. *American Journal of Public Health, 61* (1), 90–96.

Besser, L. M., & Dannenberg, A. L. (2005). Walking to public transit: Steps to help meet physical activity recommendations. *American Journal of Preventive Medicine, 29* (4), 273–80.

Branche, C. M., & Stevens, J. A. (2003). Injury prevention: An important component of the built environment. *Atlanta Medicine,* 3(77), 23–25.

Brison, R. J., Wicklund, K., & Mueller, B. A. (1988). Fatal pedestrian injuries to young children: A different pattern of injury. *American Journal of Public Health, 78* (7), 793–795.

Bunn, F., Collier, T., Frost, C., Ker, K., Roberts, I., & Wentz, R. (2003). Area-wide traffic calming for preventing traffic related injuries. *The Cochrane Database of Systematic Reviews, 1* (1), 1–21.

Bureau of Transportation Statistics. (2004). *Transportation Statistics Annual Report.* Washington, DC: U.S. Department of Transportation.

Cayless, S. M. (2001). Slip, trip and fall accidents: Relationship to building features and use of coroners' reports in ascribing cause. *Applied Ergonomics, 32* (2), 155–162.

Centers for Disease Control and Prevention. (1994). Injuries associated with soccer goalposts—United States, 1979–1993. *Morbidity & Mortality Weekly Report, 43* (9), 153–155.

Centers for Disease Control and Prevention. (1999). Motor-vehicle safety: A 20th century public health achievement. *Morbidity & Mortality Weekly Report, 48* (18), 369–374.

Centers for Disease Control and Prevention, National Center for Injury Prevention and Control. Web-based Injury Statistics Query and Reporting System (WISQARS) (2005a). Retrieved December 10, 2005, from www.cdc.gov/ncipc/wisqars.

Centers for Disease Control and Prevention (2005b). Barriers to children walking to or from school—United States, 2004. *Morbidity & Mortality Weekly Report, 54* (38), 949–952.

Chalmers, D., & Morrison, L. (2003). Epidemiology of non-submersion injuries in aquatic sporting and recreational activities. *Sports Medicine, 33* (10), 745–770.

Cheng, T. L., Fields, C. B., Brenner, R. A., Wright, J. L., Lomax, T., & Scheidt, P. C. (2000). Sports injuries: An important cause of morbidity in urban youth. District of Columbia Child/Adolescent Injury Research Network. *Pediatrics, 105* (3), E32.

Cote, A. (1984). Field test and evaluation of residential sprinkler system: Part III. *Fire Technology, 20,* 41–46.

Crowe, T. (1991). *Crime prevention through environmental design: Applications of architectural design and space management concepts.* Boston: Butterworth-Heinemann.

Cubbin, C., LeClere, F. B., & Smith, G. S. (2000). Socioeconomic status and injury mortality: Individual and neighbourhood determinants. *Journal of Epidemiology & Community Health, 54* (7), 517–524.

Dellinger, A., Sleet, D.A., & Jones, B. (2006). Motor vehicle injury prevention. In J. Ward and C. Warren (Eds). *Silent victories: Public health triumphs of the 20th century*. New York: Oxford University Press.

Dugan, J., Fowler, C. J., & Bolton, P. A. (2000). Assessing the opportunity for sexual violence against women and children in refugee camps. *Journal of Humanitarian Assistance, Document Posted: 22 August 2000*, Retrieved January 14, 2004, from www.jha.ac/.

Elvik, R. & Vaa, T. (2004). The handbook of road safety measures. New York: Elsevier.

Erdmann, T. C., Feldman, K. W., Rivara, F. P., Heimbach, D. M., & Wall, H. A. (1991). Tap water burn prevention: The effect of legislation. *Pediatrics, 88* (3), 572–577.

Ernst, M. (2004). *Mean streets 2004 how far have we come?* Washington, DC: U.S. Surface Transportation Policy Project. Retrieved December 9, 2005, from www.transact.org.

Evans, L. E. (2004). *Traffic Safety*. Bloomfield Hills, Michigan: Science Serving Society.

Ewing, R., Schieber, R. A., & Zegeer, C. V. (2003). Urban sprawl as a risk factor in motor vehicle occupant and pedestrian fatalities. *American Journal of Public Health, 93* (9), 1541–1545.

Farmer, C. M., & Lund, A. K. (2002). Rollover risk of cars and light trucks after accounting for driver and environmental factors. *Accident Analysis & Prevention, 34* (2), 163–173.

Federal Highway Administration. (2001). *Summary of travel trends*. Washington, DC: U.S. Department of Transportation.

Feldman, K. W., Schaller, R. T., Feldman, J. A., & McMillon, M. (1978). Tap water scald burns in children. *Pediatrics, 62* (1), 1–7.

Gill, T. M., Williams, C. S., Robison, J. T., & Tinetti, M. E. (1999). A population-based study of environmental hazards in the homes of older persons. *American Journal of Public Health, 89* (4), 553–556.

Gillespie, L. D., Gillespie, W. J., Robertson, M. C., Lamb, S. E., Cumming, R. G., & Rowe, B. H. (2003). Interventions for preventing falls in elderly people. *The Cochrane Database of Systematic Reviews*, (4). CD00340.

Home Safety Council. (2004). *The state of home safety in America*. Washington, DC: University of North Carolina Injury Prevention Research Center.

Houk, V. N., Millar, J. D., Rosenberg, M. L., & Waxweiler, R. J. (1992). Setting the national agenda for injury control in the 1990s. *Annals of Emergency Medicine, 21* (2), 201–206.

Idris, A. H., Berg, R. A., Bierens, J., Bossaert, L., Branche, C. M., Gabrielli, A., Graves, S. A., Handley, A. J., Hoelle, R., Morley, P. T., Papa, L., Pepe, P. E., Quan, L., Szpilman, D., Wigginton, J. G., Modell, J. H., & American Heart Association. (2003). Recommended guidelines for uniform reporting of data from drowning: The "Utstein style". *Circulation, 108* (20), 2565–2574.

Illingworth, C., Brennan, P., Jay, A., Al-Rawi, F., & Collick, M. (1975). 200 injuries caused by playground equipment. *British Medical Journal, 4* (5992), 332–334.

Insurance Institute for Highway Safety. (1999). Putting the crash compatibility issue in perspective. *Status Report, 34* (9), 1–11.

Istre, G. R., McCoy, M. A., Stowe, M., Davies, K., Zane, D., Anderson, R. J., & Wiebe, P. (2003). Childhood injuries due to falls from apartment balconies and windows. *Injury Prevention, 9* (4), 349–352.

Jacobs, J. (1961). *The death and life of great American cities*. New York: Random House.

Jacobsen, P. L. (2003). Safety in numbers: More walkers and bicyclists, safer walking and bicycling. *Injury Prevention, 9* (3), 205–209.

Jagger, J. (1992). Prevention of brain trauma by legislation, regulation, and improved technology: A focus on motor vehicles. *Journal of Neurotrauma, 9* (suppl. 1), S313–316.

Janda, D. H., Bir, C., Wild, B., Olson, S., & Hensinger, R. N. (1995). Goal post injuries in soccer. A laboratory and field testing analysis of a preventive intervention. *American Journal of Sports Medicine, 23* (3), 340–344.

Janda, D. H., Hankin, F. M., & Wojtys, E. M. (1986). Softball injuries: Cost, cause and prevention. *American Family Physician, 33* (6), 143–144.

Kelter, A. (2001). *The experience of the adoption of CPSC guidelines by California*. Paper presented at the United States Summit for Playground Safety, Des Moines, IA.

Koepsell, T., McCloskey, L., Wolf, M., Moudon, A. V., Buchner, D., Kraus, J., & Patterson, M. (2002). Crosswalk markings and the risk of pedestrian-motor vehicle collisions in older pedestrians. *Journal of the American Medical Association, 288* (17), 2136–2143.

Leden, L. (2002). Pedestrian risk decrease with pedestrian flow. A case study based on data from signalized intersections in Hamilton, Ontario. *Accident Analysis & Prevention, 34* (4), 457–464.

Leyden, K. M. (2003). Social capital and the built environment: The importance of walkable neighborhoods. *American Journal of Public Health, 93* (9), 1546–1551.

Loomis, D., Marshall, S. W., Wolf, S. H., Runyan, C. W., & Butts, J. D. (2002). Effectiveness of safety measures recommended for prevention of workplace homicide. *Journal of the American Medical Association, 287* (8), 1011–1017.

Lucy, W. H. (2003). Mortality risk associated with leaving home: Recognizing the relevance of the built environment. *American Journal of Public Health, 93* (9), 1564–1569.

Lyons, R. A., Sander, L. V., Weightman, A. L., Patterson, J., Jones, S. A., Rolfe, B., Kemp, A., & Johansen, A. (2003). Modification of the home environment for the reduction of injuries (CD003600). *The Cochrane Database of Systematic Reviews* (4).

MacKay, M. (2003). Playground injuries. *Injury Prevention, 9* (3), 194–196.

Mair, J. S., & Mair, M. (2003). Violence prevention and control through environmental modifications. *Annual Review of Public Health, 24*, 209–225.

Moritz, A. R., & Henriques, F. C. (1947). Studies of thermal injury: The relative importance of time and surface temperature in the causation of cutaneous burns. *American Journal of Pathology, 23*, 695–720.

Moore, R. C., Goltsman, S. M., & Iacofano, D. S. (1992). *Play for all guidelines: Planning, design and management of outdoor play settings for all children* (2nd ed.). Berkeley CA: MIG Communications.

Moulton, R. (1943). *The Coconut Grove Night Club fire, Boston, 28 November 1942.* Boston: National Fire Protection Association.

Nantulya, V. M., & Reich, M. R. (2002). The neglected epidemic: Road traffic injuries in developing countries. *British Medical Journal, 324* (7346), 1139–1141.

National Highway Traffic Safety Administration. (2005). Buying a safer car 2005. Retrieved January 6, 2005, from www.safecar.gov.

National SAFE KIDS Campaign. (2004). *Drowning fact sheet.* Washington, DC: Author.

National Safety Council. (2002). *Playground safety fact sheet.* Retrieved April 9, 2005, from www.nsc.org/library/facts/plgrdgen-old.htm.

National Safety Council. (2003). *Injury facts.* Itasca, IL: Author.

Newgard, C. D., & Lewis, R. J. (2005). Effects of child age and body size on serious injury from passenger air-bag presence in motor vehicle crashes. *Pediatrics, 115* (6), 1579–1585.

Nolan, D. (2001). *Encyclopedia of fire protection.* Albany, NY: Thomson Learning.

Norton, C., Nixon, J., & Sibert, J. R. (2004). Playground injuries to children. *Archives of Disease in Childhood, 89* (2), 103–108.

Peden, M., McGee, K. S., & Sharma, G. (2002). *The injury chart book: A graphical overview of the global burden of injuries.* Geneva: World Health Organization.

Peden, M., Scurfield, R., Sleet, D. A., Mohan, D., Hyder, A. A., Jarawan, E., & Mathers, C. (Eds). (2004). *World report on road traffic injury prevention.* Geneva: World Health Organization.

Pucher, J., & Dijkstra, L. (2003). Promoting safe walking and cycling to improve public health: Lessons from the Netherlands and Germany. *American Journal of Public Health, 93* (9), 1509–1516.

Retting, R. A., Ferguson, S. A., & Hakkert, A. S. (2003). Effects of red light cameras on violations and crashes: A review of the international literature. *Traffic Injury Prevention, 4* (1), 17–23.

Retting, R. A., Ferguson, S. A., & McCartt, A. T. (2003). A review of evidence-based traffic engineering measures designed to reduce pedestrian-motor vehicle crashes. *American Journal of Public Health, 93* (9), 1456–1463.

Retting, R. A., Persaud, B. N., Garder, P. E., & Lord, D. (2001). Crash and injury reduction following installation of roundabouts in the United States. *American Journal of Public Health, 91* (4), 628–631.

Retting, R. A., Weinstein, H. B., & Solomon, M. G. (2003). Analysis of motor-vehicle crashes at stop signs in four U.S. cities. *Journal of Safety Research, 34* (5), 485–489.

Rivers, R. P., Boyd, R. D., & Baderman, H. (1978). Falls from equipment as a cause of playground injury. *Community Health (Bristol), 9* (3), 178–179.

Roudsari, B. S., Mock, C. N., Kaufman, R., Grossman, D., Henary, B. Y., & Crandall, J. (2004). Pedestrian crashes: Higher injury severity and mortality rate for light truck vehicles compared with passenger vehicles. *Injury Prevention, 10* (3), 154–158.

Runyan, C. W., Johnson, R. M., Yang, J., Waller, A. E., Perkis, D., Marshall, S. W., Coyne-Beasley, T., & McGee, K. S. (2005). Risk and protective factors for fires, burns, and carbon monoxide poisoning in U.S. households. *American Journal of Preventive Medicine, 28* (1), 102–108.

Salmon, P. (2001). Effects of physical exercise on anxiety, depression, and sensitivity to stress: A unifying theory. *Clinical Psychology Review, 21* (1), 33–61.

Sattin, R. W., Rodriguez, J. G., DeVito, C. A., & Wingo, P. A. (1998). Home environmental hazards and the risk of fall injury events among community-dwelling older persons. Study to assess falls among the elderly (SAFE) Group. *Journal of the American Geriatrics Society, 46* (6), 669–676.

Schneider, T. (2006). Crime and violence prevention through environmental design. In Frumph, Geller, R., Rubin, L., & Nodvin, J. (Eds.). *Safe and healthy school environments.* New York: University Press.

Scott, I. (2003). Prevention of drowning in home pools—Lessons from Australia. *Injury Control & Promotion, 10* (4), 227–236.

Suecoff, S. A., Avner, J. R., Chou, K. J., & Crain, E. F. (1999). A comparison of New York City ground hazards in high- and low-income areas. *Archives of Pediatric & Adolescent Medicine, 1* 363–366.

Shenassa, E. D., Stubbendick, A., & Brown, M. J. (2004). Social disparities in housing and related atric injury: A multilevel study. *American Journal of Public Health, 94* (4), 633–639.

Smith, C. L. (1994). *Smoke detector operability survey: Report on findings.* Bethesda, MD: U.S. Cons Product Safety Commission.

Smith, K. M., & Cummings, P. (2006). Passenger seating position and the risk of passenger dea traffic crashes: A matched cohort study. *Injury Prevention, 12* (2), 83–86.

Stevens, J. A., & Olson, S. (2000). Reducing falls and resulting hip fractures among older women. *M Recommendations & Reports, 49* (RR-2), 3–12.

Tester, J. M., Rutherford, G. W., Wald, Z., & Rutherford, M. W. (2004). A matched case-control s evaluating the effectiveness of speed humps in reducing child pedestrian injuries. *American Jo of Public Health, 94* (4), 646–650.

Thompson, D. C., & Rivara, F. P. (2000). Pool fencing for preventing drowning in children. *The Coch Database of Systematic Reviews,* (2), CO001047.

Tinsworth, D. K., & McDonald, J. F. (2001). *Special study: Injuries and deaths associated with children's ground equipment.* Washington, DC: U.S. Consumer Product Safety Commission.

Transportation Research Board. (1990). *Safety research for a changing highway environment* (Special Rep #229). Washington, DC: National Research Council, Transportation Research Board.

Transportation Research Board. (2002). *The relative risks of school travel* (Special Report #269). Washi ton, DC: Committee on School Transportation Safety.

Transportation Research Board. (2003). *Integrated safety management process.* Washington, DC: Instit of Medicine, National Academy of Sciences.

U.S. Environmental Protection Agency. (2004). *Fuel economy guide 2004.* Washington, DC: U.S. Depa ment of Energy, Environmental Protection Agency.

Von Drehle, D. (2003). *Triangle: The fire that changed America.* Boston: Atlantic Monthly Press.

Waller, P. F. (2002). Challenges in motor vehicle safety. *Annual Review of Public Health, 23*, 93–113.

Warda, L., Tenenbein, M., & Moffatt, M. E. (1999). House fire injury prevention update. Part I. A revie of risk factors for fatal and non-fatal house fire injury. *Injury Prevention, 5* (2), 145–150.

Wennberg, R. (2004). Collision frequency in elite hockey on North American versus international siz rinks. *Canadian Journal of Neurological Sciences, 31* (3), 373–377.

Zegeer, C. V., Seiderman, C., Lagerwey, P., Cynecki, M., Ronkin, M., & Schneider, B. (2000) *Pedestrian facilities users guide—providing safety and mobility.* Washington, DC: Federal Highwa Administration.

Zegeer, C. V., Stewart, J. R., Huang, H., & Lagerwey, P. (2001). Safety effects of marked versus unmarke crosswalks at uncontrolled locations. *Transportation Research Record, 1723*, 56–68.

Zhu, L., Gorman, D. M., & Horel, S. (2004). Alcohol outlet density and violence: A geospatial analysis. *Alcohol & Alcoholism, 39* (4), 369–375.

Dellinger, A., Sleet, D.A., & Jones, B. (2006). Motor vehicle injury prevention. In J. Ward and C. Warren (Eds). *Silent victories: Public health triumphs of the 20th century*. New York: Oxford University Press.

Dugan, J., Fowler, C. J., & Bolton, P. A. (2000). Assessing the opportunity for sexual violence against women and children in refugee camps. *Journal of Humanitarian Assistance, Document Posted: 22 August 2000*, Retrieved January 14, 2004, from www.jha.ac/.

Elvik, R. & Vaa, T. (2004). The handbook of road safety measures. New York: Elsevier.

Erdmann, T. C., Feldman, K. W., Rivara, F. P., Heimbach, D. M., & Wall, H. A. (1991). Tap water burn prevention: The effect of legislation. *Pediatrics, 88* (3), 572–577.

Ernst, M. (2004). *Mean streets 2004 how far have we come?* Washington, DC: U.S. Surface Transportation Policy Project. Retrieved December 9, 2005, from www.transact.org.

Evans, L. E. (2004). *Traffic Safety*. Bloomfield Hills, Michigan: Science Serving Society.

Ewing, R., Schieber, R. A., & Zegeer, C. V. (2003). Urban sprawl as a risk factor in motor vehicle occupant and pedestrian fatalities. *American Journal of Public Health, 93* (9), 1541–1545.

Farmer, C. M., & Lund, A. K. (2002). Rollover risk of cars and light trucks after accounting for driver and environmental factors. *Accident Analysis & Prevention, 34* (2), 163–173.

Federal Highway Administration. (2001). *Summary of travel trends*. Washington, DC: U.S. Department of Transportation.

Feldman, K. W., Schaller, R. T., Feldman, J. A., & McMillon, M. (1978). Tap water scald burns in children. *Pediatrics, 62* (1), 1–7.

Gill, T. M., Williams, C. S., Robison, J. T., & Tinetti, M. E. (1999). A population-based study of environmental hazards in the homes of older persons. *American Journal of Public Health, 89* (4), 553–556.

Gillespie, L. D., Gillespie, W. J., Robertson, M. C., Lamb, S. E., Cumming, R. G., & Rowe, B. H. (2003). Interventions for preventing falls in elderly people. *The Cochrane Database of Systematic Reviews, (4)*. CD00340.

Home Safety Council. (2004). *The state of home safety in America*. Washington, DC: University of North Carolina Injury Prevention Research Center.

Houk, V. N., Millar, J. D., Rosenberg, M. L., & Waxweiler, R. J. (1992). Setting the national agenda for injury control in the 1990s. *Annals of Emergency Medicine, 21* (2), 201–206.

Idris, A. H., Berg, R. A., Bierens, J., Bossaert, L., Branche, C. M., Gabrielli, A., Graves, S. A., Handley, A. J., Hoelle, R., Morley, P. T., Papa, L., Pepe, P. E., Quan, L., Szpilman, D., Wigginton, J. G., Modell, J. H., & American Heart Association. (2003). Recommended guidelines for uniform reporting of data from drowning: The "Utstein style". *Circulation, 108* (20), 2565–2574.

Illingworth, C., Brennan, P., Jay, A., Al-Rawi, F., & Collick, M. (1975). 200 injuries caused by playground equipment. *British Medical Journal, 4* (5992), 332–334.

Insurance Institute for Highway Safety. (1999). Putting the crash compatibility issue in perspective. *Status Report, 34* (9), 1–11.

Istre, G. R., McCoy, M. A., Stowe, M., Davies, K., Zane, D., Anderson, R. J., & Wiebe, P. (2003). Childhood injuries due to falls from apartment balconies and windows. *Injury Prevention, 9* (4), 349–352.

Jacobs, J. (1961). *The death and life of great American cities*. New York: Random House.

Jacobsen, P. L. (2003). Safety in numbers: More walkers and bicyclists, safer walking and bicycling. *Injury Prevention, 9* (3), 205–209.

Jagger, J. (1992). Prevention of brain trauma by legislation, regulation, and improved technology: A focus on motor vehicles. *Journal of Neurotrauma, 9* (suppl. 1), S313–316.

Janda, D. H., Bir, C., Wild, B., Olson, S., & Hensinger, R. N. (1995). Goal post injuries in soccer. A laboratory and field testing analysis of a preventive intervention. *American Journal of Sports Medicine, 23* (3), 340–344.

Janda, D. H., Hankin, F. M., & Wojtys, E. M. (1986). Softball injuries: Cost, cause and prevention. *American Family Physician, 33* (6), 143–144.

Kelter, A. (2001). *The experience of the adoption of CPSC guidelines by California*. Paper presented at the United States Summit for Playground Safety, Des Moines, IA.

Koepsell, T., McCloskey, L., Wolf, M., Moudon, A. V., Buchner, D., Kraus, J., & Patterson, M. (2002). Crosswalk markings and the risk of pedestrian-motor vehicle collisions in older pedestrians. *Journal of the American Medical Association, 288* (17), 2136–2143.

Leden, L. (2002). Pedestrian risk decrease with pedestrian flow. A case study based on data from signalized intersections in Hamilton, Ontario. *Accident Analysis & Prevention, 34* (4), 457–464.

Leyden, K. M. (2003). Social capital and the built environment: The importance of walkable neighborhoods. *American Journal of Public Health, 93* (9), 1546–1551.

Loomis, D., Marshall, S. W., Wolf, S. H., Runyan, C. W., & Butts, J. D. (2002). Effectiveness of safety measures recommended for prevention of workplace homicide. *Journal of the American Medical Association, 287* (8), 1011–1017.

Lucy, W. H. (2003). Mortality risk associated with leaving home: Recognizing the relevance of the built environment. *American Journal of Public Health, 93* (9), 1564–1569.

Lyons, R. A., Sander, L. V., Weightman, A. L., Patterson, J., Jones, S. A., Rolfe, B., Kemp, A., & Johansen, A. (2003). Modification of the home environment for the reduction of injuries (CD003600). *The Cochrane Database of Systematic Reviews* (4).

MacKay, M. (2003). Playground injuries. *Injury Prevention, 9* (3), 194–196.

Mair, J. S., & Mair, M. (2003). Violence prevention and control through environmental modifications. *Annual Review of Public Health, 24,* 209–225.

Moritz, A. R., & Henriques, F. C. (1947). Studies of thermal injury: The relative importance of time and surface temperature in the causation of cutaneous burns. *American Journal of Pathology, 23,* 695–720.

Moore, R. C., Goltsman, S. M., & Iacofano, D. S. (1992). *Play for all guidelines: Planning, design and management of outdoor play settings for all children* (2nd ed.). Berkeley CA: MIG Communications.

Moulton, R. (1943). *The Coconut Grove Night Club fire, Boston, 28 November 1942.* Boston: National Fire Protection Association.

Nantulya, V. M., & Reich, M. R. (2002). The neglected epidemic: Road traffic injuries in developing countries. *British Medical Journal, 324* (7346), 1139–1141.

National Highway Traffic Safety Administration. (2005). Buying a safer car 2005. Retrieved January 6, 2005, from www.safecar.gov.

National SAFE KIDS Campaign. (2004). *Drowning fact sheet.* Washington, DC: Author.

National Safety Council. (2002). *Playground safety fact sheet.* Retrieved April 9, 2005, from www.nsc.org/library/facts/plgrdgen-old.htm.

National Safety Council. (2003). *Injury facts.* Itasca, IL: Author.

Newgard, C. D., & Lewis, R. J. (2005). Effects of child age and body size on serious injury from passenger air-bag presence in motor vehicle crashes. *Pediatrics, 115* (6), 1579–1585.

Nolan, D. (2001). *Encyclopedia of fire protection.* Albany, NY: Thomson Learning.

Norton, C., Nixon, J., & Sibert, J. R. (2004). Playground injuries to children. *Archives of Disease in Childhood, 89* (2), 103–108.

Peden, M., McGee, K. S., & Sharma, G. (2002). *The injury chart book: A graphical overview of the global burden of injuries.* Geneva: World Health Organization.

Peden, M., Scurfield, R., Sleet, D. A., Mohan, D., Hyder, A. A., Jarawan, E., & Mathers, C. (Eds). (2004). World report on road traffic injury prevention. Geneva: World Health Organization.

Pucher, J., & Dijkstra, L. (2003). Promoting safe walking and cycling to improve public health: Lessons from the Netherlands and Germany. *American Journal of Public Health, 93* (9), 1509–1516.

Retting, R. A., Ferguson, S. A., & Hakkert, A. S. (2003). Effects of red light cameras on violations and crashes: A review of the international literature. *Traffic Injury Prevention, 4* (1), 17–23.

Retting, R. A., Ferguson, S. A., & McCartt, A. T. (2003). A review of evidence-based traffic engineering measures designed to reduce pedestrian-motor vehicle crashes. *American Journal of Public Health, 93* (9), 1456–1463.

Retting, R. A., Persaud, B. N., Garder, P. E., & Lord, D. (2001). Crash and injury reduction following installation of roundabouts in the United States. *American Journal of Public Health, 91* (4), 628–631.

Retting, R. A., Weinstein, H. B., & Solomon, M. G. (2003). Analysis of motor-vehicle crashes at stop signs in four U.S. cities. *Journal of Safety Research, 34* (5), 485–489.

Rivers, R. P., Boyd, R. D., & Baderman, H. (1978). Falls from equipment as a cause of playground injury. *Community Health (Bristol), 9* (3), 178–179.

Roudsari, B. S., Mock, C. N., Kaufman, R., Grossman, D., Henary, B. Y., & Crandall, J. (2004). Pedestrian crashes: Higher injury severity and mortality rate for light truck vehicles compared with passenger vehicles. *Injury Prevention, 10* (3), 154–158.

Runyan, C. W., Johnson, R. M., Yang, J., Waller, A. E., Perkis, D., Marshall, S. W., Coyne-Beasley, T., & McGee, K. S. (2005). Risk and protective factors for fires, burns, and carbon monoxide poisoning in U.S. households. *American Journal of Preventive Medicine, 28* (1), 102–108.

Salmon, P. (2001). Effects of physical exercise on anxiety, depression, and sensitivity to stress: A unifying theory. *Clinical Psychology Review, 21* (1), 33–61.

Sattin, R. W., Rodriguez, J. G., DeVito, C. A., & Wingo, P. A. (1998). Home environmental hazards and the risk of fall injury events among community-dwelling older persons. Study to assess falls among the elderly (SAFE) Group. *Journal of the American Geriatrics Society, 46* (6), 669–676.

Schneider, T. (2006). Crime and violence prevention through environmental design. In Frumpkin, H., Geller, R., Rubin, L., & Nodvin, J. (Eds.). *Safe and healthy school environments.* New York: Oxford University Press.

Scott, I. (2003). Prevention of drowning in home pools—Lessons from Australia. *Injury Control & Safety Promotion, 10* (4), 227–236.

Suecoff, S. A., Avner, J. R., Chou, K. J., & Crain, E. F. (1999). A comparison of New York City playground hazards in high- and low-income areas. *Archives of Pediatric & Adolescent Medicine, 153* (4), 363–366.

Shenassa, E. D., Stubbendick, A., & Brown, M. J. (2004). Social disparities in housing and related pediatric injury: A multilevel study. *American Journal of Public Health, 94* (4), 633–639.

Smith, C. L. (1994). *Smoke detector operability survey: Report on findings.* Bethesda, MD: U.S. Consumer Product Safety Commission.

Smith, K. M., & Cummings, P. (2006). Passenger seating position and the risk of passenger death in traffic crashes: A matched cohort study. *Injury Prevention, 12* (2), 83–86.

Stevens, J. A., & Olson, S. (2000). Reducing falls and resulting hip fractures among older women. *MMWR Recommendations & Reports, 49* (RR-2), 3–12.

Tester, J. M., Rutherford, G. W., Wald, Z., & Rutherford, M. W. (2004). A matched case-control study evaluating the effectiveness of speed humps in reducing child pedestrian injuries. *American Journal of Public Health, 94* (4), 646–650.

Thompson, D. C., & Rivara, F. P. (2000). Pool fencing for preventing drowning in children. *The Cochrane Database of Systematic Reviews,* (2), CO001047.

Tinsworth, D. K., & McDonald, J. F. (2001). *Special study: Injuries and deaths associated with children's playground equipment.* Washington, DC: U.S. Consumer Product Safety Commission.

Transportation Research Board. (1990). *Safety research for a changing highway environment* (Special Report #229). Washington, DC: National Research Council, Transportation Research Board.

Transportation Research Board. (2002). *The relative risks of school travel* (Special Report #269). Washington, DC: Committee on School Transportation Safety.

Transportation Research Board. (2003). *Integrated safety management process.* Washington, DC: Institute of Medicine, National Academy of Sciences.

U.S. Environmental Protection Agency. (2004). *Fuel economy guide 2004.* Washington, DC: U.S. Department of Energy, Environmental Protection Agency.

Von Drehle, D. (2003). *Triangle: The fire that changed America.* Boston: Atlantic Monthly Press.

Waller, P. F. (2002). Challenges in motor vehicle safety. *Annual Review of Public Health, 23,* 93–113.

Warda, L., Tenenbein, M., & Moffatt, M. E. (1999). House fire injury prevention update. Part I. A review of risk factors for fatal and non-fatal house fire injury. *Injury Prevention, 5* (2), 145–150.

Wennberg, R. (2004). Collision frequency in elite hockey on North American versus international size rinks. *Canadian Journal of Neurological Sciences, 31* (3), 373–377.

Zegeer, C. V., Seiderman, C., Lagerwey, P., Cynecki, M., Ronkin, M., & Schneider, B. (2000). *Pedestrian facilities users guide—providing safety and mobility.* Washington, DC: Federal Highway Administration.

Zegeer, C. V., Stewart, J. R., Huang, H., & Lagerwey, P. (2001). Safety effects of marked versus unmarked crosswalks at uncontrolled locations. *Transportation Research Record, 1723,* 56–68.

Zhu, L., Gorman, D. M., & Horel, S. (2004). Alcohol outlet density and violence: A geospatial analysis. *Alcohol & Alcoholism, 39* (4), 369–375.